Principles & Foundations of Health Promotion and Education

THIRD EDITION

Related Benjamin Cummings Health Titles

Anspaugh/Ezell, *Teaching Today's Health*, Seventh Edition (2004)

Barr, *Introduction to US Health Policy* (2002)

Buckingham, *Primer on International Health* (2001)

Donatelle, *Access to Health*, Ninth Edition (2006)

Donatelle, *Health: The Basics*, Sixth Edition (2005)

Donnelly, Elburne, Kittleson, *Mental Health: Dimensions of Self-Esteem and Emotional Well-Being* (2001)

Girdano/Dusek/Everly, *Controlling Stress and Tension*, Seventh Edition (2005)

Karren/Hafen/Smith/Frandsen, *Mind/Body Health*, Second Edition (2002)

McKenzie/Smeltzer, *Planning, Implementing, and Evaluating Health Promotion Programs: A Primer*, Fourth Edition (2005)

Neutens/Rubinson, *Research Techniques for the Health Sciences*, Third Edition (2002)

Reagan/Brookins, *Community Health in the 21st Century*, Second Edition (2002)

Seaward, *Health of the Human Spirit: Spiritual Dimensions for Personal Health and Well-Being* (2001)

Skinner, *Promoting Health Through Organizational Change* (2002)

Check out these and other Benjamin Cummings Health titles at: www.aw-bc.com

Principles & Foundations of Health Promotion and Education

THIRD EDITION

Randall R. Cottrell, D.Ed., CHES
University of Cincinnati

James T. Girvan, Ph.D., M.P.H., CHES
Boise State University

James F. McKenzie, Ph.D., M.P.H.
Ball State University

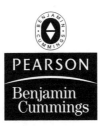

PEARSON

Benjamin
Cummings

San Francisco   Boston   New York
Cape Town   Hong Kong   London   Madrid   Mexico City
Montreal   Munich   Paris   Singapore   Sydney   Tokyo   Toronto

Publisher: *Daryl Fox*
Acquisitions Editor: *Deirdre Espinoza*
Editorial Assistants: *Sabrina Larson and Alison Rodal*
Managing Editor: *Deborah Cogan*
Production Supervisor and Photo Researcher: *Keith Ingram*
Production Management and Composition: *The Left Coast Group*
Production Editor: *David Novak*
Illustrations: *Karl Miyajima and The Left Coast Group*
Cover Designer: *Armen Kojoyian*
Copy Editor: *Anna Reynolds*
Marketing Manager: *Sandra Lindelof*
Manufacturing Buyer: *Stacey Weinberger*
Cover Photograph: *Corbis*

Library of Congress Cataloging-in-Publication Data

Cottrell, Randall R.
  Principles & foundations of health promotion and education/Randall R.
Cottrell, James T. Girvan, James F. McKenzie.—3rd ed.
      p. ; cm.
  Includes bibliographical references and index.
  ISBN 0-8053-7878-2
 1. Health education. 2. Health promotion.
  [DNLM: 1. Health Education. 2. Health Promotion. WA 590 C851pa 2006]
I. Title: Principles and foundations of health promotion and education. II.
Girvan, James T., 1946– III. McKenzie, James F., 1948– IV. Title.
  RA440.5.C685 2006
  613–dc22

                                                                    2004030923

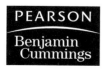

                                                        ISBN 0-8053-7878-2
                          2 3 4 5 6 7 8 9 10—MAL—09 08 07 06 05
                                                              www.aw-bc.com

CONTENTS

CHAPTER 7
The Settings for Health Education *187*

CHAPTER 8

CHAPTER 9

What is health education?" "What do health educators do?" "If I get a degree in health education, what types of jobs are available?" Many faculty members in health education professional preparation programs have heard these questions from both prospective students and current majors. Health education is often described by academicians as a "discovery major." Few students enter colleges and universities as health education majors. Students often "discover" the health education field after experiences in elective health education courses or other health-related majors, or as a result of developing an interest in health and lifestyle. Although these students often enter our programs with a high level of enthusiasm, they seldom have even a basic understanding of the profession. Even those students who began their college career as health education majors usually enter programs with a limited perspective of the profession.

Foundations and principles courses are designed to assist students in the development of an appreciation of the history, contemporary importance, and future potential of the profession of health education. Cottrell, Girvan, and McKenzie's text, *Principles & Foundations of Health Promotion and Education,* provides a teaching resource for instructors, and a learning resource for students, to actively address the key aspects of such a course.

Health educators have long recognized that learning is more than simply the acquisition of knowledge. Learning also involves instructional elements such as critical thinking, skill development, and real-life application. It is evident throughout the book that the authors have placed importance on these elements—it is more than just a reader for students. While the book serves as a repository of information in topic areas such as history, philosophy, theory, ethics, current issues, work settings, and future trends, it provides students with opportunities for involvement in activities such as online fact finding, formulation of opinions, and professional applications. This approach allows instructors to use the text for more than just assigned reading; it can also serve as a source for student-centered activities both within and outside of the classroom.

Numerous aspects of the textbook deserve special mention. Students should find the writing in each chapter both engaging and informative. The authors have done an excellent job of incorporating both "classic" and current literature from the health education field while also integrating meaningful information from other professional literature. Boxes and tables are used to clarify and enrich important information.

The beginning of each chapter includes a listing of precise objectives. These objectives clearly indicate specific expectations for students and provide a framework for assessment for course instructors. At the end of each chapter, review questions are designed to address the objectives. Critical thinking questions are also included at the end of each chapter, along with activities that provide students with application opportunities related to the content of the chapter. Each chapter's concluding activity is a case study in which the student is presented with a health education situation and asked to apply knowledge and skills learned in the chapter. Together, the end-of-chapter activities enable students to authentically demonstrate learning through a variety of methods and products.

Because of the ever-changing nature and updating of the World Wide Web, the "Activities on the Web" that appeared in the previous edition of this text have been removed and replaced with the new "Weblinks" section, a collection of Web addresses and short descriptions. The "Weblinks" can be found at the end of each chapter and allow students the opportunity to explore a number of different Web sites that are available to support the content presented in the chapter.

Another exciting and valuable feature of the book is the "Practitioner's Perspective." This feature, interspersed throughout the book, presents the opinions of practicing health educators on topics such as planning models, ethics, certification as a health education specialist (CHES), and graduate study. Background information is presented for each practitioner including his or her position, employer, and degrees. The practitioner describes the connection of each topic to specific professional responsibilities as a health educator. This feature extends the classroom to the real world, and brings the experiences of practicing health educators to students.

Girvan, Cottrell, and McKenzie have provided instructors with a source of information, instructional activities, and assessment methods to guide students toward the development of the important knowledge, appreciation, and insight that are essential for current and prospective health educators. I have no doubt that *Principles & Foundations of Health Promotion and Education* will serve as a valuable resource for both quality instruction and informed professional practice.

David A. Birch, Ph.D., CHES
Professor & Chair
Department of Health Education &
  Recreation
Southern Illinois University, Carbondale
Carbondale, IL

Many students enter the field of health promotion and education knowing only that they are interested in health and wish to help others improve their health status. Typically, students' interest in health promotion and education is derived from their own desire to live a healthy lifestyle and not from an in-depth understanding of the historical, theoretical, and philosophical foundations of this emerging profession. Other than perhaps a high school health education teacher, many students do not know any health promotion and education practitioners. In fact, most beginning students are unaware of employment opportunities, the skills needed to practice health education, and what it would be like to work in a given health education setting.

This book is written for such students. The contents will be of value to students who are undecided if health education is the major they want to pursue, as well as for new health education majors who need information about what health education is and where health educators can be employed. The book is designed for use in an entry-level health education course in which the major goal is to introduce students to health promotion and education. In addition, it may have value in introducing new health education graduate students, who have undergraduate degrees in fields other than health education, to the emerging profession of health promotion and education.

All chapters have been revised and updated for the new third edition. Chapter 1, "A Background for the Profession," provides an overview of health promotion and education and sets the stage for the remaining chapters. Chapter 2, "The History of Health and Health Education," examines the history of health and health care, as well as the history of health promotion and education. This chapter was written to help students understand the tremendous advances that have been made in keeping people healthy, and it provides perspective on the role of health promotion and education in that effort. One cannot appreciate the present without understanding the past. Chapters 3, 4, and 5 provide what might best be called the basic foundations. All professions, such as law, medicine, business, and teacher education, must provide students with information related to the philosophy, theory, and ethics inherent in the field.

Chapter 6, "The Health Educator: Roles, Responsibilities, Certifications, Advanced Study," is designed to acquaint new students with the skills that are needed to practice in the field of health promotion and education. It also explains the certification process to students and encourages them to begin thinking of graduate study very early in their undergraduate programs. Chapter 7, "The Settings for Health Education," introduces students to the job responsibilities inherent in different types of health education positions and provides a discussion of the pros and cons of working in various health education settings. With its "A Day in the Career of . . ." sections and the "Practitioner's Perspective" boxes, this chapter is unique among introductory texts and will truly provide students with important insights into the various health education settings.

Chapter 8, "Agencies/Associations/Organizations Associated with Health Education," introduces students to the many professional agencies, associations, and organizations that support health promotion and education. This is an extremely important chapter, as all health educators need to know of these resources and allies. We believe that all introductory students should be encouraged to join one or more of the professional associations described in this chapter. For that reason, contact information for all of the professional associations discussed is included in the chapter. Chapter 9, "The Literature of Health Education," directs students to the information and resources necessary to work in the field. Included in this chapter is basic information related to the Internet and the World Wide Web that should be especially helpful to new students. With the explosion of knowledge related to health, being able to locate needed resources is a critical skill for health educators. Finally, health education students need to consider what future changes in health knowledge, policy, and funding may mean to those working in health promotion and education. They must learn to project into the future and prepare themselves to meet these challenges. Chapter 10, "Future Trends in Health Education," is an attempt to provide a window into the future for today's health promotion and education students.

As one reads the book, it will be apparent that certain standard features exist in all chapters. These are designed to help the student identify important information, guide the student's learning, and extend the student's understanding beyond the memorization of content information. Each chapter in the book begins by identifying objectives. Prior to reading a chapter, students should carefully read the objectives, as they will guide the student's learning of the information contained in that chapter. After reading a chapter, it may also be helpful to review the objectives to make certain major points were understood. Following the objectives in each chapter is a list of key terms. Again, it is a good idea to examine these closely prior to reading a chapter and to review them following one's reading. Being able to respond to each objective and define each term is typically of great value in understanding the material and preparing for examinations.

Throughout the book take note of the "Practitioner's Perspective" boxes. These are boxes typically written by young health promotion and education professionals who are currently working in the field. Many of the boxes relate to working in a particular setting, while others focus on such areas as ethics, certification, and graduate study.

At the end of each chapter, the student will find a brief summary of the information contained in that chapter. Following the summary are review questions. Students are encouraged to answer these questions, as they provide an additional method for targeting learning and reviewing the chapter's contents. Critical thinking questions follow the review questions. Critical thinking questions are designed to extend readers' learning beyond what is presented in the chapter. They require readers to apply what they have learned, contemplate major events, and project their learning to the future. A short list of activities, designed to extend the reader's knowledge beyond what can be obtained by reading the chapter, is also included. In some cases, students are asked to apply or synthesize the content information. In other activities, students are encouraged to get actively involved with experiences that will help integrate learning from the text with a practical, real-world setting. By completing these activities, students should have a better understanding of health promotion and education. The activities are followed by a new feature in the third edition, Web Links. Web Links are sites students can access to read more about a topic, extend their learning, or obtain interesting resource materials. Each chapter ends with a case study. Case studies allow readers to project themselves into realistic health education situations, and problem solve how to handle them.

We readily acknowledge that the information contained in this book represents our bias regarding what material should be taught in an introductory course. There may be important introductory information we have not included, or we may have included information that may not be considered introductory by all users. We welcome and encourage comments and feedback, both positive and negative, from all users of this text. Only with such feedback can we make improvements and include the most appropriate information in future editions of the text.

Randall R. Cottrell
James T. Girvan
James F. McKenzie

Acknowledgments

First, we would like to thank all of the health education faculty who have adopted our text and all of the students who have used the text. The response we have received has been truly gratifying. Without you we would not be writing the third edition.

We would also like to thank Benjamin Cummings for producing the book. In particular, we would like to thank Alison Rodal and Sabrina Larson for their diligent work on our behalf and for their outstanding administrative and organization skills. We would also like to thank Deirdre Espinoza, Keith Ingram, and David Novak for their hard work on this project.

We would like to express our sincere appreciation to those health education professionals who served as reviewers for the third edition. They had many good ideas that we tried to incorporate whenever possible. The reviewers were M. Allison Ford of Florida Atlantic University, Mike Perko of the University of Alabama, Georgia Johnston of the University of Texas, San Antonio, Craig Huddy of Concord College, Whitney Boling of the University of Houston, and Virginia Noland of the University of Florida. We would also like to thank the reviewers of previous editions: R. Morgan Pigg, Jr. of the University of Florida, Marilyn Morrow of Illinois State University, Steve Nagy of the University of Alabama, Emily Tyler of the University of North Carolina at Greensboro (with additional helpful feedback from Julie Orta, MPH student), and Marianne Frauenknecht of Western Michigan University.

We are lucky to have had excellent secretarial assistance with this project. A big thanks goes to Billie Kennedy, Ruth Ann Duncan, Carol Carroll, Linda Miller, and Fran Floyd. We would also like to acknowledge the staff of the High Library at Elizabethtown College, especially Sylvia T. Morra and Louise Hyder-Darlington, for their assistance in making this book possible.

Finally, we would like to dedicate this book to the people in our lives who mean the most to us: our wives, Karen, Georgia, and Bonnie; our children, Kyle, Kory, Jennifer, Erik, Becky, Anne and Greg; grandchild, Mitchell; and our parents, Russell and Edith Cottrell, Terry and Margaret Girvan, and Gordon and Betty McKenzie.

CHAPTER 1

A Background for the Profession

Chapter Objectives

After reading this chapter and answering the questions at the end, you should be able to:

1. Explain why health education should be considered an emerging profession.
2. Describe the current status of health education.
3. Define the terms *health, health education, health promotion, health promotion and disease prevention, public health, community health, coordinated school health program,* and *wellness.*
4. Define *epidemiology.*
5. Explain the means by which health or health status can be measured.
6. List and explain the goal and objectives of health education.
7. Identify the practice of health education.
8. Explain the following concepts and principles:
   a. Health Field Concept
   b. levels of prevention
   c. risk factors
   d. health risk reduction
      chain of infection
      communicable disease model
      multicausation disease model
   e. Selected principles of health education—participation, empowerment, and cultural sensitivity

Key Terms

adjusted rate

advocacy

chain of infection

communicable diseases

communicable disease model

community health

coordinated school health program

crude rate

culturally competent

cultural sensitivity

death rates

continued

Key Terms, *continued*

disability-adjusted life
    expectancy (DALE)

disability-adjusted life years
    (DALYs)

disease prevention

discipline

ecological

emerging profession

empowerment

endemic

environment

epidemic

epidemiological data

epidemiology

health

health-adjusted life
    expectancy (HALE)

health behavior

health care organization

health education

health field

Health Field Concept

health promotion

health-related quality of life
    (HRQOL)

human biology

life expectancy

lifestyle

mental health

modifiable risk factors

multicausation disease model

noncommunicable diseases

nonmodifiable risk factors

ownership

pandemic

participation

physical health

population-based
    approaches

prevention

primary prevention

profession

public health

rate

risk factors

secondary prevention

social health

specific rate

spiritual health

tertiary prevention

wellness

years of potential life lost
    (YPLL)

Health education has come a long way since its early beginnings. As the profession has grown and changed, so have the role and responsibilities of health educators. The purpose of this book is to provide those new to the this profession with a sense of the past—how the profession was born and on what principles it was developed; a complete understanding of the present—what it is that health educators are expected to do, how they should do it, and what theories and models guide their work; and a look at the future—where the profession is headed, and how health educators can keep pace with the changes in order to be responsive to those whom they serve.

This first chapter provides a common background in the terminology, concepts, and principles of the profession. It briefly discusses why health education is referred to as an emerging profession, looks at the current state of the profession, defines many of the key words and terms used in the profession, shows how health and health status have been measured, outlines the goals and objectives of the profession, identifies the practice of health education, and discusses some of the basic, underlying concepts and principles of the profession.

An Emerging Profession

"Health education is eclectic in nature. As an applied science, it derives its body of knowledge from a variety of disciplines" (Galli, 1976, p. 158). More specifically, health education's "body of knowledge represents a synthesis of facts, principles, and concepts drawn from biological, behavioral, sociological, and health sciences, but interpreted in terms of human needs, human values, and human potential" (Cleary & Neiger, 1998, p. 11). As the applied science of health education has developed over the years, it has been labeled in a variety of ways as a process, a field, a discipline, and/or a profession. Most would agree health education is a process or several processes but to label it as only a process would not be accurate. The words *field* and *discipline* have been used interchangeably, so for the purposes of this discussion we will use the term *discipline*. Thus, the real question becomes, Is health education a discipline or a profession? Health education is neither but is somewhere between the two: in other words, an **emerging profession.** Though the debate may seem trivial, more technical than significant, or just a question of semantics, it is important that those studying to be health educators have an understanding of this discussion and be able to see how health education fits into the bigger picture.

One reason health education has been described in so many ways is that health educators have not been consistent in their use of labels. In the past, health educators either did not think it important to make a distinction in terminology or did not give much thought as to what the individual labels meant.

A **discipline** has been defined as "a branch of knowledge or learning" (Agnes, 2001, p. 410). Health education fits this definition, and then some. We see a discipline as something that is smaller than a **profession,** which has been defined as "a vocation or occupation requiring advanced education and training, and involving intellectual skills" (Agnes, 2001, pp. 1145–1146). Or, as Livingood (1996, p. 421) has stated, a profession is "the sociological construct for an occupation that has special status." Using these definitions, we see health education as fitting somewhere between a discipline and a profession, thus the term *emerging profession*.

To further support our claim that health education is an emerging profession, it might be helpful to present a list of characteristics of a profession. Feeney and Freeman (1999) felt that the following functions distinguish a profession. The words in the brackets are our opinions on how health education stacks up with each of these characteristics.

- A profession requires practitioner's to participate in *prolonged training* based on principles that involve judgment for their application, not a precise set of behaviors that apply in all cases. [Health educators are not in agreement over what constitutes an extensive period of preparation. Some say a bachelor's degree is necessary; others say a master's degree.]

- Professional training is delivered in accredited institutions. Rigorous *requirements for entry* to the training are controlled by members of the profession. [Health education has no requirement that training must take place in accredited institutions, nor does health education have requirements for entry into training.]

- A profession bases its work on a *specialized body of knowledge and expertise,* which is applied according to the particular needs of each case. [As noted earlier, health education's body of knowledge represents a synthesis of facts, principles, and concepts from several disciplines.]

- Members of the profession have agreed on *standards of practice*—procedures that are appropriate to the solution of ordinary predicaments that practitioners expect to encounter in their work. [Health education has identified the responsibilities and competencies for those who practice health education.]
- A profession is characterized by *autonomy*—it makes its own decisions regarding entry to the field, training, licensing, and standards. The profession exercises internal control over the quality of the services offered and regulates itself. [This is emerging, but not all of these aspects are clearly defined by health education. Currently, there is only informal control of the quality of services offered.]
- A profession has a *commitment to serving a significant social value*. It is altruistic and service oriented rather than profit oriented. Its primary goal is to meet the needs of clients. Society recognizes a profession as the only group from within the community that can perform this specialized function. [Health education has a commitment to serving a significant social value. With the acknowledgment in 1998 of the U.S. Department of Commerce and Labor formally recognizing "health educator" as a distinct occupation, health education is moving in the right direction, but there are still many, including some health professionals, who do not recognize the work of health educators.]
- A profession has a *code of ethics* that spells out its obligations to society. [Health Education has a code of ethics (see Appendix A).]

Though many of the characteristics on Feeney and Freeman's list can be met by health education, not all can be.

Further, Barber (1988) states that an emerging profession is an occupation which does not rank so clearly high or so clearly low on those attributes that distinguish an occupation from a profession. In other words, Barber indicates that an emerging profession has not been clearly defined by itself or others. We feel Feeney and Freeman's list and our comments on his list show that health education is an emerging profession.

Stating that health education is not at full profession status is not to say that those who engage in the work—health educators—are not professionals. A professional is "a person practicing a profession; a person who does something with great skill" (Agnes, 2001, p. 1146). All health educators, just like all physicians and lawyers, are professionals, regardless of the setting in which they work. Greene and Simons-Morton (1984, p. 388) have described professionals with the following descriptors.

1. They believe in what they are doing.
2. They want to see the job done properly.
3. They do their best.
4. They feel a sense of responsibility for the quality of work done by others in the field.

It is our belief that health educators meet all of these descriptors.

Have we convinced you that health education is an emerging profession? Maybe we have and maybe we have not; however, throughout the remainder of this book we use the term *profession* to represent *emerging profession*. We are also sure the debate (discipline vs. emerging profession vs. profession) will continue.

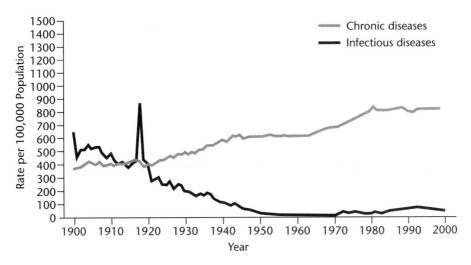

Figure 1.1   Infectious and Chronic Disease Death Rates in the United States, 1900–2000

Source: Adapted from G. L. Armstrong, L. A. Conn, and R. W. Pinner, "Trends in Infectious Disease Mortality in the United States During the 20th Century," Journal of the American Medical Association 281, no. 1 (1999): 61–66.

Current Status of Health Education

In looking back through history, there have been a number of occasions that can be pointed to as "critical" to the development of health education. (See Chapter 2 for an in-depth presentation of the history.) But there has been no time in history in which the status of the profession has been more visible to the average person or as widely accepted by other health professionals as it is today. Much of this notoriety can be attributed to the health promotion period of public health history that began about 1974 in the United States.

The United States' first public health revolution spanned the time period from the late nineteenth century through the mid-twentieth century and was aimed at controlling the harm (morbidity and mortality) that came from infectious diseases. By the mid-1950s, many of the infectious diseases in the United States were pretty much under control (see Figure 1.1). This was evidenced by the improved infant mortality rates, the reduction in the number of children who were contracting childhood diseases, the reduction in the overall death rates in the country, and the increase in life expectancy (see Table 1.1). With the control of many communicable diseases, the focus moved to the major chronic diseases such as heart disease, cancer, and strokes—diseases that were, in large part, the result of the way people lived.

By the mid-1970s, it had become apparent that the greatest potential for reducing morbidity, saving lives, and reducing health care costs in the United States was to be achieved through health promotion and disease prevention. At the core of this approach was health education. In 1980, the U.S. Department of Health, Education, and Welfare (USDHEW) presented a blueprint of the health promotion and disease prevention strategy in its first set of health objectives in the document called *Promoting Health/Preventing Disease: Objectives for a Nation* (USDHEW, 1980). This document proposed a total of 226 objectives divided into three main areas—preventive

Table 1.1   Life Expectancy at Birth, at Sixty-Five Years of Age, and at Seventy-Five Years of Age, According to Sex: United States, Selected Years 1900–2002

	At Birth			At 65 Years			At 75 Years		
Year	Both Sexes	Male	Female	Both Sexes	Male	Female	Both Sexes	Male	Female
1900	47.3	46.3	48.3	11.9	11.5	12.2	*	*	*
1950	68.2	65.6	71.1	13.9	12.8	15.0	*	*	*
1960	69.7	66.6	73.1	14.3	12.8	15.8	*	*	*
1970	70.8	67.1	74.7	15.2	13.1	17.0	*	*	*
1980	73.7	70.7	77.4	16.4	14.1	18.3	10.4	8.8	11.5
1990	75.4	71.8	78.8	17.2	15.1	18.9	10.9	9.4	12.0
1995	75.8	72.5	78.9	17.4	15.6	18.9	11.0	9.7	11.9
2000	76.9	74.1	79.5	17.9	16.3	19.2	11.3	10.1	12.1
2002[#]	77.4	74.7	79.9	18.2	16.6	19.5	11.6	10.4	12.5

* = Data not available
# = Estimate

Sources: Data from V. M. Freid, K. Prager, A. P. MacKay, and H. Xia, *Chartbook on Trends in Health of Americans. Health United States, 2003,* (Hyattsville, MD: National Center for Health Statistics, 2003), 140, and from K. D. Kochanek and B. L. Smith, *National Vital Statistics Reports, Deaths: Preliminary Data for 2002, 52* (13), (Hyattsville, MD: National Center for Health Statistics, 2004), 25.

services, health protection, and health promotion. This was the first time a comprehensive national agenda for prevention had been developed, with specific goals and objectives for anticipated gains (McGinnis, 1985). In 1985, it was apparent that only about one-half of the objectives established in 1980 would be reached by 1990, another one-fourth would not be reached, and progress on the others could not be judged because of the lack of data (Mason & McGinnis, 1990). Even though not all objectives were reached, the 1980 planning process demonstrated the value of setting goals and listing specific objectives as a means of measuring progress in the nation's health and health care services. These goals and objectives published by the U.S. Department of Health and Human Services (USDHHS), now in their third generation as *Healthy People 2010* (USDHHS, 2000), have defined the nation's health agenda and guided its health policy since their inception.

As we begin the 21st century, the health of the people in the United States is better than any time in the past. "By every measure, we are healthier, live longer, and enjoy lives that are less likely to be marked by injuries, ill health, or premature death" (Institute of Medicine [IOM], 2002, p. 2). Yet, we could do better. Much of the ill-health faced by Americans is the result of preventable conditions linked to our lifestyle.

Behavior patterns represent the single most prominent domain of influence over health prospects in the United States. The daily choices we make with respect to diet, physical activity, and sex; the substance abuse and additions to which we fall prey; our approach to safety; and our coping strategies in confronting stress are all important determinants of health (McGinnis, Williams-Russo, & Knickman, 2002, p. 82).

Clearly, there is a greater need for health education and health promotion interventions in the United States both today and in the future.

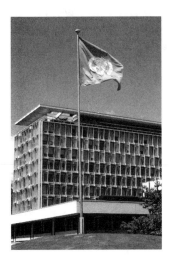

A specialized agency of the United Nations with 192 Member States, WHO promotes technical cooperation for health among nations, carries out programs to control and eradicate disease, and strives to improve the quality of human life. (World Health Organization/ Geneva, Switzerland)

Key Words, Terms, and Definitions

Each chapter introduces new terminology that is either important to the specific content presented in the chapter or used frequently in the profession. This chapter discusses the more common terms that will be used throughout this text. Like the profession, these words and definitions have evolved over the years. Over the past seventy plus years there have been several efforts to standardize the terms used in the profession. The most recent effort occurred in 2000 (Joint Terminology Committee, 2001). Every ten years the American Association for Health Education forms a task force, called the Joint Committee on Health Education and Health Promotion Terminology, to review and update the terminology of the profession (see Chapter 8 for information on this and other professional associations). The members of the 2000 Committee represented all of the professional associations within the Coalition of National Health Education Organizations (see Chapter 8), as well as key federal agencies (Joint Terminology Committee, 2001). Prior to this meeting, there have been six major terminology reports developed for the profession with the first dating back to 1927 (Johns, 1973; Joint Committee on Health Education Terminology, 1991a, 1991b; Moss, 1950; Rugen, 1972; Williams, 1934; & Yoho, 1962).

Prior to presenting some of the key terms used in the profession, an in-depth discussion of the word *health* may be helpful. Health is a difficult concept to put into words, but it is one that most people intuitively understand. The World Health Organization (WHO, 1947) has defined **health** as "the state of complete mental, physical and social well being not merely the absence of disease or infirmity." This classic definition is important, as it identifies the vital components of health. It further implies that health is a holistic concept involving an interaction and interdependence among these various components. A number of years after the writing of the WHO definition, Hanlon (1974) defined health as "a functional state which makes possible the achievement of other goals and activities. Comfort, well-being, and the distinction between physical and mental health differ in social classes, cultures, and religious groups" (p. 73). And more recently, the WHO (1986) has stated that health is a resource for everyday life, not the object of living. In other words, good health should not be the goal of life, but rather a vehicle to reaching one's goals in life. We are in agreement with these more recent definitions of health. We also believe health should still be conceptualized as a holistic concept involving mental, physical, and social components, and viewed as one's state of being. There are different levels of health, ranging from good to poor; therefore, one can be in a state of good health, a state of poor health, or anywhere in between.

To more fully understand the meaning of health, it is important to understand each of the individual components of health. Utilizing an extensive literature review, Goodstadt, Simpson, and Loranger (1987, p. 59) have aptly described each component of health:

physical health—the absence of disease and disability; functioning adequately from the perspective of physical and physiological abilities; the biological integrity of the individual

mental health—(termed *psychological health* by Goodstadt, Simpson, & Loranger, 1987)—may include emotional health; may make explicit reference to intellectual capabilities; the subjective sense of well-being

social health—the ability to interact effectively with other people and the social environment; satisfying interpersonal relationships; role fulfillment

The actual number of health components has been another point of contention. While WHO identified three components, others have separated emotional from psychological health and added spiritual health to arrive at as many as five components. In our discussions, we will maintain emotional and psychological as one domain but will add a spiritual domain. To define what is meant by spiritual, however, will be left to the individual reader. Goodstadt, Simpson, and Loranger (1987, p. 59) have noted the following description in the literature:

spiritual health—also labeled as "personal health"; it has been associated with the concept of self-actualization; it sometimes reflects a concern for issues related to one's value system; alternatively, it may be concerned with a belief in a transcending, unifying force (whether its basis is in nature, scientific law, or a godlike source).

In addition to the word *health* and its various components, it is also important to have an understanding of the following key terms and definitions:

community health—"the health status of a defined group of people and the actions and conditions to protect and improve the health of the community" (Green & McKenzie, 2002, p. 247)

health education—"any combination of planned learning experiences based on sound theories that provide individuals, groups, and communities the opportunity to acquire information and the skills needed to make quality health decisions" (Joint Committee, 2001, p. 99)

health promotion—"any planned combination of educational, political, environmental, regulatory, or organizational mechanisms that support actions and conditions of living conducive to the health of individuals, groups, and communities" (Joint Committee, 2001, p. 101) (See Figure 1.2 for the relationship between health education and health promotion.)

disease prevention—"the process of reducing risks and alleviating disease to promote, preserve, and restore health and minimize suffering and distress" (Joint Committee, 2001, p. 99)

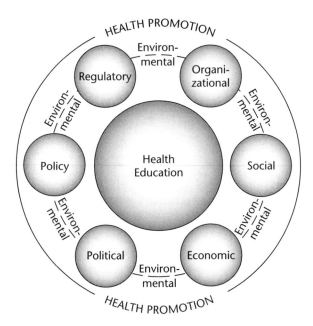

Figure 1.2   Relationship between Health Education and Health Promotion

Source: From J. F. McKenzie, B. L. Neiger, and J. L. Smeltzer, *Planning, Implementing and Evaluating Health Promotion Programs: A Primer.* 4th ed. (San Francisco: Benjamin Cummings, 2005). Reprinted by Permission.

public health—"the health status of a defined group of people and the governmental actions and conditions to promote, protect, and preserve their health" (McKenzie, Pinger, & Kotecki, 2005, p. 6).

coordinated school health program—"an organized set of policies, procedures, and activities designed to protect, promote, and improve the health and well-being of students and staff, thus improving a student's ability to learn. It includes, but is not limited to, comprehensive school health education; school health services; a healthy school environment; school counseling; psychological and social services; physical education; school nutrition services; family and community involvement in school health; and school-site health promotion for staff" (Joint Committee, 2001, p. 99) Note: In 1998, the term *coordinated school health program* replaced *comprehensive school health program* to distinguish it from comprehensive health education.

wellness—"an approach to health that focuses on balancing the many aspects, or dimensions, of a person's life through increasing the adoption of health-enhancing conditions and behaviors rather than attempting to minimize conditions of illness" (Joint Committee, 2001, p. 103)

Before we leave the discussion about key words and terms of the profession, it should be noted that there is not a complete agreement on terminology. For more on this topic, see the following two articles: Livingood, 1996; Ubbes & Watts, 1995.

Table 1.2 Estimated Death Rates for the Fifteen Leading Causes of Death: United States, 2002

Cause	Deaths per 100,000 Population
Diseases of the heart	241.3
Malignant neoplasms (cancer)	193.8
Cerebrovascular diseases (stroke)	56.5
Chronic lower respiratory diseases	43.5
Accidents (unintentional injuries)	35.5
Diabetes mellitus	25.5
Influenza and pneumonia	22.9
Alzheimer's disease	20.4
Nephritis, nephrotic syndrome, and nephrosis	14.2
Septicemia	11.7
Intentional self-harm (suicide)	10.6
Chronic liver disease and cirrhosis	9.4
Essential (primary) hypertension and hypertensive renal disease	7.0
Pneumonitis due to solids and liquids	6.1
Assault (homicide)	5.9
All other causes	144.6

Source: Data from K. D. Kochanek and B. L. Smith, *National Vital Statistics Reports, Deaths: Preliminary Data for 2002, 52* (13) (Hyattsville, MD: National Center for Health Statistics, 2004), 4.

Measuring Health or Health Status

Though the definition of *health* is easy to state, trying to quantify the amount of health an individual or a population possesses is not easy. Therefore, most measures of health are expressed using health statistics based on the traditional medical model of describing ill health (injury, disease, and death) instead of well health. Thus, the higher the presence of injury, disease, and death indicators, the lower the level of health; the lower the presence of injury, disease, and death indicators, the higher the level of health. Out of necessity we have defined the level of health with just the opposite—ill health (Cohen, 1991; McKenzie et al., 2005b).

The information gathered when measuring health is referred to as **epidemiological data**. These data are gathered at the local, state, and national levels to assist with the prevention of disease outbreaks or control those in progress and to plan and assess health education and promotion programs. Epidemiology is one of those disciplines noted earlier in the chapter that helps provide the foundation for the health education profession. **Epidemiology** is defined as "the study of the distribution and determinants of diseases and injuries in human populations" (Mausner & Kramer, 1985, p. 1). In the following sections, several of the more common epidemiological means by which health, or lack thereof, are described and quantified.

Rates

A **rate** "is a measure of some event, disease, or condition in relation to a unit of population, along with some specification of time" (Freid, Prager, MacKay, and Xia, 2003, p. 449). Rates are important because they provide an opportunity for comparison of events, diseases, or conditions that occur at different times or places. Some

Table 1.3   Selected Mortality Rates and Their Formulas

Rate	Definition	Example (U.S. 2002)*
Crude death rate =	$\dfrac{\text{Number of deaths (all causes)}}{\text{Estimated midyear population}} \times 100{,}000$	848.9/100,000
Age-specific death rate =	$\dfrac{\text{Number of deaths, 45–54}}{\text{Estimated midyear population, 45–54}} \times 100{,}000$	429.6/100,000
Cause-specific mortality rate =	$\dfrac{\text{Number of deaths (HIV)}}{\text{Estimated midyear population}} \times 100{,}000$	4.9/100,000

* = Estimate

Source: Data from K. D. Kochanek and B. L. Smith, *National Vital Statistics Reports, Deaths: Preliminary Data* for 2002, 52 (13). (Hyattsville, MD: National Center for Health Statistics, 2004) 4, 7, & 15.

of the more commonly used rates are death rates, birth rates, and morbidity rates. **Death rates** (the number of deaths per 100,000 resident population), sometimes referred to as *mortality* or *fatality rates*, are probably the most frequently used means of quantifying the seriousness of injury or disease. (See Table 1.2 for death rates and Table 1.3 for an example of a formula used to tabulate rates). "The transition from wellness to ill health is often gradual and poorly defined. Because death, in contrast, is a clearly defined event, it has continued to be the most reliable single indicator of health status of a population. Mortality statistics, however, describe only a part of the health status of a population, and often only the endpoint of an illness process" (USDHHS, 1991, p. 15). Rates can be expressed in three forms—crude, adjusted, and specific. A **crude rate** is the rate expressed for a total population. An **adjusted rate** is also expressed for a total population but is statistically adjusted for a certain characteristic such as age. A **specific rate** is a rate for a particular population subgroup such as for a particular disease (i.e., disease-specific) or for a particular age of people (i.e., age-specific) (Mausner & Kramer, 1985). Examples include calculating the death rate for heart disease in the United States, or the age-specific death rate for forty-five- to fifty-four-year-olds.

There are three other epidemiological terms that are used to describe the magnitude of a rate of some event, disease, or condition in a unit of population. They are: **endemic**—occurs regularly in a population as a matter of course; **epidemic**—an unexpectedly large number of cases of a disease in a population; and **pandemic**—an outbreak of a disease over a wide geographical area, such as a continent. As you continue your preparation to become a health educator, you will be introduced to more and more epidemiological principles and terms.

Life Expectancy

Life expectancy is another means by which health or health status has been measured. It, too, however, is based on mortality. Even with this limitation, though, life expectancy has been described as "the most comprehensive indicator of patterns of

Box 1.1 Practitioner's Perspective: Epidemiology

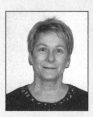

NAME: Jean Woodward, BS, CHES

CURRENT POSITION/TITLE: Manager, Idaho Asthma Prevention and Control/Health Education Specialist, Senior

EMPLOYER: Idaho Department of Health and Welfare

DEGREE/INSTITUTION/YEAR: Bachelor of Health Science/Boise State University/2001

MAJOR: Health Promotion

How I obtained my job: My diverse employment background prepared me well to be a public health educator. Prior to my public health service, I was a teacher (grades 1–12) for 10 years and an acute care nurse for 18 years. In addition, I was involved in several community-level programs, many of which I was the initiator. My background in health and education along with my community mobilization experience made public health educator a natural choice for me. I began at the local health district level and after four years moved to the state level.

While I was working at the local health district in a clinical capacity, a position in health promotion became available. Candidates for the position had to meet minimum experience and educational requirements. My background, risk communication skills, and ability to work with diverse communities were the deciding points for my being hired.

How I utilize an understanding of epidemiology in my job: Public health is a population-based practice that includes assessing health status, diagnosing and investigating health problems and health hazards, designing solutions for health problems, and evaluating the efficacy of those solutions. Epidemiology is the tool I use to perform each of these functions. Epidemiology helps me determine if a health problem exists, who has the health problem, where the health problem is located, and the severity of the health problem. It can also guide me to

an effective intervention point and potential solutions to the problem. In short, epidemiology provides the science-base for my public health interventions.

What I like most about my job: Health promotion is always challenging; no two days are ever the same. Because of its prevention focus, I believe I can truly make a difference in people's lives. Also, public health is collaborative by nature and I enjoy the synergy of team effort. By engaging and networking with community partners I am able to provide more comprehensive, effective, and efficient health promotion programs.

What I like least about my job: Health doesn't occur in a vacuum. I feel that only through utilizing an integrated systems approach to health, we can effectively support the health behavior changes that result in improved public health. Funding for public health tends to be categorical. There are separate pots of money for each health issue, no matter that most health issues are related at some level. This compartmentalization leads to inefficiency through duplication of efforts and wasting of resources.

Recommendations for those preparing to be health educators: There are four recommendations that I would make: (1) Get as much education as you can; there is no such thing as too much; (2) Get broad experience through graduate assistantships/internships/work; (3) Apply what you learn as quickly as possible; and (4) Learn to write succinctly.

Table 1.4   Age-adjusted Years of Potential Life Lost (per 100,000 population) before Age 75 for Selected Leading Causes of Death: United States, 1990 and 2000

Cause	1990	2000
Malignant neoplasms	2,003.8	1,674.1
Diseases of the heart	1,617.7	1,253.0
Accidents (unintentional injuries)	1,162.1	1,026.6
Intentional self-harm (suicide)	393.1	334.5
Assault (homicide)	417.4	266.5
Cerebrovascular diseases (stroke)	259.6	223.3
Chronic lower respiratory diseases	187.4	188.1
Diabetes mellitus	155.9	178.4
HIV	383.8	174.6
Chronic liver disease and cirrhosis	196.9	164.1
Influenza and pneumonia	141.5	87.1

Source: Data from V. M. Freid, K. Prager, A. P. MacKay, and H. Xia, *Chartbook on Trends in Health of Americans. Health United States, 2003.* (Hyattsville, MD: National Center for Health Statistics, 2003), 140.

health and disease, as well as living standards and social development" (Centers for Disease Control and Prevention [CDC], 1994, pp. 2–8). **Life expectancy** "is the average number of years of life remaining to a person at a particular age and is based on a given set of age-specific death rates, generally the mortality conditions existing in the period mentioned. Life expectancy may be determined by race, sex, or other characteristics using age-specific death rates for the population with that characteristic" (Freid et al., 2003, p. 434). The two most frequently used times to state life expectancy are at birth and at age sixty-five. These two times are used because they are means of quantifying the length of life and length of retirement, assuming most people retire at age sixty-five (see Table 1.1). In terms of evaluating the effect of chronic disease on a population, life expectancies calculated *after* birth have been found to be more useful measures than life expectancy *at* birth, because life expectancy at birth reflects infant mortality rates.

Years of Potential Life Lost

A third means by which health or health status has been measured is **years of potential life lost (YPLL).** YPLL "is a measure of premature mortality" (Freid et al., 2003, p. 454) (see Table 1.4). It is calculated by subtracting a person's age at death from seventy-five years. For example, for a person who dies at age thirty, the YPLL are forty-five. Obviously, the earlier someone dies, the greater the YPLL. Some ask why age seventy-five is used instead of a person's projected life expectancy when calculating YPLL. Until 1996, the U.S. government regularly used sixty-five for calculating YPLL because sixty-five was the standard age of retirement (McKenzie et al., 2005b). However, today people are living and working longer, thus the switch to age seventy-five.

Table 1.5   Disability-Adjusted Life Expectancy (DALE) for Selected Countries

Country	Both Sexes At birth	Males At birth	Males Age 60	Females At birth	Females Age 60
Japan	74.5	71.9	17.5	77.2	21.6
United States	70.0	67.5	15.0	72.6	18.4
Mexico	65.0	62.4	14.7	67.6	16.8
China	62.3	61.2	11.6	63.3	13.5
Malawi, Africa	29.4	29.3	6.8	29.4	8.3

Source: Data from C. D. Mathers, R. Sdana, J. A. Salomon, C. J. L. Murray and A. D. Lopez, *Estimates of DALE for 191 countries: Methods and results.* Global Programme on Evidence for Health Policy Working Paper No. 16. (Geneva, Switzerland: World Health Organization, 2000). Available at http://www3 .who.int/whosis/

Disability-Adjusted Life Years

The three measures of health and health status noted previously are commonly used in the United States and other developed countries. However, because mortality does not express the burden of living with disability (for example, the resulting paralysis from an automobile crash or the depression that often follows a stroke), the WHO and the World Bank developed a measure called **disability-adjusted life years (DALYs).** One DALY is equal to one lost year of healthy life (Murray & Lopez, 1996).

> To calculate total DALYs for a given condition in a population, years of life lost (YLL) and years lived with disability of known severity and duration (YLDs) for that condition must each be estimated, then the total summed. For example, to calculate DALYs incurred through road accidents in India in 1990, add the total years of life lost in fatal road accidents and the total years of life lived with disabilities by survivors of such accidents (Murray & Lopez, 1996, p. 7).

Disability-Adjusted Life Expectancy and Health-Adjusted Life Expectancy

Two other measurements, which are used by the WHO and are based on disability and life expectancy rather than mortality, are **disability-adjusted life expectancy** (**DALE**) and **health-adjusted life expectancy** (**HALE**). Like life expectancy, DALEs and HALEs can be calculated at birth and at other ages. Each measures approximately the same thing, namely expected remaining years of healthy life, but they are calculated differently because they differ in the way they measure disability (Mathers, Sdana, Salomon, Murray, & Lopez, 2000). Table 1.5 presents the DALE for selected countries for both sexes at birth and for males and females at birth and age sixty.

Health-Related Quality of Life

Even though DALYs, DALEs, and HALEs go beyond measuring health in terms of just mortality, they really do not get at the quality of life (QOL). That is, even though people may have a good health-adjusted life expectancy (HALE), they may not feel that their quality of life is good. "QOL is a popular term that conveys an overall sense of well-being, including aspects of happiness and satisfaction with life as a whole" (CDC, 2000, p. 5). Those aspects of people's quality of life that can be clearly shown to affect their health, either physically or mentally, make up their **health-related quality of life (HRQOL)** (McHorney, 1999).

The concept of HRQOL can be applied to both the health of an individual and the health of a community. On the individual level, HRQOL "includes physical and mental health perceptions and their correlates, including health risks and conditions, functional status, social support, and socioeconomic status" (CDC, 2000, p. 6). "On the community level, HRQOL includes resources, conditions, policies, and practices that influence a population's health perceptions and functional status" (CDC, 2000, p. 6).

In recent years, more and more health professionals have been using the concept of HRQOL to quantify and track the health status of people. Measures of HRQOL are now included on a number of different health surveys, including the Behavioral Risk Factor Surveillance Survey (BRFSS).

Health Surveys

Data collected through surveys conducted by governmental agencies are other means by which health or health status has been measured in the United States. Six examples are presented here. The first two, the National Health Interview Survey and the National Health and Nutrition Examination Survey (NHANES), are conducted by the National Center for Health Statistics. The National Health Interview Survey is a telephone interview in which respondents are asked a number of questions about their health and health behavior. One of the questions, for example, asks the respondents to describe their health status using one of five categories: excellent, very good, good, fair, or poor. The NHANES data are collected using a mobile examination center. Through direct physical examinations, clinical and laboratory testing, and related procedures, data are collected on a representative group of Americans. "These examinations result in the most authoritative source of standardized clinical, physical, and physiological data on the American people. Included in the data are the prevalence of specific conditions and diseases and data on blood pressure, serum cholesterol, body measurements, nutritional status and deficiencies, and exposure to environmental toxins" (McKenzie et al., 2005b, p. 79).

The third and fourth surveys, also conducted by the National Center for Health Statistics, are the National Hospital Discharge Survey (NHDS) and the National Hospital Ambulatory Care Survey (NHAMCS). The former survey is an important source of national data on the characteristics of patients discharged from nonfederal short-stay hospitals. Such data can be used to determine the rates for inpatient procedures, diagnoses, length of stay, and rates of discharges (Hall & DeFrances, 2003). The purpose of the NHAMCS has been to collect and disseminate data about the health care provided by hospital outpatient and emergency departments to the U.S. population (Hing & Middleton, 2003).

The fifth example of data collected through a survey is the data collected through the Behavioral Risk Factor Surveillance System (BRFSS). These data are collected by individual states, territories, and the District of Columbia through cooperative agreements with the Centers for Disease Control and Prevention (CDC). Through the use of telephone survey techniques, each state selects a probability sample from the civilian, noninstitutionalized adult population (over eighteen years of age). Those selected are asked a set of standard core questions, developed by the CDC in order to produce data about health behaviors that can be compared across states (CDC, 2003a). In addition, states may include other questions that would be useful in monitoring health in that particular state.

Because of the success of the BRFSS a similar surveillance system was begun for youth. The Youth Risk Behavior Surveillance System (YRBSS) was developed in 1990 to monitor priority health risk behaviors that contribute markedly to the leading causes of death, disability, and social problems among youth and adults in the United States. The six categories of priority health-risk behaviors include: tobacco use; dietary behaviors; inadequate physical activity; alcohol and other drug use; sexual behaviors that contribute to unintended pregnancy and sexually transmitted infections, including HIV infection; and behaviors that contribute to unintentional injuries and violence (CDC, 2003b).

The Goal and Objectives of the Profession

The ultimate goal of all service professions, including health education, is to improve the quality of life, even though the quality of life is difficult to quantify (Raphael, Brown, Renwick, and Rootman, 1997). However, many professionals feel that there is a direct relationship between quality of life and health status. Quality of life is usually improved when health status is improved, or, as Ashley Montagu (1968, p. 206) has stated, "The highest goal in life is to die young, at as old an age as possible." To that end, "the goal of health education is to promote, maintain, and improve individual and community health. The teaching-learning process is the hallmark and social agenda that differentiates the practice of health education from that of other helping professions in achieving this goal" (NCHEC, 1996, pp. 2–3).

Because quality of life and health status are complex variables, they are not usually changed in a short period of time. In order to reach these goals, people usually, over a period of time, work their way through a number of small steps that equip them with all that is necessary to impact both their health status and, in turn, their quality of life. To assist with these steps, health educators have identified a hierarchy of objectives that are useful in developing health education/promotion programs. This hierarchy is presented in Table 1.6. Please note that these objectives are presented from easiest to most difficult to achieve. For clarification, we define *easiest* as those that take the least time and resources to accomplish.

The Practice of Health Education

The practice of health education is based on the assumption "that beneficial health behavior will result from a combination of planned, consistent, integrated learning opportunities. This assumption rests on the scientific evaluations of health education programs in schools, at worksites, in medical settings, and through the mass media" (Green & Ottoson, 1999, pp. 93–94). It also rests on evidence from experiences outside the fields of health and education such as community development, social work, agricultural extension, and marketing (Green & Ottoson, 1999).

Table 1.6 Hierarchy of Objectives and Their Relation to Evaluation (Easiest to Most Difficult)

Type of Objective	Program Outcomes	Possible Evaluation Measures	Type of Evaluation
Process/Administrative Objectives	Activities presented and tasks completed	Number of sessions held, exposure, attendance participation, staff performance, appropriate materials, adequacy of resources, tasks on schedule	Process (form of formative)

Learning Objectives
  Awareness
  Knowledge
  Attitudes
  Skills
	Change in awareness
	Change in knowledge
	Change in attitude
	Change in skills
		Increase in awareness
		Increase in knowledge
		Improved attitude
		Skill development or acquisition
			Impact (form of summative)

Action/Behavioral Objectives	Change in behavior	Current behavior modified or discontinued, or new behavior adopted	Impact (form of summative)
Environmental Objectives	Change in the environment	Protection added to or hazards or barriers removed from the environment	Impact (form of summative)
Program Objectives	Change in quality of life (QOL), health status risk factors, and social benefits	QOL measures, morbidity data, mortality data, measures of risk (i.e., HRA), physiological measures, signs and symptoms	Outcome (form of summative)

Source: From J. F. McKenzie, B. L. Neiger, and J. L. Smeltzer, *Planning, Implementing and Evaluating Health Promotion Programs: A Primer,* 4th ed. (San Francisco: Benjamin Cummings, 2005), 131. Copyright © 2005 by Benjamin Cummings. Originally adapted from S. G. Deeds, *The Health Education Specialist: Self-Study for Professional Competence.* (Los Alamitos, CA: Loose Canon, 1992) and M. J. Cleary and B. L. Neiger, *The Certified Health Education Specialist: A Self-Study Guide for Professional Competency,* 3rd ed. (Allentown, Pa: The National Commission for Health Education Credentialing, 1998). Reprinted by permission.

Though the specific work of health educators is outlined in the responsibilities and competencies presented in Chapter 6, the primary role of health educators is to develop—plan, implement, and evaluate—appropriate health education/promotion programs for the people they serve. Though easily stated, this is by no means an easy task. Good health education/promotion programs do not just happen. Much time, effort, practice, and on-the-job training are required to be successful. Even the most experienced health educators find program development challenging because of the constant changes in settings, resources, and priority populations (McKenzie, Neiger, & Smeltzer, 2005).

Though the specific steps taken to develop a health education/promotion program vary based on the planning model used (see Chapter 4), most models include the following steps (McKenzie et al., 2005a) (see Figure 4.4):

1. Understanding the community and engaging the priority population
2. Assessing the needs of the priority population
3. Setting goals and objectives
4. Developing an intervention that considers the peculiarities of the setting
5. Implementing the intervention
6. Evaluating the results

Therefore, it becomes the practice of health educators to be able to carry out all that is associated with these tasks.

Basic Underlying Concepts of the Profession

As was noted earlier in this chapter and discussed in greater detail in Chapter 2, the profession of health education is one that has been built on the principles and concepts of a number of disciplines and professions. Within health education can be found pieces of community development and organizing, education, epidemiology, medicine, psychology, and sociology. In the sections that follow, we present some of the basic underlying concepts of the profession. Please note that we have not exhausted the discussion of each of these topics but, rather, present sufficient information to allow a basic understanding of each.

The Health Field Concept

Shortly after the Canadian government implemented its national health plan in 1973 that insured health care for all Canadians, it began to look more closely at the health field as a way of improving Canadians' health. The **health field** is a term the government described as being far more encompassing than the "health care system." This term was much broader and included all matters that affected health (Lalonde, 1974). Since the health field was such a broad concept, it was felt that there was a need to develop a framework that would subdivide the concept into principal elements so that the elements could be studied. Such a framework was developed and called the **Health Field Concept** (Laframboise, 1973).

The Health Field Concept divided the health field into four elements: human biology, environment, lifestyle, and health care organization. "These four elements were identified through an examination of the causes and underlying factors of sickness and death in Canada, and from an assessment of the parts the elements play in affecting the level of health in Canada" (Lalonde, 1974, p. 31). **Human biology** "includes all those aspects of health, both physical and mental, which are developed within the human body as a consequence of the basic biology of man [sic] and the organic make-up of an individual" (Lalonde, 1974, p. 31). This includes not only the genetic inheritance of an individual but also the processes of maturation and aging and the complex interaction of the various systems of the human body (Lalonde, 1974). The element of **environment** "includes all those matters related to health which are external to the human body and over which the individual has little or no control" (Lalonde, 1974, p. 32). Some examples of things often included in the element of environment are geography, climate, community size, industrial development, economy, and social norms.

The element of **lifestyle** is comprised of the "aggregation of decisions by individuals which affect their health and over which they more or less have control" (Lalonde, 1974, p. 32). In more recent times, lifestyle has been more commonly referred to as **health behavior** (those behaviors that impact a person's health). The fourth element in the Health Field Concept is health care organization. **Health care organization** "consists of the quantity, quality, arrangement, nature and relationships of people and resources in the provision of health care" (Lalonde, 1974, p. 32). This fourth element is often referred to as the health care system.

The utility of the Health Field Concept has proved to be very helpful over the years, both in Canada and the United States. Its greatest importance may have been to bring attention to the concept of health promotion and disease prevention. Prior to this point in history, the primary focus of health care had been on the cure of disease, not the prevention of disease. In fact, it was stated that the Health Field Concept put human biology, environment, and lifestyle on equal footing with health care organization (Lalonde, 1974). Since its development, studies using this concept in both Canada and the United States have provided a greater understanding of what contributes to morbidity and mortality, and what health professionals can do to help improve the health of those whom they serve.

Using a similar framework as that of the elements of the Health Field Concept, it is now believed that the health of populations is shaped by five intersecting domains: genetics, social circumstances, environmental conditions, behavioral choices, and medical care (IOM, 2001; McGinnis, 2001). Further, these domains are dynamic and vary in impact depending on where one is in the life cycle (IOM, 2001). For example, we know that genetics play a big part in late onset diseases such as diabetes, cancer, and cardiovascular disease, while employment and income (social circumstances) have a significant influence on health and health care throughout life.

> On a population basis, using the best available estimates, the impacts of various domains on early deaths in the United States distribute roughly as follows: genetic predispositions, about 30%, social circumstances, 15%, environmental exposures, 5%, behavioral patterns, 40%; and shortfalls in medical care about 10%. But more important than these proportions is the nature of the influences in play where the domains intersect. Ultimately, the health fate of each of us is determined by factors acting not mostly in isolation but by our experience where domains interconnect. Whether a gene is expressed can be determined by environmental exposures or behavioral patterns. The nature and consequences of behavioral choices are affected by our social circumstances. Our genetic predispositions affect the health care we need, and our social circumstances affect the health care we receive (McGinnis, et al., 2002, p. 83).

The Levels and Limitations of Prevention

The word *prevention* has already been used several times in this chapter. We now want to formally define the term, present the different levels of prevention, and briefly discuss the limitations of prevention. **Prevention,** as it relates to health, has

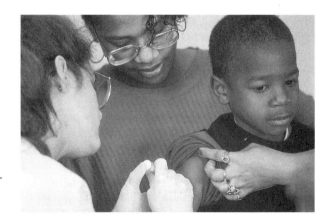

Vaccination is an example of primary prevention. (F. Hoffman/ The Image Works)

been defined as the planning for and the measures taken to forestall the onset of a disease or other health problem before the occurrence of undesirable health events. This definition presents three distinct levels of prevention: primary, secondary, and tertiary prevention. **Primary prevention** is comprised of those preventive measures that forestall the onset of illness or injury during the prepathogenesis period (before the disease process begins) (McKenzie et al., 2005b). Examples of primary prevention measures include wearing a safety belt, using rubber gloves when there is potential for the spread of disease, immunizing against specific diseases, exercising, and brushing one's teeth. And any health education/promotion program aimed specifically at forestalling the onset of illness or injury is also an example of primary prevention.

Illness and injury cannot always be prevented. In fact, many diseases, such as cancer and heart disease, can establish themselves in humans and cause considerable damage before they are detected and treated. In such cases, the sooner a condition is detected and medical personnel intervene, the greater the chances of limiting disability and preventing death. Such identification and intervention are known as secondary prevention. More specifically, **secondary prevention** includes the preventive measures that lead to an early diagnosis and prompt treatment of a disease or an injury to limit disability and prevent more serious pathogenesis. Good examples of secondary prevention include personal and clinical screenings and exams such as blood pressure, cholesterol, and hemocult (hidden blood) screenings; breast self-exams (BSE); and testicle self-exams (TSE). The goal of such screenings and exams "is not to prevent the onset of the disease but rather to detect its presence during early pathogenesis, thus permitting early intervention (treatment) and limiting disability" (McKenzie et al., 2005b, p. 104).

The final level of prevention is **tertiary prevention.** It is at this level that health educators work to retrain, reeducate, and rehabilitate the individual who has already incurred disability, impairment, or dependency. Examples of some tertiary measures include educating a patient after lung cancer surgery or working with an individual who has diabetes to ensure that the daily insulin injections are taken. Figure 1.3 provides a visual representation of the levels of prevention in relation to health status.

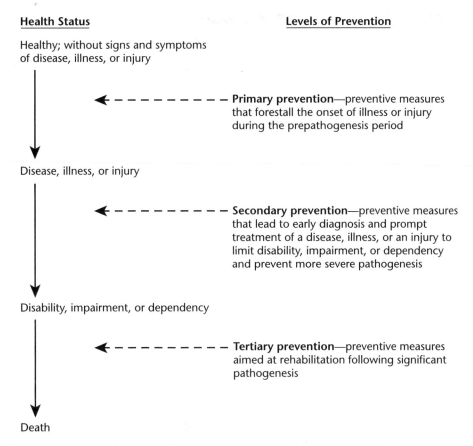

Figure 1.3   Levels of Prevention

Source: From J. F. McKenzie, B. L. Neiger, and J. L. Smeltzer, *Planning, Implementing and Evaluating Health Promotion Programs: A Primer.* 4th ed., (San Francisco: Benjamin Cummings 2005), 6. Originally adapted from G. E. Pickett and J. J. Hanlon, *Public Health: Administration and Practice.* (St. Louis: Mosby-Year Book, Inc., 1990). Reprinted by Permission.

Though health educators can intervene at any of the three levels of prevention, and can have a great deal of success in halting or reversing the disease process, it should be obvious from the earlier discussion of the Health Field Concept that prevention is not the "magic bullet" for an endless life. Prevention does have its limits. McGinnis (1985) has noted four major categories of limitations: biological, technological, ethical, and economic. Biological limitations center around life span. How long should individuals expect to live healthy lives or, for that matter, how long should they expect to live at all? Even with the very best inputs and a bit of luck, one should not expect to live longer than 80 to 110 years. Body parts will eventually wear out from use.

Technological advances also have their limitations. Today, health care workers have a vast array of technical equipment available to help them care for their patients, but technology still has not been able to eradicate AIDS or malaria, or to explain the causes of arthritis or Alzheimer's disease.

Prevention is also limited by ethical concerns (see Chapter 5). Even though helmets would increase the chances of survival in automobile crashes, is it ethical to have a law that says all drivers and passengers in automobiles must wear them? Or is it ethical to penalize people via fines, taxes, or surcharges for acting in unhealthy ways, such as driving an automobile without a safety belt on, buying and using tobacco products, or for not having a smoke detector and fire extinguisher in the home?

Finally, prevention has economic limitations. Prevention is limited by the amount of money that is put into it. Though the exact figures are difficult to determine, it is commonly understood that less than 5% of all dollars spent on health in the United States each year are spent on prevention. Stated another way, approximately 95% of the trillion plus dollars spent on health in the United States each year are spent on curing ill health, not on preventing it (IOM, 2000; 2002).

Risk Factors

The Health Field Concept has provided those interested in health issues with a framework from which the health field can be studied. The levels of prevention and their limitations have provided this same group of people with a time frame from which to plan to help forestall the onset of, limit the spread of, and rehabilitate after pathogenesis or another health problem. What neither of these concepts fully discloses is the focus at which health promotion and disease prevention programming should be aimed. The targets of such programming are **risk factors,** those inherited, environmental, and behavioral influences "capable of provoking ill health with or without previous disposition" (USDHEW, 1979, p. 13). Risk factors increase the probability of morbidity and premature mortality but do not guarantee that people with a risk factor will suffer the consequences.

Risk factors can be divided into two categories: **modifiable** (changeable or controllable) and **nonmodifiable** (nonchangeable or noncontrollable) **risk factors.** The former include such factors as sedentary lifestyle, smoking, and poor dietary habits—things that individuals can change or control while the latter group includes factors such as age, sex, and inherited genes—things that individuals cannot change or do not have control over. Note that these two categories of risk factors are often interrelated. In fact, the combined potential for harm from a number of risk factors is greater than the sum of their individual potentials. For example, asbestos workers have an increased risk for cancer because of their exposure to this carcinogen. Further, if they smoke, they have a thirty times greater chance of developing lung cancer than do their nonsmoking coworkers and a ninety times greater chance of getting lung cancer than do people who neither work with asbestos nor smoke (USDHEW, 1979). The risks increase if they have an inherited respiratory disease.

Over the years, knowledge about the impact of risk behaviors has continued to grow. In looking back over the 20th century, we have seen disease prevention change "from focusing on reducing environmental exposures over which the individual had little control, such as providing potable water, to emphasizing behaviors such as avoiding use of tobacco, fatty foods, and a sedentary lifestyle" (Breslow, 1999, p. 1030). As noted earlier, approximately 40% of the deaths in the United States each year are caused by these behavior patterns that could be modified by preventive interventions (McGinnis et al., 2002). Therefore, much of the focus of the work of health educators has been to help individuals identify and control their modifiable risk factors.

Table 1.7   Leading Causes of Death and Associated Risk Factors for All Ages: United States, 2002

Rank	Cause	Risk Factors
1	Diseases of the heart	Tobacco use, high blood pressure, elevated serum cholesterol, diet, diabetes, obesity, lack of exercise, alcohol abuse, biological factors
2	Malignant neoplasms (cancer)	Tobacco use, alcohol misuse, diet, solar radiation, ionizing radiation, worksite hazards, environmental pollution, biological factors
3	Cerebrovascular diseases (stroke)	Tobacco use, high blood pressure, elevated serum cholesterol, diabetes, obesity, biological factors
4	Chronic lower respiratory diseases	Tobacco use diseases
5	Accidents (unintentional injuries)	Alcohol misuse, tobacco use (fires), product design, home hazards, handgun availability, lack of safety restraints, excessive speed, automobile design, roadway design
6	Diabetes mellitus	Obesity (for type II diabetes), diet, lack of exercise, biological factors
7	Pneumonia and influenza	Tobacco use, infectious agents, biological factors
8	Alzheimer's disease	Age, family history[a]
9	Nephritis, nephrotic syndrome, and nephrosis	Infectious agents, drug hypersensitivity, biological factors, trauma
10	Septicemia	Infectious agents[b]
11	Intentional self-harm (suicide)	Handgun availability, alcohol or drug misuse, stress, biological factors
12	Chronic liver disease and cirrhosis	Alcohol misuse, infectious agents

Source: [a]Alzheimer's Association (2004). *Facts: About Genes and Alzheimer's Disease.* Retrieved March 26, 2004 from http://www.alz.org/

Source: [b]National Library of Medicine and the National Institutes of Health (2003). *Medical Encyclopedia: Septicemia.* Retrieved March 26, 2004 from http://www.nlm.nih.gov/medlineplus/print/ency/article/001355.htm

Health Risk Reduction

In order to be able to take aim at specific risk factors, health educators must have a basic understanding of both communicable (infectious) and noncommunicable (noninfectious) diseases. "**Communicable diseases** are those diseases for which biological agents or their products are the cause and that are transmissible from one individual to another" (McKenzie et al., 2005b, pp. 92–93), while "**noncommunicable diseases** or illnesses are those that cannot be transmitted from an infected person to a susceptible, healthy one" (McKenzie et al., 2005, p. 93). Our intent in this section and the ones that follow is not to present information on all possible diseases and their related risk factors that a health educator may have to develop programs for, but rather to provide a general understanding of the spread and cause of disease. (See Table 1.7 for leading causes of death and their risk factors.)

Table 1.8   Actual Causes of Death in the United States, 1990 and 2000

	1990		2000	
Actual Cause	Number	%[a]	Number	%[a]
Tobacco	400,000	19	435,000	18.1
Poor diet and physical inactivity	300,000	14	400,000	16.6
Alcohol consumption	100,000	5	85,000	3.5
Microbial agents	90,000	4	75,000	3.1
Toxic agents	60,000	3	55,000	2.3
Motor vehicle	25,000	1	43,000	1.8
Firearms	35,000	2	29,000	1.2
Sexual behavior	30,000	1	20,000	0.8
Illicit drug use	20,000	<1	17,000	0.7
Total	1,060,000	50	1,159,000	48.2

[a]= The percentages are for all deaths

Sources: The 1990 data from J. M. McGinnis and W. H. Foege, "Actual Causes of Death in the United States." *Journal of the American Medical Association* 270 18 (1993): 2207–2212. The 2000 data from A. H. Mokdad et al., "Actual Causes of Death in the United States, 2000." *Journal of the American Medical Association* 29, 10 (2004): 1238–1245.

Before moving on, we would like to make a special note about one of the terms presented in Table 1.7. The term *leading causes of death* is used in this table. That term refers to "the primary pathophysiological conditions identified at the time of death, as opposed to the root causes" (McGinnis & Foege, 1993, p. 2207). In 1993 McGinnis and Foege conducted a study to see if they could identify the root causes of death. What they found was that the leading *actual causes of death* were modifiable behaviors; behaviors that people could change. The behavior that was the leading actual cause of death was tobacco use, accounting for some 400,000, or 19%, of the mortality in 1990. A similar study to that of McGinnis and Foege (1993) was conducted by Mokdad, Marks, Stroup, and Gerberding in 2004 using 2000 mortality data. They also found tobacco to be the leading actual cause of death, but that poor diet and physical inactivity killed almost as many (see Table 1.8). "These findings, along with escalating health care costs and aging population, argue persuasively that the need to establish a more preventive orientation in the U.S. health care and public health systems has become more urgent" (Mokdad et al., 2004, p. 1238).

The Chain of Infection.   The **chain of infection** (see Figure 1.4) is a model used to explain the spread of a communicable disease from one host to another. The basic premise represented in the chain of infection is that individuals can break the chain (reduce the risk) at any point; thus, the spread of disease can be stopped. For example, the spread of some waterborne diseases are stopped when the first link of the chain is broken with the chlorination of the water supply, thus killing the pathogens that cause a disease. The risk is reduced because the pathogen is destroyed before it is consumed. The chain can also be broken by placing a barrier between the means of transmission and the portal of entry, as when health care providers protect themselves with surgical masks and rubber

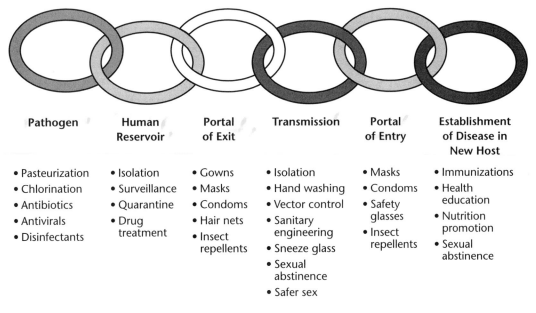

Pathogen	Human Reservoir	Portal of Exit	Transmission	Portal of Entry	Establishment of Disease in New Host
• Pasteurization	• Isolation	• Gowns	• Isolation	• Masks	• Immunizations
• Chlorination	• Surveillance	• Masks	• Hand washing	• Condoms	• Health education
• Antibiotics	• Quarantine	• Condoms	• Vector control	• Safety glasses	• Nutrition promotion
• Antivirals	• Drug treatment	• Hair nets	• Sanitary engineering	• Insect repellents	• Sexual abstinence
• Disinfectants		• Insect repellents	• Sneeze glass		
			• Sexual abstinence		
			• Safer sex		

Figure 1.4   Chain of Infection Model and Strategies for Disease Prevention and Control

Source: J. F. McKenzie, R. R. Pinger, and J. E. Kotecki. *An Introduction to Community Health.* 5th ed. (Sudbury, MA: Jones and Bartlett Publishers, 2005). Reprinted by permission.

gloves. In this case, the risk is reduced because individuals are not exposing themselves to the pathogen. With such information, health educators can help create programs that are aimed at "breaking" the chain and reducing the risks.

Communicable Disease Model.   A second model used to describe the spread of a communicable disease is the **communicable disease model.** Figure 1.5 presents the elements of this model—agent, host, and environment. These three elements summarize the minimal requirements for the presence and spread of a communicable disease in a population. The agent is the element (or, using the chain of infection labels, the pathogen) that must be present for a disease to spread—for example, bacteria or a virus. The host is any susceptible organism that can be invaded by the agent. Examples include plants, animals, and humans. The environment includes all other factors that either prohibit or promote disease transmission. Thus, communicable disease transmission occurs when a susceptible host and a pathogenic agent exist in an environment conducive to disease transmission.

Multicausation Disease Model.   Obviously, the chain of infection and communicable disease models are most helpful in trying to prevent disease caused by a pathogen. However, they are not applicable to noncommunicable diseases, which include many of the chronic diseases such as heart disease and cancer. Most of these diseases manifest themselves in people over a period of time and

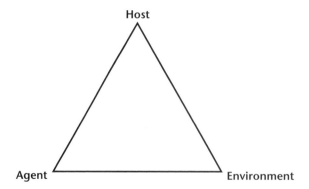

Figure 1.5 Communicable Disease Model

are not caused by a single factor but by combined factors. The concept of "caused by many factors" is referred to as the **multicausation disease model** (see Figure 1.6). For example, it is known that heart disease is more likely to manifest itself in individuals who are older, who smoke, who do not exercise, who are overweight, who have high blood pressure, who have high cholesterol, and who have immediate family members who have had heart disease. Note that within this list of factors there are both modifiable and nonmodifiable risk factors. As when using the chain of infection model, the work of health educators is to create programs to help people reduce the risk of disease and injury by helping those in the priority population identify and control as many of the multicausative factors as possible.

Other Selected Principles

Several other principles of health education have been noted by Cleary and Neiger (1998). They have identified via the work of others that health educators must address the principles of participation, empowerment, and cultural sensitivity if health education is to be successful. We would like to add two other principles to this list, ecological approach and advocacy. **Participation** refers to the active involvement of those in the priority population in helping identify, plan, and implement programs to address the health problems they face. Without such participation, ethical issues associated with program development come into play, and the priority population probably will not support and feel **ownership** of (responsibility for) the program. For example, if the health educators for a large corporation are creating a health promotion program for all employees, they should not begin to plan without the participation of (or at least representation by) each of the segments (clerical, labor, and management) of the employee population.

During the 1990s, health education/promotion initiatives placed more emphasis on ecological approaches to improving health. **Ecological** "refers to the social, political, economic, organizational, policy, regulatory, and other environmental circumstances interacting with behavior in affecting health" (Green & Kreuter, 1999, p. 27). Because of the movement toward an ecological approach, health educators

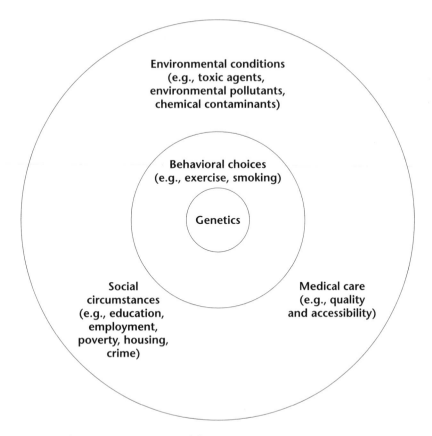

Figure 1.6   Multicausation Disease Model

must do more than just educate to help to change behavior. They must now work in new ways and develop new skills. As a group these new skills are often called **population-based approaches.** They include policy development, policy advocacy, organizational change, community development, empowerment of individuals, and economic supports.

To more clearly see how a population based approach works, consider the following example. A state-level voluntary health organization was spending most of its time and resources helping individuals quit smoking or preventing others from starting to smoke. Recently the organization has developed a state-wide advocacy network to respond to tobacco-related legislation. They are using a population-based approach to influence legislation and policy that will ultimately impact individual smoking behaviors. They still maintain the more individual approaches to dealing with the tobacco issue but have added the population-based approach.

Advocacy is another principle in which health educators have become more involved. **Advocacy** is defined "as the actions or endeavors individuals or groups engage in order to alter public opinion in favor or in opposition to a certain policy" (Pinzon-Perez & Perez, 1999, p. 29). Professional associations encourage health educators to get more involved in advocacy for the profession and for health-related issues. As an example, the Coalition of National Health Education Organizations (CNHEO) (see Chapter 8 for more on this organization) sponsors the Health Education Advocate Web site (see the Weblink at the end of this chapter for the URL for this site). This site provides health education professionals with an easy link to contact their legislators whenever health education-related bills or concerns are considered by Congress.

If health education is going to create lasting change, then those in the priority population must be empowered as a result of the health education/promotion programming. **Empowerment** is "a social action process that promotes participation of people, organizations, and communities in gaining control over their lives in their community and larger society. With this perspective, empowerment is not characterized as achieving power to dominate others, but rather power to act with others to affect change" (Wallerstein & Bernstein, 1988, p. 380). The neighborhood watch program provides a good example of empowerment. Obviously, police can make a neighborhood safer by regularly patrolling the area. However, because of limited resources, the police cannot be present in every neighborhood. Empowering neighborhood residents, however, with the knowledge and skills (empowered) to provide an effective "watch" (be the eyes and ears of the police), can decrease crime and improve safety.

Health education/promotion programming cannot be effective unless it is sensitive to the culture, beliefs, and concerns of those for whom the program is intended. **Cultural sensitivity** is having and showing respect for cultures other than one's own. This is an important health education principle because of the close relationship that often exists between health and culture. Cultural factors arise from guidelines (both explicit and implicit) that individuals "inherit" from being a part of a particular society, ethnic group, race, or other group (Helman, 1984). Examples include the various beliefs, traditions, and prejudices held by individuals. In order for health educators to be effective in a variety of communities, they need to strive to be **culturally competent.** This means having the knowledge and interpersonal skills to understand, appreciate, and work with individuals from cultures other than their own. It involves an awareness and acceptance of cultural differences; self-awareness; knowledge of the culture of those in the priority population; and the adaptation of professional skills to respond to the priority population's cultural differences (McManus, 1988). Even services that are provided to all in an equal and nondiscriminatory manner may not take into account the needs of those in the priority population and therefore be culturally inappropriate (Davis & Voegtle, 1994).

SUMMARY

In this introductory chapter, many of the basic principles of the profession of health education were presented including a brief discussion of why health education is referred to as an emerging profession; a look at the current status of health education; definitions of many of the key words and terms used in the profession, including *health, health education, health promotion,* and *wellness;* an explanation of how health or health status has been measured, including mortality rates, life expectancy, YPLL,

DALYs, DALEs, HALEs, HRQOL, and health surveys; an outline of the goal and objectives of the profession; the practice of health education, including planning, implementing, and evaluating programs; some of the basic underlying concepts and principles of the profession, including the health field concept, levels of prevention, risk factors, health risk reduction via understanding disease; and the principles of participation, empowerment, cultural sensitivity, ecological approach, and advocacy.

REVIEW QUESTIONS

1. Why have the authors chosen to describe health education as an emerging profession?
2. What is the current status of health education?
3. Define—*health, health education, health promotion, disease prevention, public health, community health, coordinated school health program,* and *wellness.* ·
4. Explain each of the following means of measuring health or health status.
   - Mortality rates. What is the difference among crude, adjusted, and specific rates?
   - Life expectancy
   - Years of potential life lost (YPLL)
   - Disability-adjusted life years (DALYs)
   - Disability-adjusted life expectancy (DALE), and health-adjusted life expectancy (HALE)
   - Health-related quality of life (HRQOL)
   - Health surveys
5. Of all the different measures of health presented in this chapter, which one do you think is the best indicator of health? Why?
6. Why is epidemiology such an important discipline for health education?
7. In a given community with a midyear population estimate of 50,000, there were twenty-one deaths due to strokes in the year. What is the rate of stroke deaths per 100,000 population?
8. What is the goal of health education?
9. Name the different levels of objectives of health education.
10. What constitutes the basic practice of health education?
11. Briefly explain the following concepts and principles of health education.
    - Health Field Concept
    - Levels of prevention
    - Risk factors
    - Health risk reduction
    - Chain of infection
    - Communicable disease model
    - Multicausation disease model
    - Selected principles of health education—participation, ecological approach, advocacy, empowerment, and cultural sensitivity

CRITICAL THINKING QUESTIONS

1. In this chapter, the term *public health* was defined. To what extent do you think that the government, at any level, has the right to legislate good health? For example, do you think a governmental body has the responsibility (or right) to require all motorcycle drivers to wear helmets because statistics show that wearing helmets can save lives? Defend your answer.

2. If you were asked by the Centers for Disease Control and Prevention to come up with a new measure to describe the health status of an individual, what would you include in such a measure and why?

3. If you had the opportunity to develop three new health education programs, one at each level of the three levels of prevention (primary, secondary, and tertiary) for the community in which you live, what would they be? Who would be the priority audience? Why did you pick the three that you did?

ACTIVITIES

1. If you have not already done so, locate and read a copy of the government document *Healthy People: The Surgeon General's Report on Health Promotion and Disease Prevention* (USDHEW, 1979). It provides a good background on the health promotion era in the United States.

2. Do you agree with the authors that health education is an emerging profession? Defend your response in a one- to two-page paper.

3. Write your own definitions for *health, health education,* and *health promotion* using the concepts presented in the chapter.

4. Write one paragraph for each of the following:
   • Why do you think the Health Field Concept was so important in getting people to think about health promotion?
   • At what level of prevention do you think it would be most difficult to change health behavior? Why?

5. In a one-page paper, use the chain of infection to outline three different means for preventing the spread of HIV.

6. In a one-page paper, use the multicausation disease model to explain how a person develops heart disease.

WEBLINKS

1. **http://www.aahperd.org/aahe/template.cfm**

   American Association for Health Education (AAHE)

   This association has been instrumental in the development of the health profession over the years. Every ten years, the AAHE forms a task force (the Joint Terminology Committee) of experienced health educators to evaluate the current terminology in the field of health education.

2. **http://www.cdc.gov/nchs/default.htm**

   National Center for Health Statistics (NCHS)

   This site is a rich source of data about health in the United States and the instruments used to collect the data.

3. **http://www.cdc.gov/brfss/#about_BRFSS**

   Behavioral Risk Factor Surveillance Survey (BRFSS)

   The BRFSS, the world's largest telephone survey, tracks health risks in the United States. Information from the survey is used to improve the health of U.S. citizens. At this site, you will find general information about the BRFSS, data generated by the BRFSS, copies of the data collection instruments, and more.

4. **http://www.cdc.gov/nccdphp/dash/yrbs/index.htm**

   Youth Risk Behavioral Surveillance Survey (YRBSS)

   At this site, you will find general information about the YRBSS, data generated by the YRBSS, copies of the data collection instruments, and more.

5. **http://www.iom.edu/**

   Institute of Medicine's (IOM)

   The IOM is a nonprofit organization specifically created to provide science-based advice on matters of biomedical science and medicine and health, as well as an honorific membership organization that was chartered in 1970 as a component of the National Academy of Sciences. The IOM's mission is to serve as adviser to the nation to improve health. The Institute provides unbiased, evidence-based, and authoritative information and advice concerning health and science for all. At this site you can find many of their reports cited in this chapter.

6. **http://www.healtheducationadvocate.org**

   Health Education Advocate

   The Health Education Advocate site is sponsored by the Coalition of National Health Education Organizations (CNHEO). It was designed to provide a timely source of advocacy information related to the field of health education and promotion. It also includes a number of items to health planners with advocacy activities. The site includes, but is not limited to, information about how to identify and contact senators and congressional representatives, the status of specific bills, health resolutions and policy statements of sponsoring agencies, and advocacy resources.

7. **http://www.omhrc.gov/cultural/index.htm**

   Office of Minority Health (OMH)

   This site presents information on cultural competence. The OMH mandate is to develop the capacity of health care professionals to address the cultural and linguistic barriers to health care delivery and increase access to health care for limited English–proficient people. This site provides many resources including, but not limited to, standards, materials, and links to other Web sites to assist health professionals to become more culturally competent.

CASE STUDY

As a health educator with the Delaware County Health Department, Matt has been asked by a local religious leader to give a presentation on HIV/AIDS to the ecumenical youth group (ninth to twelfth graders) of the community. The request has taken Matt by surprise because for the past couple of years he has attempted to make similar presentations in the local schools but has been turned away because the superintendent said "the community was too conservative for such matters." Knowing that at least some of the people in the community think HIV/AIDS is too controversial to talk about, but also knowing the information is important for youth to have, Matt wants to make sure he prepares and delivers a program that is well received. This is finally the chance he has been waiting for to make his entry into the youth population of the community. Matt has decided to create a presentation on HIV/AIDS that incorporates information on both risk factors and the chain of infection. To make sure that his presentation is on target he has asked several other employees of the health department to sit down with him and brainstorm some ideas for his presentation. He begins his session with his colleagues by asking them all to write down information they think he should include in his presentation. Assume that you are one of these other employees of the health department in this meeting. What would you include on your list for Matt? What would you advise Matt not to include? Why? He then asks his colleagues for ideas on how to present the information (e.g., lecture, video, role playing). What do you think would be the best method to use? Why did you select this method? How long do you think Matt's presentation should be? Why?

REFERENCES

Agnes, M. (Ed.). (2001). *Webster's new world college dictionary* (4th ed.). Cleveland, OH: IDG Books Worldwide, Inc.

Alzheimer's Association. (2004). *Facts: About genes and Alzheimer's disease.* Retrieved March 26, 2004 from http://www.alz.org/

Barber, B. (1988). Professions and emerging professions. In J. C. Callahan (Ed.), *Ethical issues in professional life* (pp. 35–39). New York: Oxford University Press.

Breslow, L. (1999). From disease prevention to health promotion. *Journal of the American Medical Association, 281* (11), 1030–1033.

Centers for Disease Control and Prevention (CDC). (1994). *Chronic disease in minority populations.* Atlanta, GA: Author.

Centers for Disease Control and Prevention (CDC) (2003a*). Behavioral Risk Factor Surveillance Survey.* Retrieved March 26, 2004 from http://www.cdc.gov/brfss/about.htm

Centers for Disease Control and Prevention (CDC). (2000). *Measuring healthy days.* Atlanta, GA: Author.

Centers for Disease Control and Prevention (CDC). (2003b). *Youth Risk Behavior Surveillance Survey.* Retrieved March 26, 2004 from http://www.cdc.gov/nccdphp/dash/yrbs/index.htm

Cleary, M. J., & Neiger, B. L. (1998). *The certified health education specialist: A self- study guide for professional competency* (3rd ed.). Allentown, PA: The National Commission for Health Education Credentialing.

Cohen, H. J. (1991). My grandmother said, "If you had your health, you have everything." What did she mean? In M. Feinleib (Ed.), *Vital and health statistics: Proceedings of 1988 international symposium on data on aging* (USDHHS pub. no. PHS-91-1482) (pp. 5–9). Washington, DC: U.S. Government Printing Office.

Davis, B. J., & Voegtle, K. H. (1994). *Culturally competent health care for adolescents.* Chicago, IL: American Medical Association.

Feeney, S., & Freeman, N. K. (1999). *Ethics and the early childhood educators: Using the NAEYC code.* Washington, DC: National Association for the Education of Young Children.

Freid, V. M., Prager, K., MacKay, A. P., & Xia, H. (2003). *Chartbook on trends in health of Americans. Health United States, 2003.* Hyattsville, MD: National Center for Health Statistics.

Galli, N. (1976). Foundations of health education. *The Journal of School Health, 46* (3), 158–165.

Goodstadt, M. S., Simpson, R. I., & Loranger, P. O. (1987). Health promotion: A conceptual integration. *American Journal of Health Promotion, 1*(3), 58–63.

Green, L. W., & Kreuter, M. W. (1999). *Health promotion planning: An educational and ecological approach* (3rd ed.). San Francisco, CA: Mayfield.

Green, L. W., & McKenzie, J. F. (2002). Community and Population HealthIn L. Breslow, L. Green, W. Keck, J. Last, & J. M. McGinnis (Eds.) *Encyclopedia of Public Health* (pp. 247–255). New York: Macmillan Reference.

Green, L. W., & Ottoson, J. M. (1999). *Community and population health* (8th ed.). Boston: WCB/McGraw-Hill.

Greene, W. H., & Simons-Morton, B. G. (1984). *Introduction to health education.* New York: Macmillan.

Hall, M. J., & DeFrances, C. J. (2003). 2001 National Hospital Discharge Survey. *Advance Data from Vital and Health Statistics, No. 332.* Hyattsville, MD: National Center for Health Statistics.

Hanlon, J. J. (1974). *Public Health.* St. Louis, MO: Mosby.

Helman, C. (1984). *Culture, health and illness: An introduction for health professions.* Bristol, England: John Wright & Son, Stonebridge Press.

Hing, E., & Middleton, K. (2003). National Hospital Ambulatory Medical Care Survey: 2001 Outpatient Department Summary. *Advance Data from Vital and Health Statistics, No. 338.* Hyattsville, MD: National Center for Health Statistics.

Institute of Medicine (IOM). (2000). *Brief Report. Promoting health: Intervention strategies from social and behavioral research.* Retrieved March 25, 2004 from http://www.iom.edu/includes/dbfile.asp?id=4121

Institute of Medicine (IOM). (2001). *Health and behavior: The interplay of biological, behavioral, and societal influences.* Washington, DC: Academy Press.

Institute of Medicine (IOM). (2002). *Brief Report. The future of the public's health in the 21st century.* Retrieved March 25, 2004 from http://www.iom.edu/file.asp?id=4165

Johns, E. B. (1973). Joint Committee on Health Education Terminology: Report of the joint committee on health education terminology. *Health Education, 4* (6), 25.

Joint Committee on Health Education Terminology. (1991a). Report of the 1990 Joint Committee on Health Education Terminology. *Journal of Health Education, 22* (2), 105–106.

Joint Committee on Health Education Terminology. (1991b). Report of the 1990 Joint Committee on Health Education Terminology. *Journal of School Health, 61* (6), 251–254.

Joint Committee on Health Education and Health Promotion Terminology. (2001). Report of the 2000 Joint Committee on Health Education and Health Promotion Terminology. *American Journal of Health Education, 32* (2), 89–103.

Kochanek, K. D., & Smith, B. L. (2004). *National Vital Statistics Reports, Deaths: Preliminary Data for 2002, 52* (13). Hyattsville, MD: National Center for Health Statistics.

Laframboise, H. L. (1973). Health policy: Breaking it down into more manageable segments. *Journal of the Canadian Medical Association, 108* (Feb. 3), 388–393.

Lalonde, M. (1974). *A new perspective on the health of Canadians: A working document.* Ottawa, Canada: Ministry of National Health and Welfare.

Landau, S. I. (Ed.). (1979). *Funk and Wagnalls standard desk dictionary.* New York: Funk and Wagnalls.

Livingood, W. C. (1996). Becoming a health education profession: Key to societal influence—1995 SOPHE presidential address. *Health Education Quarterly, 23* (4), 421–430.

Mason, J. O., & McGinnis, J. M. (1990). Healthy people 2000: An overview of the national health promotion disease prevention objectives. *Public Health Reports, 105*(5), 441–446.

Mathers, C. C., Sdana, R., Salomon, Murray, C. J. L., & Lopez, A. D. (2000). *Estimates of DALE for 191 countries: Methods and results. Global programme on evidence for health policy working paper no. 16.* Retrieved February 27, 2004 from http://www3.who .int/whosis/

Mausner, J. S., & Kramer, S. (1985). *Epidemiology—An introductory text.* Philadelphia: W. B. Saunders.

McGinnis, J. M. (1985). The limits of prevention. *Public Health Reports, 100* (3), 255–260.

McGinnis, J. M. (2001). United States. In C. E. Koop (Ed.), *Critical issues in global health* (pp. 80–90). San Francisco: Jossey-Bass.

McGinnis, J. M., & Foege, W. H. (1993). Actual causes of death in the United States. *Journal of the American Medical Association, 270* (18), 2207–2212.

McGinnis, J. M., Williams-Russo, & Knickman, J. R. (2002). The case for more active policy attention to health promotion. *Health Affairs, 21* (2), 78–93.

McHorney, C. A. (1999). Health status assessment methods for adults: Past accomplishments and future challenges. *Annual Review of Public Health, 20,* 309–335.

McKenzie, J. F., Neiger, B. L., & Smeltzer, J. L. (2005a). *Planning, implementing, and evaluating, health promotion programs: A primer* (4th ed.). San Francisco, CA: Benjamin Cummings.

McKenzie, J. F., Pinger, R. R., & Kotecki, J. E. (2005b). *An introduction to community health* (5th ed.). Boston: Jones and Bartlett Publishers.

McManus, M. C. (Ed.) (1988). Services to minority populations: Cross cultural competence continuum. *Focal Point, 3* (1), 1–4. Portland, OR: Research and Training Center, Regional Research Institute for Human Services, Portland State University.

Mokdad, A. H., Marks, J. S., Stroup, D. F., & Gerberding, J. L. (2004). Actual causes of death, in the United States, 2000. *Journal of the American Medical Association, 291* (10), 1238–1245.

Montagu, A. (1968). *Man observed.* New York: G. P. Putnam.

Moss, B. (1950). Joint Committee on Health Education Terminology. *Journal of Physical Education, 21,* 41.

Murray, C. J. L., & Lopez, A. D. (Eds.). (1996). *Summary of the global burden of disease: A comprehensive assessment of mortality and disability from diseases, injuries, and risk factors in 1990 and projected to 2020.* Geneva, Switzerland: World Health Organization.

Murray, C. J. L., Salomon, J. A., Mathers, C. D., & Lopez, A. D. (Eds.). (2002). *Summary measures of population health: Concepts, ethics, measurement, and application.* Geneva: World Health Organization.

National Commission for Health Education Credentialing, Inc. (NCHEC). (1996). *A competency-based framework for professional development of certified health education specialists.* Allentown, PA: Author.

National Library of Medicine and the National Institutes of Health (2003). *Medical Encyclopedia: Septicemia.* Retrieved March 26, 2004 from http://www.nlm.nih.gov /medlineplus/print/ency/article/001355.htm

Pinzon-Perez, H., & Perez, M. A. (1999). Advocacy groups for Hispanic/Latino health issues. *The Health Educator Monograph Series, 17* (2), 29–31.

Raphael, D., Brown, I., Renwick, R., & Rootman, I. (1997). Quality of life: What are the implications for health promotion? *American Journal of Health Behavior, 21* (2), 118–128.

Rugen, M. (1972). *A fifty year history of the public health section of American Public Health Association; 1922–1972.* Washington, DC: American Public Health Association, Inc.

Ubbes, V. A., & Watts, P. R. (1995). Terminology, tolerance, and flexibility: Communication challenges for health education. *Journal of Health Education, 26* (4), 251–253.

Upton, L. A. (1970). *A study of secondary school counselors' perceptions of school counseling as a profession and their desires for professionalization of school counseling.* Doctoral dissertation. State University of New York at Buffalo.

U.S. Department of Health, Education, and Welfare (Public Health Service) (USDHEW). (1979). *Healthy people: The Surgeon General's report on health promotion and disease prevention.* (Publication No. 79-55071). Washington, DC: U.S. Government Printing Office.

U.S. Department of Health, Education, and Welfare (USDHEW). (1980). *Promoting health/preventing disease: Objectives for the nation.* Washington, DC: U.S. Government Printing Office.

U.S. Department of Health and Human Services (USDHHS). (1991). *Health status of minorities and low-income groups* (3rd ed.). Washington, DC: U.S. Government Printing Office.

U.S. Department of Health and Human Services (USDHHS) (2000). *Healthy People 2010.* (Conference Edition, in Two Volumes). Washington, DC: U.S. Government Printing Office.

Wallerstein, N., & Bernstein, E. (1988). Empowerment education: Freier's ideas adapted to health education. *Health Education Quarterly, 15* (4), 379–394.

Williams, J. F. (1934). Report of the Health Education Section of the American Physical Education Association: Definitions of terms in health education. *Journal of Physical Education, 5* (16–17), 50–51.

World Health Organization (WHO). (1947). Constitution of the World Health Organization. *Chronicle of the World Health Organization 1.* Geneva, Switzerland: Author.

World Health Organization (WHO). (1986). *Ottawa Charter for Health Promotion.* Retrieved February 27, 2004 from http://www.who.int/hpr/NPH/docs/ottawa_charter _hp.pdf

Yoho, R. (1962). Joint Committee on Health Education Terminology: Health education terminology. *Journal of Physical Education and Recreation, 33* (Nov.), 27–28.

CHAPTER 2

The History of Health and Health Education

Chapter Objectives

After reading this chapter and answering the questions at the end, you should be able to:

1. Discuss health beliefs and practices from earliest humans to present day.
2. Identify the dual roots of modern health education.
3. Explain why a need for professional health educators emerged.
4. Trace the history of public health in the United States.
5. Relate the history of school health from the mid-1800s to the present.
6. Identify important governmental publications from 1975 to the present, and describe how these publications have impacted health promotion and education.

Key Terms

A New Perspective on the Health of Canadians

Asclepiads

Asclepius

atomic theory

bacteriological period of public health

caduceus

Code of Hammurabi

comprehensive school health instruction

coordinated school health program

health literacy

Healthy People

Healthy People 2010

Hippocrates

Hygeia

life expectancy

Medicaid

Medicare

miasmas theory

Panacea

Promoting Health/Preventing Disease: Objectives for the Nation

school health advisory council

School Health Education Evaluation Study

School Health Education Study

Smith Papyri

W hile the history of health education as an emerging profession is just over 100 years old, the concept of educating about health has been around since the dawn of humans. This chapter chronicles human knowledge of health, health care, and health education from the earliest records to the present. It will focus primarily on Northern Africa and Europe, as these were the areas of greatest influence on the development of health knowledge and health care in the United States. This does not mean that other parts of the world—for example, the Far East, Central America, and South America—did not contribute to the history of health and health care. However, to review the history of all societies is beyond the scope of this book and would not be as directly relevant to the history of health, health care, and health education in the United States as is the health history of Western societies.

As one reads through this chapter, it should become clear that the need for professional health educators emerged as human knowledge of health and health care increased. Particular emphasis will be placed on the history of health education during the past 150 years as it evolved to its present status from the dual roots of school health and public health.

This information should be of particular interest to those new to health education, as one cannot fully appreciate the profession without understanding its origin. Historical study allows one to see the progress made and to ascertain trends over time. It also depicts the difficulties and obstacles faced by those persons interested in promoting health throughout the years and enhances appreciation of their efforts. "At the same time, historical study shows us that despite the difficulties, change is possible, given dedication, organization and persistence. . . . Historical case studies may be able to teach us useful lessons about successful strategies used by public health reformers in the past" (Fee & Brown, 1997, p. 1763).

Early Humans

It must be assumed that the earliest humans learned by trial and error to distinguish those things that were good for them and would enhance health from those that were harmful and would impair health. Goerke and Stebbins (1968) noted, "By observing animals he learned that bathing not only cooled and refreshed his body, but helped remove external parasites; he learned that application of mud assuaged insect bites; and by determining the actions of certain herbs, he learned their various medicinal or poisonous characteristics" (p. 5).

It does not stretch the imagination too far to see how health education first took place. Someone may have eaten a particular plant or herb and become ill. That person would then warn (educate) others against eating the same substance. Conversely, someone may have ingested a plant or an herb that produced a desired effect. That person would then encourage (educate) others to use this substance. Through observation, trial, and error, other types of health-related knowledge would be discovered. Eventually, this knowledge would be transformed into rules or taboos for a given society. Rules about preserving food and how to bury the dead may have been implemented. Perhaps taboos against defecation within the tribe's communal area or near sources of drinking water were established (McKenzie, Pinger, & Kotecki, 2005). Over time and as knowledge increased, there would be less need for the trial and error method, which undoubtedly produced serious illness and even death among some of these early humans. Knowledge would be passed from one generation to the next, thus preventing at least some of the potential ill effects of everyday life.

There was still much more that was unknown than was known about how to protect health. Disease and death were probably much more common than health

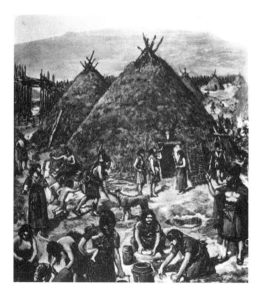

People have always been concerned about their health. This picture shows a reconstruction of life on the Sussex Downs in the late Bronze Age. (Corbis)

and longevity. To early humans, it was puzzling when disease and death occurred for no apparent reason. In an attempt to make these events seem more rational, "disease and infirmity were believed to be caused by the influence of magic or malevolent spirits that inhabited streams, trees, animals, the earth, and the air. Purposively or accidentally provoking any of the spirits, it was thought, would result in dire consequences for the individual or his/her community" (Goerke & Stebbins, 1968, p. 5). To prevent disease, sacrifices were made to the gods, taboos were obeyed, amulets were worn, and haunted places were avoided. Charms, spells, and chants were also used to protect one from disease (Duncan, 1988). Again, it is not too hard to imagine that there was some form of rudimentary health education taking place to inform people about what they needed to do to keep from provoking the spirits and, thus, prevent disease.

Early Efforts at Community Health

Evidence of broad-scale community health activity has been found in the very earliest of civilizations. In India, sites excavated at Mohenjo-Daro and Harappa dating back 4,000 years indicate that bathrooms and drains were common. The streets were broad, paved, and drained by covered sewers (Rosen, 1958). Archeological evidence also shows that the Minoans (3000–1430 B.C.) and Myceneans (1430–1150 B.C.) built drainage systems, toilets, and water flushing systems (Pickett & Hanlon, 1990). The oldest written documents related to health care are the **Smith Papyri,** dating from 1600 B.C., which describe various surgical techniques. The earliest written record concerning public health is the **Code of Hammurabi,** named after the king of Babylon. It contained laws pertaining to health practices and physicians, including the first known fee schedule (Rubinson & Alles, 1984).

Box 2.1 The Rights and Duties of the Surgeon of 2080 B.C.: From the Code of Hammurabi

"If a physician operate on a man for a severe wound (or make a severe wound upon a man), with a bronze lancet, and save the man's life; or if he open an abscess (in the eye) of a man, with a bronze lancet, and save the man's eye, he shall receive ten shekels of silver (as his fee)."

"If he be a freeman,[1] he shall receive five shekels."

"If it be a man's slave, the owner of the slave shall give two shekels of silver to the physician."

"If a physician operate on a man for a severe wound, with a bronze lancet, and cause the man's death; or open an abscess (in the eye) of a man with a bronze lancet, and destroy the man's eye, they shall cut off his hands."

"If a physician operate on a slave of a freeman for a severe wound, with a bronze lancet, and cause his death, he shall restore a slave of equal value."

"If he open an abscess (in his eye), with a bronze lancet, and destroy his eye, he shall pay silver to the extent of one half of his price."

"If a physician set a broken bone for a man or cure his diseased bowels, the patient shall give five shekels of silver to the physician."

"If he be a freeman,* he shall give three shekels."

"If it be a man's slave, the owner of the slave shall give two shekels of silver to the physician."

"If a veterinary physician operate on an ox or ass for a severe wound and save its life, the owner of the ox or ass shall give the physician, as his fee, one sixth of a shekel of silver."

"If he operate on an ox or an ass for a severe wound, and cause its death, he shall give to the owner of the ox or ass one fourth its value."

Freeman indicates a rank intermediate between that of "man" (or gentleman) and that of "slave."

Source: From R. F. Harper, *The Code of Hammurabi,* 1904, Chicago.

Egyptians

The medical lore of the distant past was handed down from generation to generation. In virtually every culture for which there are documented historical accounts, it appears there existed some type of a physician or medicine man to which people turned for health information, treatments, and cures (Green & Simons-Morton, 1990). In Egypt, as in many other cultures, this role was held by the priests. Eventually, the various incantations, spells, exorcisms, prescriptions, and clinical observations were compiled into written format, some of which survive in our museums and libraries (Libby, 1922).

Due at least in part to the conservatism of the priest-physicians, "Egyptian medicine never advanced far beyond primitive medicine with its simple faith in magic spells and the virtue of a rich pharmacopoeia, and its belief that the cause of disease was the malice of a demon, the justice of an avenging god, the ill-will of an enemy, or the anger of the dead" (Libby, 1922, p. 4). Some of the more disgusting substances the Egyptians used as remedies included "dung of the gazelle and the

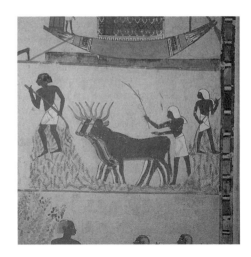

The Egyptians were known for their cleanliness and were considered the healthiest people of the time. ("Tomb Menna"/The Ancient Art & Architecture Collection)

crocodile, the fat of a serpent, mammalian entrails and other excreta, tissues and organs. In some cases the object seems to have been to wheedle, in other cases to repel, the evil spirits that had taken possession of the patient" (Libby, 1922, p. 6).

Still, the Egyptians made substantial progress in the area of public health. They possessed a strong sense of personal cleanliness and were considered to be the healthiest people of their time. They used numerous pharmaceutic preparations and constructed earth privies for sewage, as well as public drainage pipes (Pickett & Hanlon, 1990).

In approximately 1500 B.C. the Hebrews extended Egyptian hygienic thought and formulated (in the biblical book of Leviticus) what is probably the world's first written hygienic code. It dealt with a variety of personal and community responsibilities, including cleanliness of the body, protection against the spread of contagious diseases, isolation of lepers, disinfection of dwellings after illness, sanitation of campsites, disposal of excreta and refuse, protection of water and food supplies, and specific hygiene rules for menstruating women and women who had recently delivered a child.

Greeks

The history of health and health care in the Greek culture (1000–400 B.C.) is intriguing as well as relevant to modern health care philosophy. The Greeks were perhaps the first people to put as much emphasis on prevention of disease as on the treatment of disease conditions. Balance among the physical, mental, and spiritual aspects of the person was emphasized. Among the early Greeks, religion played an important role in health care; however, the role of physician began to take more defined shape, and a more scientific view of medicine emerged.

In the early stages of Greek culture, as represented in the *Iliad* and the *Odyssey*, the priesthood played a role in the healing arts. In the *Iliad*, **Asclepius** was a Thessalian chief who had received instruction in the use of drugs. By the beginning of the eighth century B.C., tradition had endowed him as the god of medicine. He had two daughters, who also had health-related powers. **Hygeia** was given the power to

---

Box 2.2 The Story of Asclepius

"According to Greek mythology, Asclepius, the son of Apollo, was a god of healing whose powers were so great that he could bring the dead back to life. When Hades, the god of the dead, jealously complained to Zeus that Asclepius was cheating the kingdom of the dead, Zeus agreed with Hades that Asclepius had violated a basic law of nature by saving mortals from death. Consequently, Asclepius was killed with a thunderbolt.

Before he died, however, he gave his healing powers to two of his daughters: Panacea, goddess of healing, who administered medication to the sick, and Hygeia, goddess of health, who taught mortals to live wisely and preserve their bodies."

Source: Bates, I. J., & Winder, A. E. *Introduction to Health Education,* 1984, San Francisco: Mayfield Publishing.

---

prevent disease, while **Panacea** was given the ability to treat disease. Hygeia was the more prominent figure and was often pictured with her father in sculptures and illustrations of the time (Schouten, 1967). The words *hygiene* and *panacea* can be traced back to these daughters of Asclepius (Libby, 1922).

Eventually, hundreds of elaborate temples were built throughout Greece to worship Asclepius. These temples were typically on beautiful sites overlooking the sea or beside healing fountains. The temple priests practiced their healing arts, which often involved fraud. The priests played on the superstitions of the sufferers through the use of sacrificial rites and purifications, tame snakes, and dream interpretation. In fact, sleep and dreams were a major aspect of the Asclepian temples. Sufferers were often allowed to sleep near the temple. Priests would imper-

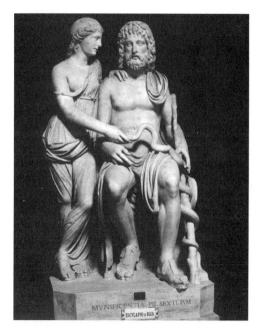

Asclepius and Hygeia (Museo Vaticano/Art Resource)

sonate Asclepius and appear to the sufferers while they slept. Those who believed they had benefited from the suggestions and worship left tablets telling of their cure or other remembrances such as gold, silver, or marble models of the cured body part. The priests always made sure all knew of the therapeutic value of a substantial fee (Libby, 1922). These ancient temples of Asclepius left their symbol as a permanent reminder of the past—the staff and serpent of the physician, known as the **caduceus** (Rubinson & Alles, 1984).

The temple priests should not be confused with the **Asclepiads.** The Asclepiads were a brotherhood of men present at the temples who initially claimed descent

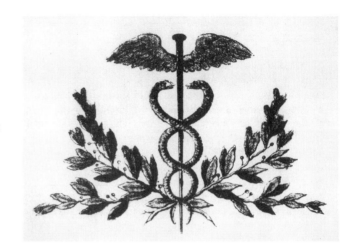

Illustration of a caduceus, a symbol which shows two snakes braided around a staff. It is representative of the medical profession and has its earliest association with Asclepius, the Greek healer. (Corbis)

from Asclepius. While some of the Asclepiads probably helped the priests with their chicanery, others broke away from the priests and began to practice medicine based on more rational principles.

The famous Greek physician **Hippocrates** came from the Asclepian tradition. He lived from about 460 B.C. until 377 B.C. and developed a theory of disease causation consistent with the philosophy of nature held by leading philosophers of his day. Essentially, he believed all things were composed of different combinations of particles too small to be seen. He called these particles *atoms*; thus, his theory became known as the **atomic theory.** Hippocrates believed there were only four kinds of atoms: earth, air, fire, and water. Each atom retained two of the four qualities of wetness, dryness, warmth, and coldness. Earth was cold and dry; air was hot and wet; water was cold and wet; and fire was hot and dry. Hippocrates further believed that the human body was made up of four substances, which he called the four *humours.* The humours were blood, phlegm, yellow bile, and black bile. Each humour was made up of one type of atom. Blood was made up of air and possessed the properties of being hot and wet; phlegm was made up of water and was cold and wet; yellow bile was compared to fire, so it was hot and dry; and black bile was similar to earth, which meant it was cold and dry (Duncan, 1988). Table 2.1 provides a visual depiction of Hippocrates' theory.

Hippocrates taught that health was the result of balance of the four humours; conversely, disease was the result of an imbalance of the four humours. An excess of hot, wet blood, for example, resulted in fever, sweating, and diarrhea and could be treated by bleeding the sufferer. Colds, which were associated with cold, wet phlegm, were treated with hot, spicy foods and applications of mustard or other irritants to the chest to produce a feeling of warmth. Excess phlegm or black bile, both cold, could be sweated out in a steam bath or eliminated by vomiting. Excess yellow bile could be eliminated by enemas (Duncan, 1988).

To the Greeks, the ideal person was perfectly balanced in mind, body, and spirit. Thus, study and practice related to philosophy, athletics, and theology were all important to maintain balance. To do this, however, took a tremendous commitment of time and energy. Each day required physical activity, study, and philosophical

Table 2.1   Hippocrates' Atomic Theory

Body Parts (Humours)	Atoms	Properties
Blood	Air	Hot and wet
Phlegm	Water	Cold and wet
Yellow bile	Fire	Hot and dry
Black bile	Earth	Cold and dry

discussion while maintaining proper nutrition and rest. Few people could afford to lead such a life. Those who did were the aristocratic upper class leading a life of leisure supported by a slave economy (Rosen, 1958). The ideal Greek human being that is so often mentioned was, in fact, a small percentage of the Greek population.

Hippocrates holds an important place in the history of medicine. While his atomic theory seems simplistic and of little value in the world of modern medicine, it is important to remember that the atomic theory was still being taught in medical schools as a valid theory of disease causation as recently as the first quarter of the twentieth century. Hippocrates, however, did more than just theorize about disease. He carefully observed and recorded associations between certain diseases and such factors as geography, climate, diet, and living conditions. Duncan (1988) noted, "One of his [Hippocrates'] most noteworthy contributions is the distinction between 'endemic' diseases, which vary in prevalence from place to place, and 'epidemic' diseases, which vary in prevalence over time" (p. 12). The traditional Hippocratic Oath is still used today and is the basis for medical ethics. Hippocrates and the Asclepiads moved health care away from religion and priests and attempted to establish a more rational basis to explain health and disease. Hippocrates' concept of balance in life is still promoted today as the best means for maintaining health and well-being.

Hippocrates has been credited as being the first epidemiologist and the father of modern medicine (Duncan, 1988). It is not hard to imagine that he was also a health educator. One can easily see Hippocrates educating his friends and patients about diet, exercise, rest, and the importance of balance in preventing disease and promoting health.

Romans

The Romans conquered the Mediterranean world, including the Greeks. In doing so, however, the Romans did not destroy the cultures they conquered but learned from them. The Romans accepted many of the Greek ideas, including those related to health and medicine. "As clinicians, the Romans were hardly more than imitators of the Greeks, but as engineers and administrators, as builders of sewerage systems and baths, and as providers of water supplies and other health facilities, they set the world a great example and left their mark in history" (Rosen, 1958, p. 38).

The Roman Empire (500 B.C.–A.D. 500) built an extensive and efficient aqueduct system. "Evidence of some 200 Roman aqueducts remains today, from Spain to Syria and from northern Europe to North Africa" (McKenzie, Pinger, & Kotecki, 2005, p. 11). The total capacity of the thirteen aqueducts delivering water to the city of Rome has been estimated at 222 million gallons per twenty-four hours. At the height of the

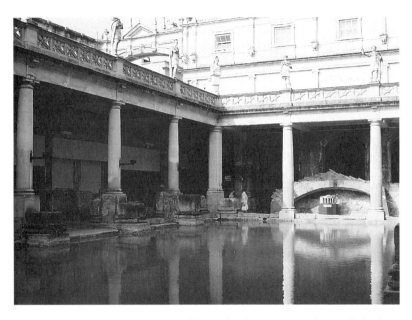

The Romans enjoyed a system of public baths that were supplied with fresh water. This picture shows the Roman baths in Bath, England. (Pierre Berger/ Photo Researchers)

empire, this would have been enough water to provide each citizen of Rome with at least forty gallons of fresh water per day. Additionally, attention was paid to water purity. At specific points along the aqueduct, generally near the middle and end, settling basins were located, in which sediment might be deposited (Rosen, 1958).

The Romans also developed an extensive system of underground sewers. These served to carry off both surface water and sewage. The main sewer in Rome that emptied into the Tiber River was 10 feet wide and 12 feet high; it was still part of the Roman sewer system during the 20th century.

Romans had a great appreciation for hygiene and developed an extensive system of private and public baths. Rosen (1958) notes,

> A census of baths was taken by Agrippa in 33 B.C. At that time there were 170. The number grew steadily and later approached a thousand. The fee generally charged was about half a cent and children entered free. Up to the time of Trajan, mixed bathing was not formally prohibited, although there were balneae exclusively for women. Sometime between 117 and 138, Hadrian issued a decree separating the sexes in the baths. (p. 48)

The Romans made other health advancements. They learned to locate new towns on salubrious sites, giving considerable attention to the position, orientation, and drainage of dwellings. The Romans observed the effect of occupational hazards on health, and they were the first to build hospitals. By the second century A.D., a public medical service was constituted whereby physicians were appointed to various towns and institutions. A system of private medical practice also developed during the Roman era (Rosen, 1958).

The Romans furthered the work of the Greeks in the study of human anatomy and the practice of surgery. Some Roman anatomists even dissected living human beings to further their knowledge of anatomy (Libby, 1922). In quoting the Latin writer Cornelius, Libby found that these anatomists "procured criminals out of prison, by royal permission, and dissecting them alive, contemplated, while they were still breathing, the parts which nature had before concealed, considering their position, color, figure, size, order, hardness, softness, smoothness, and asperity" (Libby, 1922, p. 54). While some opposed this hideous practice, others supported it, holding "it is by no means cruel as most people represent it, by the tortures of a few guilty, to search after remedies for the whole innocent race of mankind in all ages" (Libby, 1922, p. 54).

Middle Ages

The era from the collapse of the Roman Empire to about A.D. 1500 is known as the Middle Ages or Dark Ages. This was a time of political and social unrest, when many of the advancements related to health were lost. Rosen (1958) notes that "the problem that confronted the medieval world was to weld together the culture of the barbarian invaders with the classical heritage of the defunct [Roman] Empire and with the beliefs and teachings of the Christian religion" (p. 52). This proved to be no easy task.

With the Roman Empire no longer able to protect the settlements, each city had to defend itself against its enemies. Security rested on its citizens and its encircling fortifications. For safety, one lived within the walls of the city. Domesticated animals were also kept inside the city walls. Many public health problems were simply the result of too many people and animals living within a confined area. As the population grew, expansion was difficult and overcrowding common (Rosen, 1958) and the public health advancements of the Roman Empire were lost. Lack of fresh water and sewage removal was a major problem for many of these medieval cities.

To make matters worse, there was little emphasis on cleanliness or hygiene. The new religion, Christianity,

> found its disciples among the lower classes, where personal hygiene was not practiced, and as a consequence, an entirely different attitude toward the human body developed. Excessive care of the body, that is, man's earthly and mutable part, was unimportant in the Christian dualistic concept, which separated body from soul. For some Eastern churchmen and holy men, living in filth was regarded as evidence of sanctity: cleanliness was thought to betoken pride, and filthiness humility. (Goerke & Stebbins, 1968, p. 9)

Fortunately, as Christianity matured so did its concept of the human body. Eventually, Christians came to understand that the body is the abode for the soul on earth, therefore permitting one to preserve and take care of it.

Early Christians also reinforced the earlier notion that disease was caused by sin or disobeying God. This propelled the priests and religious leaders back into the position of preventing and treating disease. The health-related advancements of the Greco-Roman era were abandoned and shunned. Entire libraries were burned, and knowledge about the human body was seen as sinful.

The Middle Ages were characterized by great epidemics. Perhaps the cruelest of these was leprosy, a disease characterized by severe facial disfigurement. A highly contagious and virulent disease, all Western countries issued edicts against anyone suspected of having leprosy and regulated every aspect of the sufferer's life. In some communities lepers were given the last rites of the church and were forced to leave the city, were made to wear identifying clothing, and were required to carry a rod identifying them as lepers. Others were forced to wear a bell around their necks and to ring it as a warning when others came near. Such isolation usually brought about a relatively quick death due to hunger and exposure (Goerke & Stebbins, 1968). Eventually, leprosy hospitals were founded to treat the inflicted. It has been estimated that by A.D. 1200 there were 1,900 leper houses and leprosaria in Europe (Rosen, 1958).

The bubonic plague, known as the Black Death, may have been the most severe epidemic the world has ever known. The death toll was higher and the disruption of society greater than from any war, famine, or natural disaster in history. "At Constantinople, the plague raged with such violence that 5,000, and even 10,000 persons are said to have died in a single day" (Donan, 1898, p. 94). Estimates of casualties vary from 20 to 35 million, with Europe losing one quarter to one third of its entire population. In Avignon, France, 60,000 people died and the pope was forced to consecrate the Rhone River in order that bodies might be thrown into it, because the churchyards were filled (Goerke & Stebbins, 1968).

Imagine what it must have been like to live through the plague. Literally one out of every three or four people you knew would have contracted the disease and died. The cause of the disease was unknown; thus, fear and superstition were rampant. Often religious leaders and doctors were some of the first victims, since they were exposed to the disease early in the epidemic through their contact with infected sufferers. This left many communities with no religious or medical leadership.

Goerke and Stebbins (1968) note, "Many people reacted to the plague either by becoming licentious and hedonistic or by becoming severely ascetic, such as those who formed the sect known as the Flagellants. Jews were burned or exiled not so much because they were thought to have caused the epidemic, but rather because the nobles and communities were heavily indebted to them, and the deteriorated moral and ethical practices which accompanied the plague sanctioned escaping the debts in this way" (p. 11).

The Brotherhood of the Flagellants was a group of religious zealots who believed the plague could be avoided by admitting to their sins and then ritualistically beating themselves in atonement. Today, such a group would most likely be labeled a religious cult. Members of this group marched in long, two-column lines from city to city. In each city, they would chant a litany and conduct their ritualistic ceremony. At a signal from the group's master, the Flagellants would strip to the waist and march in a circle until they received another signal from the master. Upon receiving the second signal, they would throw themselves to the ground with their position indicating the specific sin they had committed. The master would move among the bodies thrashing those that had committed certain sins or had offended the discipline of the Flagellants in some way. This would be followed by a collective flagellation whereby each group member would rhythmically beat their own backs and breasts with a heavy scourge made of three or four leather thongs tipped with metal studs. According to eyewitness accounts, the Flagellants lashed themselves until their bodies became swollen and blue, and blood dripped to the ground. Further complicating the health consequences of such punishment was a rule prohibiting bathing, washing, or changing clothes. When joining the Brotherhood, group members had to pledge to scourge themselves three times daily for thirty-three days and eight hours, which represented one day for each year of Christ's earthly life (Ziegler, 1969).

Debate existed during the Middle Ages concerning the cause of the plague. In 1348, Jehan Jacme wrote that the disease was caused by five factors: the wrath of God, the corruption of dead bodies, waters and vapors formed in the interior of the earth, unnatural hot and humid winds, and the conjunction of stars and planets (Winslow, 1944). Another story concerning the origins of the disease had Italian merchants trapped in a city on the Black Sea that was under siege by a local Mongol prince. The prince was forced to call off the siege because large numbers of his army were dying of a strange disease. Before leaving, the prince ordered his army to catapult the dead, diseased bodies into the city. Within days, the people inside the city began to die. Afraid, the Italian merchants set sail for Italy, but not before infected rats had boarded the ship. Soon many of the sailors became sick. The ship tried to dock in several cities but was denied permission because of the illness. Finally permission was granted to dock in Sicily where the rats came on shore and the plague began (De'ath, 1995). Despite the disagreement that existed on the cause of the disease, contemporaries believed that the disease was contagious. In other words, it was passed from person to person in some unknown way. While this concept of contagion had been around for many years and was discussed in the Bible, it was not until the Middle Ages and the epidemics of leprosy and bubonic plague that it started to become more universally accepted. The contagion concept opened the door to new interest in science and severely weakened the argument of those promoting the sin-disease theory.

The Middle Ages also saw epidemics of other communicable diseases, including smallpox, diphtheria, measles, influenza, tuberculosis, anthrax, and trachoma. The last major epidemic disease of this period was syphilis, which appeared in 1492. As with other epidemics, syphilis killed thousands of people (McKenzie, Pinger, & Kotecki, 2005).

While there were no professional health educators during the Middle Ages, education about health continued to exist. It seems priests, medical doctors, and community leaders all had ideas about health and, in particular, the prevention of disease. They proceeded to "educate" all those who would listen and who agreed with their point of view. Given the rudimentary level of health knowledge and the lack of consensus on prevention and causation of disease, a professional health educator would probably have contributed little to the health of the populous in the Middle Ages.

Renaissance

The Renaissance, which means rebirth, was roughly from A.D. 1500 to 1700. It is characterized by a gradual rebirth of thinking about the world and humankind in a more naturalistic and holistic fashion. Science again emerged as a legitimate field of inquiry, and numerous scientific advancements were made.

It must be stressed, however, that progress was slow. The world did not change overnight from the superstitious and backward beliefs of the Dark Ages to a completely enlightened society in the Renaissance.

Disease and plague still ravaged Europe and overall medical care was still rudimentary. Bloodletting was a major form of treatment for everything from the common cold to tuberculosis. Popular remedies included crabs' eyes, foxes' lungs, oil of anise, oil of spiders, and oil of earthworms. A major means of diagnosing a patient's condition consisted of examining the urine for changes in color. The inspection of a patient's urine by a true physician was known as "water casting." For many years, this was the principal occupation of the medical profession. This technique was combined with crude estimates of the balance of four "humours," or fluids, in the body as had originally been theorized by Hippocrates (Hansen, 1980).

Much surgery and dentistry was performed by barbers, because they had the best chairs and sharpest instruments available. Some barbers took their role as physician seriously and dispensed health information, as can be seen in the following example from a Danish barber-surgeon: "It is very good for persons to drink themselves intoxicated once a month for the excellent reasons that it frees their strength, furthers sound sleep, eases the passing of water, increases perspiration, and stimulates general well-being" (Durant, 1961, pp. 495–496). Unfortunately, few were probably so continent as to restrict their binges to once a month.

Rosen (1958) notes that, while the Renaissance "is characterized by the rapid growth and spread of science in various fields, public health as a practiced activity received very little, if any, direct benefit from these advances" (p. 84). Evidence of the poor public health conditions is this note describing the average English household floor of the sixteenth century:

> As to floors, they are usually made with clay, covered with rushes that grow in the fens and which are so seldom removed that the lower part remains sometimes for twenty years and has in it a collection of spittle, vomit, urine of dogs and humans, beer, scraps of fish and other filthiness not to be named. (Pickett & Hanlon, 1990, p. 25)

While living conditions among the English royalty were certainly better than for those of the laboring class, health-related problems still were prevalent. Disposal of human waste was a major problem. Those who lived in old castles located their latrines in large projections on the face of walls. The excrement was discharged from these projections into deep-walled pits, moats, or streams near the walls of the castle. Those less fortunate used chamber pots and simply tossed their contents out the nearest window (Hansen, 1980).

Even among royalty basic hygiene left much to be desired. Beneath the elaborate and costly garments of royalty was often a severe condition of uncleanliness. Few monarchs bathed more frequently than once a week. Much of the material used in royal apparel, such as silk, velvet, and ermine, could not be washed; thus, it simply accumulated dirt and perspiration. Cloaking scents were used to try to renew the clothing, but it was not effective (Hansen, 1980).

Health problems resulting from sexual indiscretions were prevalent among royalty. It was common practice for the kings and queens of the sixteenth century to look outside of marriage to satisfy their sexual appetites. There were several reasons for this; one of which was they simply had the power and money to do so. Beyond this, it must be remembered that royal couples were matched without regard for personal compatibility or mutual attraction. Language and cultural differences must have strained sexual relations. There was also tremendous pressure on these couples to produce royal offspring; thus, the royal bedroom was a place where duty and responsibility were carried out instead of a place for love and passion. Further, many of the royal family were not physically attractive. Hansen (1980) was blunt in his description of royalty when he noted, "Another problem was the extreme ugliness, even deformity, of the marriageable progeny of sixteenth-century royal families. The portraits we have do not tell the true story, painted as they were to the satisfaction of the royal subject" (p. 262). The deformities, as well as mental retardation, were probably the result of genetic inbreeding from marrying within family bloodlines over many generations.

No doubt this overall lack of physical attraction and personal appeal, combined with power and money, contributed to extramarital sexual affairs, which in turn contributed to the incidence of sexually transmitted diseases. "Venereal disease was as common as the flux at most royal courts, and the malady ruined many a promising prince. . . . It was a horrible, virulent, disfiguring, and chronic malady" (Hansen, 1980, p. 260).

Disfigurement also was caused by the use of caustic cosmetics, which were actually supposed to improve looks:

> On top of natural, exculpable flaws, the princesses of Europe defiled themselves further with the most scarifying cosmetics. The ingredients of these paints were harmful; "fucus," a red paint, was actually mercuric sulfide. This ate into flesh and left trenches if used heavily, which it often was. "Cerusa," a whitening agent, was still more toxic, being white lead. Heavy use of this substance, quite popular in an era that held pallor in the highest regard, mummified the skin, turned hair white, and caused intestinal problems. Many a young woman's early death was at least partly attributable to lead poisoning. (Hansen, 1980, p. 263)

On the positive side, the Renaissance was a period of exploration and expanded trade. The search for knowledge characteristic of the Greek and Roman eras was revitalized. Superstitions of the Middle Ages were slowly replaced with a more systematic inquiry into cause and effect. A great impetus toward the revival of learning was Johannes Gutenberg's invention of the printing press from moveable type in the middle of the fifteenth century. This allowed the great classical works of Hippocrates and Galen to be reproduced and distributed to larger audiences (Gordon, 1959).

There were also scientific advancements during the Renaissance. The human body was again considered appropriate for study, and realistic anatomical drawings were produced. John Hunter, the father of modern surgery, undertook a more orderly exploration of the workings of the human body. Antonie van Leeuwenhoek discovered the microscope and proved there were life forms too small for the human eye to see. These life forms, however, were not yet associated with disease. John Graunt forwarded the fields of statistics and epidemiology. Through studying the *Bills of Mortality*, published weekly in London, "he determined the excess of male over female births, the high rate of mortality during the earlier years of life, the approximate numerical equality of the sexes, and the excess of urban over the rural death rate" (Goerke & Stebbins, 1968, p. 16).

In Italy, numerous cities had instituted health boards to fight the plague. It did not take long, however, for their responsibilities to be expanded. By the middle of the sixteenth century, numerous matters had fallen under the control and jurisdiction of these health boards. These included "the marketing of meat, fish, shellfish, game, fruit, grain, sausages, oil, wine and water; the sewage system; the activity of the hospitals; beggars and prostitutes; burials, cemeteries, and pesthouses; the professional activity of physicians, surgeons and apothecaries; the preparation and sale of drugs; the activity of hostelries and the Jewish community" (Cipolla, 1976, p. 32).

Age of Enlightenment

The 1700s was a period of revolution, industrialization, and growth of cities. Both the French and American Revolutions took place during this period. Plague and disease still continued to be a problem; science had not yet discovered that these diseases were produced by microscopic organisms. Terrible epidemics were still frequent. It was the general belief that disease was formed in filth and that epidemics were caused by some type of poison that developed in the putrefaction process. The vapors, or "miasmas," rising from this rotting refuse could travel through the air for great distances and resulted in disease when inhaled. Known as the **miasmas theory,** it remained popular throughout much of the nineteenth century. As preventive measures, herbs and incense were often used to perfume the air supposedly filling the nose and crowding out any miasmas (Duncan, 1988). It was still not known that contaminated water could cause disease infection.

Scientific advancements continued throughout the period. Dr. James Lind, a Royal Navy surgeon, discovered that scurvy could be controlled on long sea voyages by having sailors consume lime juice. To this day, British sailors are known as limeys. Edward Jenner discovered a vaccine procedure against smallpox. Bernardino Ramazzini wrote on trade and industrial diseases. Theorists of the time conceived of the mind and body not as separate entities, but as dependent on one other. Eighteenth-century philosophers such as Diderot, Locke, Rousseau, and Voltaire, all "promoted the worth of each human life and the importance of individual health for the well being of society" (Rubinson & Alles, 1984, p. 5).

Although progress was made during this time, health education per se still did not emerge as a profession. With the rudimentary state of medical knowledge in the sixteenth, seventeenth, and even eighteenth centuries, there would have been little for a health educator to do other than promote the misconceptions and half-truths that predominated during the time period; however, with the increases in scientific and medical knowledge and the development of health boards, which were the forerunner of today's health departments, the roots of modern health education had been planted, and the first sprouts would soon emerge.

The 1800s

In the first half of the 1800s, little happened to improve the public's health. In England, the streets of London were filthy with animal and human waste. Overcrowding and industrialization added to the problem. These conditions, under which so many people lived and worked, had dire results: Smallpox, cholera, typhoid, tuberculosis, and many other diseases reached high endemic levels (Pickett & Hanlon, 1990).

In 1842, a momentous event occurred in the history of public health when Edwin Chadwick published his *Report on an Inquiry into the Sanitary Conditions of the Labouring Population of Great Britain*. In the report, he documented the deplorable living conditions of the laboring class in Great Britain, made a strong case that these conditions were the cause of much disease and suffering, and called for government intervention. This report eventually led to the formation of a General Board of Health for England in 1848 (Goerke & Stebbins, 1968).

Extraordinary advancements in biology and bacteriology took place by the middle of the nineteenth century in England and throughout Europe. In 1849, Dr. John Snow, who laboriously studied epidemiological data related to a cholera epidemic in London, hypothesized that the disease was caused by microorganisms in the drinking water from one particular water pump located on Broad Street. He removed the pump's handle to keep people from using the water source, and the epidemic abated. Snow's action was remarkable, as it predated the discovery that microorganisms cause disease and was in opposition to the miasmas theory prevailing at the time.

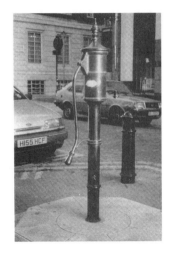

By removing the handle of this pump, which is still in place on Broad Street in London, John Snow interrupted a cholera epidemic. (Robert Hardy Picture Library Ltd., London)

In 1862, Louis Pasteur of France proposed his germ theory of disease. After this, advancements in bacteriology greatly accelerated. Over the next twenty years, Pasteur discovered how microorganisms reproduce, he introduced the first scientific approach to immunization, and he developed a technique to pasteurize milk. Robert Koch, a German scientist, developed the criteria and procedures necessary to establish that a particular microbe, and no other, caused a particular disease. Joseph Lister, an English surgeon, developed the antiseptic method of treating wounds by using carbolic acid, and he introduced the principle of asepsis to surgery. These are just a few of the tremendous advancements in bacteriology made during the second half of the nineteenth century. So great were these advancements in the study of bacteria that the period from 1875 to 1900 is known as the **bacteriological period of public health** (McKenzie, Pinger, & Kotecki, 2002).

Public Health in the United States

population growth!

1700s

During the 1700s, health conditions in the United States were similar to those in Europe—deplorable. Diseases such as smallpox, cholera, and diphtheria were prevalent. Because of the slave trade, diseases such as yaws, yellow fever, and malaria were common in southern states (Marr, 1982). Large numbers of immigrants were entering the ports, cities were growing, overcrowding was common, and the Industrial Revolution was on the verge of getting started.

Table 2.2   Expectation of Life According to Wigglesworth Life Table—1789

Expectation	Years	Expectation	Years
At birth	28.15	At age 50	21.16
At age 5	40.87	At age 55	18.35
At age 10	39.23	At age 60	15.43
At age 15	36.16	At age 65	12.43
At age 20	34.21	At age 70	10.06
At age 25	32.32	At age 75	7.83
At age 30	30.24	At age 80	5.85
At age 35	28.22	At age 85	4.57
At age 40	26.04	At age 90	3.73
At age 45	23.92	At age 95	1.62

Source: Ravenel, M. P. (Ed.). (1970). *A half century of public health.* New York: Arno Press & the New York Times.

The primary means of controlling disease were quarantine and regulations on environmental cleanliness. For example, as early as 1647, the Massachusetts Bay Colony enacted regulations to prevent pollution of Boston Harbor. In 1701, Massachusetts passed laws allowing for the isolation of smallpox patients and for ship quarantine, to be used whenever needed but there was no overseeing body or agency to enforce compliance.

In an attempt to address health problems, some cities formed local health boards (Pickett & Hanlon, 1990). Prominent citizens who were to advise elected officials on health-related matters made up these boards. They had no paid staff, no budget, and no authority to enforce regulations. Tradition has it that the first health board was formed in Boston in 1799, with Paul Revere as its chairman. This is contested, however, by other cities claiming earlier health boards, including Petersburg, Virginia (1780), Baltimore (1793), Philadelphia (1794), and New York (1796).

Life expectancy is one measure of health status for a given population. It is defined as "the average number of years a person from a specific cohort is projected to live from a given point in time" (McKenzie, Pinger, & Kotecki, 2005, p. 70). The first life expectancy tables were developed for the United States in 1789 by Dr. Edward Wigglesworth (Ravenel, 1970). Table 2.2 shows Wigglesworth's table. It provides strong evidence of the prevailing health conditions in that, in 1789, life expectancy at birth was only 28.15 years; in 2002, life expectancy at birth was 77.8—the highest ever in the United States (Kochanek & Smith, 2004).

1800s

From 1800 to 1850, health status improved little. The conditions of overcrowding, poverty, and filth worsened as the Industrial Revolution encouraged more and more people to move to the cities. Epidemics of smallpox, yellow fever, cholera, typhoid, and typhus were common. Tuberculosis and malaria also reached exceptionally high levels. For example, in Massachusetts in 1850, the tuberculosis death rate was 300 per 100,000 population, and infant mortality was about 200 per 1,000 live births. Indeed, the conditions were so bad that life expectancy actually decreased in some cities during this period of time. In Boston, the average age at death dropped from 27.85 years in 1820–1825 to 21.43 in 1840–1845. In New York during the same period, the average age of death decreased from 26.15 to 19.69 (Shattuck, 1850).

Public health reform in the United States was slow in getting started. It is interesting to note, however, that a major report helped jump-start the public health reform movement in the United States, just as Chadwick's landmark report stimulated public health reform in Britain. In the United States, the impetus was Lemuel Shattuck's *Report of the Sanitary Commission of Massachusetts*. His report contained remarkable insight into the public health problems of Massachusetts and equally remarkable foresight as to how these problems should be approached and solved. In describing the content of this famous report, Pickett and Hanlon (1990) noted:

> Among the many recommendations made by Shattuck were those for the establishment of state and local boards of health; a system of sanitary police or inspectors; the collection and analysis of vital statistics; a routine system for exchanging data and information; sanitation programs for towns and buildings; studies of the health of school children; studies of tuberculosis; the control of alcoholism; the supervision of mental disease; the sanitary supervision and study of problems of immigrants; the erection of model tenements, public bathhouses, and washhouses; the control of smoke nuisances; the control of food adulteration; the exposure of nostrums; the preaching of health from pulpits; the establishment of nurses' training schools; the teaching of sanitary science in medical schools; and the inclusion of preventive medicine in clinical practice, with routine physical examinations and family records of illness. (p.31)

This report is remarkable because no national or state public health programs existed at the time, and local health agencies that did exist were functioning at a minimal level. Shattuck visualized how to improve the public's health. "Of the 50 recommendations which Shattuck listed, 36 have become accepted principles of public health practice" (Goerke & Stebbins, 1968, p. 28).

The publication of Shattuck's report did not mean an end to the public health problems in the United States. In fact, the report went unnoticed for nineteen years until 1869, when the Commonwealth of Massachusetts established a state board of health made up of physicians and laymen exactly as Shattuck had envisioned. Following the lead of Massachusetts, Virginia and California formed their own state boards of health one year later (Ravenel, 1970). By 1900, thirty-eight states had established state boards of health. Today, every U.S. state has a state board or department of health.

Despite the formation of state boards of health, state-level health departments could not meet health needs on a more local level. With limited resources, there was simply too much to accomplish. As a result, the first full-time county health departments were formed in Guilford County, North Carolina, and Yakima County, Washington, in 1911. Some sources have cited Jefferson County, Kentucky, as the first county health department, set up in 1908 (Pickett & Hanlon, 1990).

As states initiated boards of health, the American Public Health Association was founded. (See Chapter 8 for more information on the APHA.) Following a series of national conventions on quarantine held from 1857 through 1860, "Stephen Smith invited a group of 'refined gentlemen' to discuss informally the possibility of a national sanitary association" (Bernstein, 1972, p. 2). Smith's suggestion of an association for health officials and interested citizens was well received and a decision was made to establish a committee to work on a permanent organization. One year later, in 1873, the first annual meeting was held in Cincinnati, and seventy new members were elected. Smith remained active in the association throughout his life. At the age of ninety-nine he walked to the podium unassisted to speak at the fiftieth anniversary celebration of APHA.

In addition to the state and county departments of health, the federal government had in operation the beginnings of what became the U.S. Public Health Service. The history of this illustrious organization dates back to 1798, when Congress passed the Marine Hospital Service Act. Previously, sailors in the merchant marine had nowhere to turn for health care. They paid no local or state taxes and generally were not particularly welcomed in any port city where they happened to become ill or were injured. The Marine Hospital Service Act required the owners of every ship to pay the tax collector twenty cents per month for every seaman they employed. This money was used to build hospitals and provide medical services in all major seaport cities. This is of particular importance, as "it represented the first prepaid medical and hospital insurance plan in the world, under the administrative supervision of what eventually became a public health agency" (Pickett & Hanlon, 1990, p. 34).

Successive legislation throughout the nineteenth century gradually expanded the scope of the Marine Hospital Service. In 1902, Congress retitled it the Public Health and Marine Hospital Service and provided it with a definite organizational form under the direction of the surgeon general. In 1912, "Marine Hospital" was dropped from the name, and the service became the U.S. Public Health Service.

In 1879, Congress created the National Board of Health. The board was comprised of seven members appointed by the president, including representatives of the army, navy, Marine Hospital Service, and Justice Department. Its functions were to obtain information on all matters related to public health and to provide grants-in-aid to state boards of health. The National Board also provided money to university scientists to conduct research on topics of health-related interest. Unfortunately, the board was short-lived. In administering quarantine functions, the board had incurred opposition from state agencies and private shipping concerns. Others in positions of power were not in favor of the research grant program and felt such expenditures were extravagant. Thus, in 1882, the board's appropriations were transferred to the Marine Hospital Service, which carried on with the quarantine functions but discontinued the grant program (USDHEW, 1976). With this, "the National Board of Health died, and the United States has never had a cabinet level health department or an official comparable to the minister of health in most other countries" (Pickett & Hanlon, 1990, p. 36).

1900 to Present

The period from 1900 to 1920 is known as the reform phase of public health (McKenzie, Pinger, & Kotecki, 2005). A growing concern for the many social problems facing the United States marked this period. Urban areas expanded, and many people lived and worked in deplorable conditions. To address these concerns, federal regulations were passed concerning the food industry; states passed workers' compensation laws; the U.S. Bureau of Mines was created, as was the U.S.

Department of Labor; and the first clinic for occupational diseases was established. By the end of this period, the movement for healthier conditions in the workplace was well established.

It was also during this period that the first national voluntary agencies were formed. These agencies were designed to address a specific health problem and were run primarily by volunteers. For example, the National Association for the Study and Prevention of Tuberculosis was established in 1902, and the American Cancer Society was founded in 1913. Today, volunteer agencies continue to be important players in the prevention of disease and the promotion of health (McKenzie, Pinger, & Kotecki, 2005).

The 1920s was a relatively quiet period in public health. Progress continued but at a slower pace. By the end of the decade, average life expectancy had risen to 59.7 years. Of importance to health education professionals is the founding of the Public Health Education Section of the American Public Health Association in 1922 (Bernstein, 1972).

The need for health education existed in the early years of the twentieth century. Moore (1923) included an entire chapter in his book on public health in the United States on "nostrums and quackery" and another chapter on health activities he described as "more or less misdirected." One of the most interesting examples involved a cure-all product known as Tanlac. The May 11, 1917, edition of the *Holyoke Daily Transcript* contained both an advertisement for Tanlac featuring a testimonial by a Fred Wicks and Mr. Wicks's obituary (Moore, 1923, pp. 173–174).

Other examples also abound. William Harvey Kellogg and his younger brother W.K., founded the Kellogg cereal company but were best known in the early 1900s for the sanitarium they established and operated in Battle Creek, Michigan. The rich and famous came from all over the world to be treated at the sanitarium. Many of the treatment modalities, however, would be considered questionable and even quackery by today's standards. For example, they utilized some 200 different types of hydrotherapy along with therapeutic enemas, electric horses, vibrators, and cold air (Butler, Thornton, & Stoltz, 1994). Despite the use of these questionable treatments, the sanitarium did promote exercise and good nutrition as ways to prevent and treat disease. The concept of prevention was beginning to take hold.

Evidence of differences between those people more concerned with treatment and those more concerned with prevention began to appear. Moore (1923) related a story about a town in which public health work had banished malaria. A physician was asked how his profession had been affected by this public health advancement. He replied, "If it hadn't been for the influenza, I'd have gone broke. That saved us" (p. 373). As this off-handed and jocular reply suggests, tension between preventive medicine and curative medicine in the United States has existed since at least the early part of the twentieth century.

In explaining the emphasis on treatment over prevention in a more rational manner, Newsholme (1936) noted three reasons that treatment formed a larger part of public health efforts and why it would continue to do so in the future. First, the knowledge to prevent "a large proportion of the total sickness and mortality in the community is only partial" (p. 169). Second, "even when knowledge exists which if applied would reduce avoidable illness, it has not become vitally realized by most of us, and many among us are completely ignorant concerning it. Many more are unwilling to live in accord with this knowledge or are so circumstanced that their knowledge cannot be applied in their lives" (p. 169). Third, "physicians, hygienists, and Public Health Authorities find themselves confronted by an embarrassing multitude of sick people needing immediate aid; and their primary duty obviously is to give adequate and complete treatment of already existent sickness. Ambulance work must precede work to prevent future accidents, though no ambulance work is fully satisfactory which does not include thorough investigation of the origin of the accident and the full application of the conclusions from inquiry to the prevention of recurrent accidents" (pp. 169–170). Many of the same arguments are used today to account for the emphasis on traditional medical interventions instead of prevention.

From 1930 through World War II, the role of federal government in social programs expanded. Prior to the Great Depression of 1929, medical services were provided by relatives and friends, as well as by religious organizations and some voluntary agencies. During the Depression, however, private resources could not meet the demands of those requiring assistance. In 1933, President Franklin D. Roosevelt created numerous agencies and programs as part of his New Deal, that improved the plight of the disadvantaged. Much of the money was used for public health efforts, including the control of malaria, the building of hospitals, and the construction of municipal water and sewage systems.

The Social Security Act of 1935 was a real milestone and the beginning of the federal government's involvement in social issues, including health. The act provided support for state health departments and their programs. Funding was made available to develop sanitary facilities and to improve maternal and child health.

Two major public health agencies were formed at this time. On May 26, 1930, the Ransdell Act converted the Hygienic Laboratory to the National Institute of Health (now called the National Institutes of Health), with a broad mandate to ascertain the cause, prevention, and cure of disease (USDHEW, 1976). The National Institutes of Health is now one of the premiere—if not *the* premiere—medical research facilities in the world. In 1946, the Communicable Disease Center was established in Atlanta, Georgia. Now called the Centers for Disease Control and Prevention (CDC), it has become one of the world's leading epidemiological centers and a major training facility for health communications and educational methods (Pickett & Hanlon, 1990). The CDC has as its Vision for the 21st Century, "Healthy People in a Healthy World—Through Prevention" (CDC, 2002a, p. 1), and its mission is, "To promote health and quality of life by preventing and controlling disease, injury and disability" (CDC, 2002a, p. 2).

Following World War II, concern rose over the number of health care facilities and the adequacy of the care they provided. In 1946, Congress passed the National Hospital Survey and Construction Act, also known as the Hill-Burton Act to improve the distribution and enhance the quality of hospitals. From the passage of the Hill-Burton Act through the 1960s, new hospital construction occurred rapidly. Little thought, however, was given to planning. As a result, hospitals were built too close together and provided overlapping and unnecessary services (McKenzie, Pinger, & Kotecki, 2005).

In 1954, Dr. Mayhew Derryberry, the first chief of health education in the federal government, noted, "The health problems of greatest significance today are the chronic diseases. . . . The extent of chronic diseases, various disabling conditions, and the economic burden that they impose have been thoroughly documented" (*Voices From the Past,* 2004, p. 368). Prior to the 1950s, the major emphasis of public health had been on communicable or contagious diseases. However, through improved public health services, medical care and immunization programs, many contagious diseases no longer threatened as they once had, and the focus shifted ever so slowly to the prevention of chronic diseases. Derryberry predicted how this change of focus would impact health education: "Health education and health educators will be expected to contribute to the reduction of the negative impact of such major health problems as heart disease, cancer, dental disease, mental illness and other neurological disturbances, obesity, accidents and the adjustments necessary to a productive old age" (*Voices From the Past,* 2004, p. 368). While the seed may have been planted for health educators to play a greater role in the prevention of chronic diseases, it was not until the 1970s that the seed finally sprouted.

In 1965, the federal government again passed major legislation designed to improve the health of the U.S. population. While major improvements were made in health facilities and the quality of health care, there were still many underserved people. Most of these people were either poor or elderly. In response, Congress passed the Medicare and Medicaid bills as amendments to the Social Security Act of 1935. **Medicare** was created to assist in the payment of medical bills for the elderly, while **Medicaid** did the same for the poor. These bills provided medical care for millions of people who could not otherwise have obtained such services. Unfortunately, these bills also created an influx of federal dollars to the health care system, with the ultimate result of increasing the cost of health care for everyone.

It was evident by the 1970s that providing facilities and access to care was not enough to significantly influence the health status of the U.S. population. Prevention held the greatest potential for improving health and reducing health care costs lay in prevention. The first national effort to promote the health of citizens through a more preventive approach took place in Canada. In 1974, the Canadian Ministry of Health and Welfare released a publication entitled *A New Perspective on the Health of Canadians* (Lalonde, 1974). This document, often called the Lalonde Report, presented the epidemiological evidence supporting the importance of lifestyle and environmental factors to health and sickness and called for numerous national health promotion strategies to encourage Canadians to become more responsible for their own health. (See Chapter 1 for information on the Health Field Concept associated with this publication.) This highly influential report persuaded numerous U.S. health professionals to rethink current assumptions based on high-technology, treatment-focused medicine. So important was this report that Bates and Winder (1984) likened it to a reemergence of Hygeia and the beginning of the second public health revolution (p. 24).

In the United States, the governmental publication *Healthy People* was the first major recognition of the importance of lifestyle in promoting health and well-being (U.S. Public Health Service, 1979). This publication contained strong support for shifting emphasis away from the traditional medical model and toward lifestyle and environmental strategies in order to prevent many modern-day illnesses.

In 1980, another federal document called *Promoting Health/Preventing Disease: Objectives for the Nation* was released. This document contained 226 health objectives for the United States, which were divided into three areas: preventive services, health protection, and health promotion. These objectives provided the framework for public health efforts during the 1980s. They allowed public health professionals to focus attention on the most important areas and provided baseline data for measuring progress (USDHHS, 1980).

By the end of the decade, however, only about half of the objectives had been met or were close to being met. Nevertheless, the planning and evaluation process used in developing these objectives demonstrated the value of setting goals and listing specific objectives as a means of measuring progress in U.S. health and health care services. Thus, the process was repeated in the late 1980s, and a new publication released in 1990 titled *Healthy People 2000: National Health Promotion and Disease Prevention Objectives.* Its purpose was to commit the nation to the attainment of three broad goals: (1) increase the span of healthy life for the U.S. population, (2) reduce health disparities among the U.S. population, and (3) achieve access to preventive services for all the U.S. population. To assist in meeting these goals, 332 specific objectives were written in twenty-two priority areas (USDHHS, 1990).

As of the 1998–99 *Healthy People 2000* review, 15% of the 332 objectives had been met or exceeded. For example, death rates for children 1–14 years of age had declined 26% to a rate of 25 deaths per 100,000 population. This exceeded the year 2000 target objective of 28 deaths per 100,000. In another 44% of the objectives, progress was being made toward the year 2000 objective. These included areas such as prenatal care, child immunizations and mammography. Eighteen percent of the objectives indicate movement away from the objective. Diabetes prevalence and obesity however, are notable examples of health problems that are moving in the wrong direction, or increasing. Data for 6% of the objectives indicated mixed results, 2% showed no change from baseline, and 11% had no data available to compare to baseline (USDHHS, 2000a).

On January 25, 2000, *Healthy People 2010: Understanding and Improving Health* was released at a special conference held in Washington, D.C. Building on two decades of success in Healthy People initiatives, **Healthy People 2010** is poised to address the concerns of the twenty-first century. The two major goals of the document reflect the nation's changing demographics. The first goal, which addresses the fact that we are growing older as a nation, is to increase the quality and years of healthy life. The second goal, which addresses the diversity of our population, is to eliminate health disparities. Figure 2.1 displays how the 2010 objectives are derived from these goals and are designed to impact the determinants of health and ultimately health status. In her introductory message to *Healthy People 2010*, Secretary of Health and Human Services, Donna Shalala states,

> *Healthy People 2010* provides our nation with the wide range of public health opportunities that exist in the first decade of the twenty-first century. With 467 objectives in 28 focus areas, *Healthy People 2010* will be a tremendously valuable asset to health planners, medical practitioners, educators, elected officials, and all of us who work to improve health. *Healthy People 2010* reflects the very best in public health planning—it is comprehensive, it was created by a broad coalition of experts from many sectors, it has been designed to measure progress over time, and, most important, it clearly lays out a series of objectives to bring better health to all people in this country (USDHHS, 2000b, p. iii).

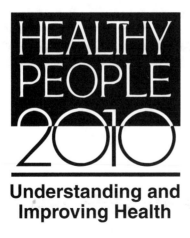

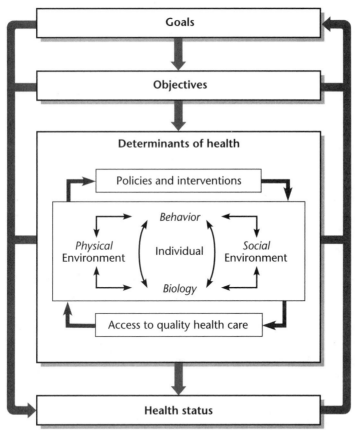

Figure 2.1   Healthy People in Healthy Communities: A Systematic Approach to Health Improvement

Source: United States Department of Health and Human Services. (2000b). *Healthy People 2010—Volume 1*. Washington, D.C.

The Healthy People initiative has evolved into an important strategic planning tool for public health professionals at the federal, state, and local level. Most individual states have developed Healthy People plans tailored to best meet their specific needs. A 1993 National Association of County and City Health Officials' survey showed that 70% of local health departments used the Healthy People objectives in their program planning. Healthy People identifies priority areas for public health efforts and provides a structure for evaluating performance and progress (USDHHS, 2000a). All health educators, regardless of the setting in which they are employed, should be familiar with these objectives.

An initiative that is designed, in part, to improve the effectiveness of public health departments working on Healthy People objectives is the National Public Health Performance Standards Program (NPHPSP). This is a partnership initiative to develop performance standards; collect, monitor, and analyze data; and ultimately improve public health performance. It is the first time that a common, systematic strategy for measuring public health performance has been available. Three instruments were developed to provide training and technical assistance related to the performance standards:

- State Public Health System Performance Standards Assessment
- Local Public Health Systems Performance Standards Assessment
- Local Public Health Governance Performance Standards Assessment

Local and state health departments have been encouraged to utilize these performance standard assessments to conduct their own self-assessments. Through this process, weaknesses can be identified and improvements made to enhance the overall performance of public health departments (CDC, 2003).

One more event important for health education occurred on October 27, 1997, when the Standard Occupational Classification (SOC) Policy Review Committee approved the creation of a new, distinct classification for the occupation of health educator (Auld, 1997/1998). Health educators have pursued this goal for over twenty-five years. Health educators were included in the category "Instructional Coordinator," a broad, primarily education-related category that failed to consider the many varied and unique responsibilities of health educators. Approval of health education as a separate occupational classification means that the Department of Labor's Bureau of Labor Statistics, Department of Commerce's Bureau of the Census, and all other federal agencies that collect occupational data now collect data on health educators. In addition, many state and local governments follow suit and maintain data on health education as well. For the first time, it is possible to determine the number of health educators employed and the outlook for future health education positions. This approval is one more sign that health education is gaining the respect and recognition it deserves.

It could reasonably be argued that the total number of advancements in public health during the twentieth century were equal to or greater than the total number of public health advancements prior to this time. In reflecting on these great successes of public health, the Department of Health and Human Services identified ten public health achievements they believed had the greatest impact on major causes of morbidity and mortality of the twentieth century. Box 2.3 lists these ten achievements. Imagine what life would be like today if none of these achievements had been realized.

> ### Box 2.3 Ten Great Public Health Achievements— United States, 1900–1999
>
> - Vaccination
> - Motor vehicle safety
> - Safer workplaces
> - Control of infectious diseases
> - Decline in deaths from coronary (heart) disease and stroke
> - Safer and healthier foods
> - Healthier mothers and babies
>
> - Family planning
> - Fluoridation of drinking water
> - Recognition of tobacco use as a health hazard
>
> *Source:* U.S. Department of Health & Human Services; Centers for Disease Control (1999). Changes in the Public Health System. *Morbidity and Mortality Weekly Report, 48* (50), 1141.

School Health in the United States

Life in early America was hard, and there was little time for education. The labor of building homes, clearing forests, tilling fields, hunting, and preparing food filled the days and most lived under primitive conditions. Settlements were few and far apart. Travel and transportation were costly, slow, and limited to foot, horseback, boat, or wagon.

In the mid-1600s, as communities became more established, the call for education was soon heard. Religion had always been an important part of life in America, and it was the religious leaders who led the drive for education. They believed that Satan benefited when people were illiterate, because they could not read the Scriptures. In 1647 Massachusetts passed the "Old Deluder" law to prevent Satan from deluding the people by keeping them from reading the Bible. The law specified that a town with fifty families should establish an elementary school and a town with one hundred households a Latin grammar secondary school (Means, 1962).

The curriculum in these early schools was largely derived from the educational practices in England. Essentially, reading, as the avenue to religious understanding, was the primary subject. Writing, spelling, grammar, and arithmetic supplemented reading. Later, geography and history were added, but the teaching of health was not part of the early education system in the United States.

Since only boys attended these early schools and working for the family was still a major concern, daily sessions were by necessity of short duration; the length of the school term was usually only a few months. Teachers were lacking in preparation, with their basic qualifications as being able to (1) read, (2) know more of the Bible than the students, (3) work cheap, and (4) keep the students under control. Teachers were totally dependent on the rod for classroom management (Means, 1962).

School buildings typically were inadequate. They were poorly built, inaccessible, and sometimes temporary structures. Their interiors were inadequately lighted, were furnished with uncomfortable seating, had no sanitary facilities, and were heated with wood-burning stoves. These schools were not even close to meeting modern standards for school construction (Means, 1962).

The schools and their curricula remained much the same until the 1800s. By the mid-1800s, most schools had become tax supported, and attendance was compulsory. Those concerned about public health pointed out the numerous health and safety problems in the schools. These concerns helped bring attention to the conditions of the schools and ultimately paved the way for health instruction in the curriculum (Means, 1962).

Horace Mann, whose writings and speeches promoted the importance of education in general, was perhaps the first spokesperson for teaching health in schools. He was elected secretary of the Massachusetts State Board of Education in 1837. Beginning in 1837 with the publication of his *First Annual Report* and continuing through the publication of the *Sixth Annual Report* in 1843, Mann called for mandatory hygiene programs that would help students understand their bodies and the relationship between their behaviors and health (Rubinson & Alles, 1984).

Another momentous event in the development of school health occurred in 1850, when Lemuel Shattuck from Massachusetts wrote his *Report on the Sanitary Commission of Massachusetts* (1850). (This is the same report discussed earlier in reference to public health.) While the report has become a classic in the field of public health, it also provided strong support for school health (Means, 1975). In the report, Shattuck (1850) eloquently supports the teaching of physiology, as the term *health education* had yet to be coined:

> It has recently been recommended that the science of physiology be taught in the public schools; and the recommendation should be universally approved and carried into effect as soon as persons can be found capable of teaching it. . . . Every child should be taught early in life, that to preserve his own life and his own health and the lives and health of others, is one of the most important and constantly abiding duties. By obeying certain laws or performing certain acts, his life and health may be preserved; by disobedience, or performing certain other acts, they will both be destroyed. By knowing and avoiding the causes of disease, disease itself will be avoided, and he may enjoy health and live; by ignorance of these causes and exposure to them, he may contract disease, ruin his health, and die. Every thing connected with wealth, happiness and long life depend upon health; and even the great duties of morals and religion are performed more acceptably in a healthy than a sickly condition. (pp. 178–179)

Aside from local and state attempts to promote the teaching of health-related curricula in the schools, no concerted national effort existed until that of the Women's Christian Temperance Union. Originally founded in 1874, the union expounded on the evils of alcohol, narcotics, and tobacco through every conceivable means and was one of the most effective lobbying organizations ever (Means, 1962). Between 1880 and 1890, every state in the union passed a law requiring instruction concerning the effects of alcohol and narcotics due to stimulus from the Temperance Movement (Turner, Sellery, & Smith, 1957).

Other national movements soon followed. In 1915, the National Tuberculosis Association introduced the "Modern Health Crusade" as a device for promoting the health of school children. It was based on promotion to "knighthood" on the basis of having followed certain health habits. The Child Health Organization of America encouraged the nation to adopt more functional health education programs. One of its active leaders, Sally Lucas Jean, was ultimately responsible for changing the name from hygiene education to health education (Means, 1962). With this name change, the focus of health education shifted from that of physiology and hygiene, which was factual and unrelated to everyday living, to an emphasis on healthy living and health behavior.

Despite these advancements, health education from 1900 to 1920 was generally characterized by inconsistency and awkward progress. World War I provided the impetus for widespread acceptance of school health education as a discipline in its own right (Turner, Sellery, & Smith, 1957). Out of 2,510,706 men who were examined to be drafted into the military at the time of World War I, 730,756 were rejected on physical grounds. A large portion of these physical deficiencies could have been prevented if the schools had been doing their part to train children concerning health and fitness (Andress & Bragg, 1922). In the immediate postwar years, sixteen states required hygiene instruction in their public schools, and twelve of these states made provisions for the preparation of health teachers in the teacher training schools supported by the state (Rogers, 1936).

Significant research and demonstration projects related to school health education were conducted in the 1920s and 1930s; for example, the Malden, Massachusetts, project, done in cooperation with the Massachusetts Institute of Technology; the Mansfield, Ohio, project supported by the American Red Cross; the Fargo, North Dakota, project sponsored by the Commonwealth Fund; and the Cattaraugus County, New York, project financed by the Milband Memorial Fund. According to Turner, Sellery, and Smith (1957), "these programs showed that habits could be changed and health improved through health education" (p. 27).

In the 1930s, the impetus for health education from the public waned. Health education continued to address the major health issues of the time but without the enthusiasm brought on by World War I. Notable research studies supplemented authoritative opinion in helping to point out difficulties and offer solutions related to the teaching of health education. Several important conferences were held on health education and youth health at the national level (Means, 1962). The profession was moving forward.

Professional organizations emerged during the 1900s that still exist today. School health education, long associated with physical education, received official recognition in 1937, when the American Physical Education Association became the American Association for Health and Physical Education. One year later, recreation was added to the association, and the name changed to the American Association for Health, Physical Education and Recreation (AAHPER).

The American Association of School Physicians, founded in 1927, had expanded its functions, interests, and scope of activity. As a result, it broadened its membership to include school health personnel other than physicians. In 1938, the name was changed to the American School Health Association to reflect these changes.

The American Public Health Association had long been an organization interested in and supportive of school health. In fact, many of the earliest supporters of health education in the schools had been leaders in public health. Appropriately, the organization established a separate section within its administrative structure to focus on school health interests. In 1942, the School Health Section of the American Public Health Association was formed. (Chapter 8 discusses in greater detail these professional associations.)

With the bombing of Pearl Harbor, on December 7, 1941, the United States found itself at war. Once again, national focus turned to physical fitness and health. With no major threats of war in the previous twenty years, the physical status of young American men had again degenerated. Of the approximately 2 million men examined for induction into the nation's armed forces, almost 50% were disqualified. Of those disqualified, 90% were found to be physically or mentally unfit (American Youth Commission, 1942). This unfortunate situation helped greatly to stimulate interest in the health of high school students and provided strong impetus for health education classes.

Following the war years, many demonstration projects and studies were completed to examine the impact of health education. The Massachusetts High School Study, the Astoria Study, The New York City Study, and the Denver Study were just a few of the efforts that provided valuable information on school health education (Means, 1975).

The **School Health Education Study** was one study of significance to health education. Directed by Dr. Elena M. Sliepcevich (1964), the study included 135 randomly selected school systems involving 1,460 schools and 840,832 students in thirty-eight states. Health behavior inventories were administered to students in grades 6, 9 and 12. Results were appalling. Health misconceptions among students at all levels prevailed. Questionnaires were distributed to school administrators throughout the country to obtain data on organizational procedures and instructional practices related to health education. Again the results indicated major problems in the organization and administration of health programs. Cortese (1993) noted, ". . . some health topics were omitted while others were repeated grade after grade at the same level of sophistication. No logical rationale placed learning exercises at various grade levels, and a need existed for a challenging and meaningful curriculum" (p. 21). The **School Health Education Evaluation Study** of the Los Angeles Area was one more important study. Its purpose was to evaluate the effectiveness of school health work in selected schools and colleges of the area. More specifically, the project aimed at the appraisal of the entire school health program, including administrative organization, school health services, health instruction, and healthful school environment. Further, it examined the students' health knowledge, attitudes, and behavior. The study resulted in eleven conclusions and seventeen important recommendations for the field. Of equal importance, the study's planning, design, and operational process established a research pattern that has provided a model for the development of subsequent similar studies (Means, 1975).

The second phase of the School Health Education Study established a curriculum writing team to develop a health education curriculum based on needs identified from the first phase of the study. The team consisted of prominent names in health education, including Gus T. Dalis, Edward B. Johns, Richard K. Means, Ann E. Nolte, Marion B. Pollock, and Robert D. Russell (Means, 1975). Over the next eight years, the writing team developed a comprehensive curriculum package that still influences school health curricula today.

After World War II, health education continued to grow as a profession. As Means (1975) observed, "This period from 1940 into the 1970s was one of appraisal, re-evaluation, and consolidation with respect to research accomplished in school health education. During this time leaders in the field attempted to look back, review, and take stock of what was known as a determinant of future action" (p. 107).

School health programs have continued to evolve from the mid-1970s to the present time. Several important events and trends have impacted school health

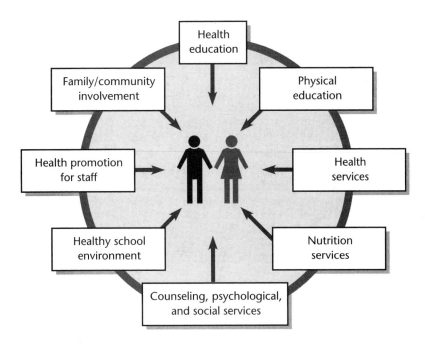

Figure 2.2   CDC Diagram of Coordinated School Health

education and overall school health programs. In 1978, the Office of Comprehensive School Health was established within the U.S. Department of Education. The primary purpose of the office was policy development for health education issues that affected children and youth. Although the office held great promise for school health education efforts, unfortunately, it was never fully funded. A director was named, Peter Cortese, but the office was finally deactivated with the budget cuts during President Ronald Reagan's administration (Rubinson & Alles, 1984).

The 1980s saw the emergence of two important concepts: coordinated school health programs and comprehensive school health instruction. Based on the initial ideas of Turner, Sellery and Smith (1957), and later refined by Allensworth and Kolbe (1987), a **coordinated school health program** consists of eight interactive components that work together to enhance the health and well-being of the students, faculty, staff, and community (see Figure 2.2). Leaders involved in each of these eight components work as an integrated team to coordinate the program. Outside leadership is provided by a **school health advisory council** (SHAC). The SHAC is formed by community members (such as parents; medical, health, and safety professionals; and political, religious, and corporate or business leaders) to assist with the planning and promotion of school health initiatives.

Comprehensive school health instruction is actually the health education component of the coordinated school health program (see Box 2.4). It refers to the development and delivery of a planned, sequential grades K–12 health curriculum. Topics include, but are not limited to personal health, family health, community

---

Box 2.4 Key Elements of Comprehensive Health Education

1. A documented, planned, and sequential program of health instruction for students in grades kindergarten through twelve.

2. A curriculum that addresses and integrates education about a range of categorical health problems and issues at developmentally appropriate ages.

3. Activities that help young people develop the skills they need to avoid: tobacco use; dietary patterns that contribute to disease; sedentary lifestyle; sexual behaviors that result in HIV infection, other sexually transmitted infections (STIs) and unintended pregnancy; alcohol and other drug use; and behaviors that result in unintentional and intentional injuries.

4. Instruction provided for a prescribed amount of time at each grade level.

5. Management and coordination by an education professional trained to implement the program.

6. Instruction from teachers who are trained to teach the subject.

7. Involvement of parents, health professionals, and other concerned community members.

8. Periodic evaluation, updating, and improvement.

Source: Centers for Disease Control (CDC). (2004). *Key elements of comprehensive health education.* Available at: http://www.cdc.gov /nccdphp/dash/about/comprehensive_ed .htm

---

health, consumer health, environmental health, sexuality education, mental and emotional health, injury prevention and safety, nutrition, prevention and control of disease, and substance use and abuse (CDC, 2004a).

In 1995, another milestone event occurred when the Joint Committee on National Health Education Standards issued the National Health Education Standards (see Box 2.5). The committee was comprised of representatives from the major health professional associations and the American Cancer Society. The standards were designed to promote **health literacy**, the capacity of individuals to access, interpret, and understand basic health information and services and the skills to use the information and services to promote health. The standards serve as a framework for organizing knowledge and skills into curricula at the state and local levels. They were not intended to be a federal mandate for a specific health curriculum (Joint Committee on Health Education Standards, 1995). As the third edition of this text goes to press, efforts are underway between The American Association for Health Education and the American Cancer Society to review and update these National Health Education Standards.

Since 1987, the concept of a coordinated school health program has dominated the school health arena. At first glance, it would seem that schools would be excited to initiate comprehensive school health programs. How could one not embrace a concept that would bring together multiple components of the school in an integrated attempt to improve the health of faculty, staff, students, and the community? A healthy child taught by a healthy teacher in a health-conscious community should forward the school's overall mission to provide each child with the best education

---

Box 2.5 National Health Education Standards

1. Students will comprehend concepts related to health promotion and disease prevention.

2. Students will demonstrate the ability to access valid health information and health promoting products and services.

3. Students will demonstrate the ability to practice health-enhancing behaviors and reduce health risks.

4. Students will analyze the influence of culture, media, technology, and other factors on health.

5. Students will demonstrate the ability to use interpersonal communication skills to enhance health.

6. Students will demonstrate the ability to use goal-setting and decision-making skills to enhance health.

7. Students will demonstrate the ability to advocate for personal, family, and community health.

Source: From Joint Committee on National Health Education Standards (1995). National Health Education Standards: Achieving Health Literacy. Athens, GA: American Cancer Society.

---

possible. Unfortunately, the full potential of coordinated school health programs has never been realized in most school districts. Many factors may be at play here, such as the low priority placed on health by many school administrators, a lack of leadership to coordinate and oversee school health programs, an overemphasis on competency testing, and adverse reactions from conservative groups that perceive coordinated school health as a means of incorporating sex education into the curriculum.

Despite the apparent lack of success with coordinated school health programs, schools still hold tremendous promise for health education efforts. With 52 million young people attending more than 100,000 schools and 14 million students attending the nation's colleges and universities (CDC, 2000c), health educators must remain diligent in their effort to bring health promotion and education programs to this population. For this reason the CDC has invested considerable time and effort into developing health education guidelines that address the six critical behaviors research shows contribute to the leading causes of death and disability among adults and youth. These six areas are alcohol and drug use, injury and violence (including suicide), tobacco use, nutrition, physical activity, and sexual behaviors (CDC, 2004a).

SUMMARY

The history of health and health education is important to professional development in health education. By understanding the past, students can appreciate the present and evolve into future leaders in this emerging profession.

The concept of health education as understood today is relatively new, dating back only to the middle to late 1800s. From the times of earliest intelligence, however, humans have been searching for ways to keep themselves healthy and free of disease. Without knowledge of disease causation or medical treatment, it was only natural to rely on superstition and spiritualism for answers. The concept of prevention was intriguing, but the knowledge and skills to prevent disease were unknown.

As one examines the great civilizations of Egypt, Greece, and Rome, progress in preventing and treating disease is evident. These early cultures recognized a need for humans to maintain sound minds and sound bodies. Systems of rudimentary pharmacology and advancements in the areas of waste disposal and the provision of safe drinking water were among some of the most noteworthy improvements.

During the Middle Ages, much of what had been learned was lost; it was as if society had taken a giant step backward. Science and knowledge were shunned, while religion gained new favor as the preferred means of preventing and treating disease. Great epidemics struck the European continent, and millions of people lost their lives.

The Renaissance witnessed a rebirth of interest in knowledge. Science again flourished, and health care advancements were made. Understanding of disease, however, was still rudimentary, and treatment was often worse than the effects of the disease. Sanitary conditions were deplorable and would remain so through the 1800s. The emergence of health education as a profession was still more than a century away.

The era of Enlightenment saw tremendous growth in cities as the industrial movement got underway in both England and the United States. Unfortunately, this population growth compounded sanitation problems related to overcrowding. Epidemics were still prevalent. In addition, the employment conditions of the working class were frequently unsafe and unhealthy.

By the mid-1850s, conditions were ripe for the birth of public health in the United States. The contagion theory of disease was emerging, and early reformers called for the government to step in and take control of environmental conditions that led to disease. Health departments at the city, state, and county level were established and began to monitor and regulate food safety, water safety, and waste disposal. Professional organizations for health personnel emerged, and voluntary agencies were formed. Major pieces of legislation were passed as government sought to improve working conditions and took greater responsibility for the poor and infirm. During the mid-1900s, emphasis was placed on building new medical facilities and enhancing the technology required to treat disease.

By the 1970s the cost of medical treatment had escalated, and concern had shifted to prevention. This set the stage for the development of national health objectives for the decades of the 1980s and 1990s. Health education made great strides as an emerging profession.

In the mid-1800s, as public health was starting to make important strides, school health education was also emerging. In addition to reading, writing, and arithmetic, early pioneers saw the need to educate students about health-related matters. In the early 1900s, groups such as the National Tuberculosis Association, the American Cancer Society, and the Women's Christian Temperance Union were strongly supporting the need to educate school children about health. Both World War I and World War II provided important impetus for health-related instruction and physical training in the schools.

The 1960s and 1970s saw several important studies completed that supported the need for health education and documented its effectiveness. Coordinated school health programs emerged in the 1980s and are still an important focus for school health. The Centers for Disease Control has promoted the notion of school health programs through the development of their School Health Program Guidelines, national health education standards, and identification of the six leading causes of death and disability.

While health and health education have made great strides since the first humans contemplated how to treat and prevent disease, there is still a long way to go. Both in the United States and worldwide there are many people who do not have access to medical care or the important information and skills of professionally trained health educators. Heart disease, cancers, diabetes, obesity, and HIV are prevalent in developed countries, while the traditional infectious diseases, parasitic infections, and malnutrition continue to affect those in developing countries.

As in the past, health professionals must envision what *can* be and strive to make that vision a reality. Turner, Sellery, and Smith (1957) noted,

> As society looks ahead, it can conceive the hope that some day almost every human being will be well, intelligent, physically vigorous, mentally alert, emotionally stable, socially reasonable and ethically sound. At least, society must concern itself with progress toward that goal. (p. 18)

Health educators must be important players in this process.

REVIEW QUESTIONS

1. Describe the earliest efforts at health care and informal health education.

2. Compare and contrast the great societies of Egypt, Greece, and Rome. How are these cultures similar in relation to health? How are they different?

3. What were the major epidemics of the Middle Ages? Why were they so feared? What factors contributed to their spread? What were some strategies people used to prevent these diseases?

4. Discuss the Renaissance and why it is important to the history of health and health care.

5. Who wrote the *Report of the Sanitary Commission of Massachusetts* (1850)? Explain how this report was important to the history of both school health and public health.

6. Identify at least five major groups or events that forwarded school health programs.

7. What Canadian publication and its U.S. counterpart helped focus attention on the importance of disease prevention and health promotion?

8. What are *national health objectives*? Where can they be found? Why are they so important?

9. Describe the initiatives that have shaped school health education programs over the past ten years.

10. Explain why it is important for health education professionals to understand the history of health, health education, and health care.

CRITICAL THINKING QUESTIONS

1. If one thinks of a health educator as simply someone who educates others about health, who would be considered humanity's first health educators? Defend your answer.

2. If a health educator trained in the year 2000 could time-travel back to the Middle Ages, what impact could such a health educator have on the health problems of that era? What positive factors would have worked in the health educator's favor? What negative factors would have worked against the health educator?

3. When the very first schools were being started in Massachusetts, do you believe health education would have been accepted as an academic subject? Why or why not? Do you believe health education is accepted as an academic subject at the present time? Why or why not?

4. Select one of the twenty-eight focus areas in *Healthy People* 2010, and find the objectives for that focus area. Select one of the objectives and explain why you feel it will or will not be met by the year 2010. What role might a health educator have in meeting the objective you selected?

ACTIVITIES

1. Develop a timeline using one hundred-year increments from the early Egyptians to the year 2000. Mark all of the important health-related events as they occurred along the timeline.

2. Imagine what it would have been like to live through an outbreak of the Black Death in the Middle Ages. Write a thirty-day personal diary, with daily entries depicting what you might have seen or heard and how you might have felt.

3. Interview several individuals who are at least eighty years old concerning the health care they received as young children. Ask them to describe any health education they can remember. When was it? Where did it take place? Who provided the education? Was it effective?

WEBLINKS

1. **http://www.cdc.gov/maso/factbook/Fact%20Book.pdf**

   Centers for Disease Control

   This CDC Web site contains the *CDC Fact Book 2000/2001*. On page 135 of this document, you will find the brief history of the CDC. This is a concise but informative overview of the most important events in the illustrious history of this organization.

2. **http://history.nih.gov/exhibits/history/**

   National Institutes of Health

   This National Institutes of Health (NIH) Web site provides a brief history of this organization highlighting some of its more important accomplishments.

3. **http://www.kented.org.uk/medhist/**

   Ian Coulson

   Interesting website that chronicles the history of health and medicine in Kent, England, from prehistoric times to the present.

4. **http://www.library.vcu.edu/tml/speccoll/musstateco.html**

Virginia Commonwealth University

This site provides a list of "History of Health" science museums in the United States and around the world. These are fascinating places to visit and provide useful information for understanding how health knowledge has developed and been disseminated throughout history.

CASE STUDY

John is a health education professor employed by a state university. He feels his health education students are often frustrated by the way health information and health education practice are constantly changing. For example, one day margarine is better than butter; the next day margarine is just as bad as butter. One day health educators are supposed to work with individuals to change health behavior; now with the social ecological model, health educators are supposed to also enter the political arena and advocate for community-wide changes in policy and law. John wants to make the point with his students that such change is nothing new—and in actuality it is a positive thing. What we learn from the past helps us to evolve and better understand what is happening today. Your task is to help John develop a lesson that will use historical examples to show how health information and health education practice has evolved over time. Identify what you consider to be the five best examples John could use to demonstrate the evolution of health information and health education practice.

REFERENCES

Allensworth, D., & Kolbe, L. (1987). The comprehensive school health program: Exploring an expanded concept. *Journal of School Health, 57,* 409–412.

American Youth Commission. (1942). *"Health and fitness," youth and the future.* Washington, DC: American Council on Education.

Andress, M. J., & Bragg, M. C. (1922). *Suggestions for a program for health teaching in the elementary schools.* U.S. Department of the Interior, Bureau of Education, Health Education No. 10, Washington, DC: U.S. Government Printing Office.

Auld, E. (Winter 1997/1998). Executive edge. *SOPHE News & Views, 24* (4), 4.

Bates, I. J., & Winder, A. E. (1984). *Introduction to health education.* San Francisco: Mayfield.

Bernstein, N. R. (1972). *APHA: The first one hundred years.* Washington, DC: American Public Health Association.

Butler, M., Thornton, F., & Stoltz, D. (1994). *The Battle Creek Idea.* Battle Creek, MI: Heritage Publications.

Centers for Disease Control. (CDC). (2000a). *Fact Book 2000/2001.* Retrieved August 31, 2004, from: http://www.cdc.gov/maso/factbook/main.htm

Centers for Disease Control (CDC). (2000b). *National School Health Strategies.* Retrieved March 1, 2004 from: http://www.cdc.gov/nccdphp/dash/coordinated.htm

Centers for Disease Control (CDC). (2003) The National Public Health Performance Standards Program Technical Assistance and Training Resources for Users. Retrieved April 9, 2004 from http://www.phppo.cdc.gov/nphpsp/documents/TA_Fact_Sheet.pdf

Centers for Disease Control. (2004a). *Health Topics.* Retrieved March 1, 2004 from: http://www.cdc.gov/nccdphp/dash/healthtopics/index.htm

Centers for Disease Control. (2004b). *Key elements of comprehensive health education.* Retrieved March 1, 2004 from: http://www.cdc.gov/nccdphp/dash/about/comprehensive_ed.htm

Centers for Disease Control. (2004c). *School health defined.* Retrieved March 1, 2004, from: http://www.cdc.gov/nccdphp/dash/about/school_health.htm#1

Cipolla, C. M. (1976). *Public health and the medical profession in the Renaissance.* Cambridge, England: Cambridge University Press.

Cortese, P. A. (1993). Accomplishments in comprehensive school health education. *Journal of School Health, 63* (1), 21–23.

De'ath, E. (1995). *The Black Death—1347 AD.* [Film]. (Available from Ambrose Video Publishing Inc., 1290 Avenue of the Americas, Suite 2245, New York, NY 10104)

Donan, C. (1898). *The Dark Ages 476–918.* London: Rivingtons.

Duncan, D. (1988). *Epidemiology: Basis for disease prevention and health promotion.* New York: Macmillan.

Durant, W. (1961). *The Age of Reason begins.* Vol. 7. *The story of civilization.* New York: Simon and Schuster.

Fee, E., & Brown, T. M. (1997). Editorial: Why history? *American Journal of Public Health, 87* (11), 1763–1764.

Goerke, L. S., & Stebbins, E. L. (1968). *Mustard's introduction to public health* (5th ed.). New York: Macmillan.

Gordon, B. (1959). *Medieval and Renaissance medicine.* New York: Philosophical Library.

Green, W. H., & Simons-Morton, B. G. (1990). *Introduction to health education.* Prospect Heights, IL: Waveland Press.

Hansen, M. (1980). *The royal facts of life.* Metuchen, NJ: The Scarecrow Press.

Joint Committee on Health Education Standards. (1995). *National health education standards: Achieving health literacy.* Atlanta, GA: American Cancer Society.

Kochanek, K. D., & Smith, B. L. (2004). Deaths: Preliminary data for 2002. *National Vital Statistics Reports. 52*(13), 1–48. Retrieved March 1, 2004, from http://www.cdc.gov/nchs/releases/04news/infantmort.htm.

Lalonde, M. (1974). *A new perspective on the health of Canadians.* Ottawa: Government of Canada.

Libby, W. (1922). *The history of medicine in its salient features.* Boston: Houghton Mifflin.

Marr, J. (Winter, 1982). Merchants of death: The role of the slave trade in the transmission of disease from Africa to the Americas. *Pharos, 31.*

McKenzie, J. F., Pinger, R. R., & Kotecki, J. E. (2005). *An introduction to community health.* Boston: Jones and Bartlett.

Means, R. K. (1962). *A history of health education in the United States.* Philadelphia: Lea & Febiger.

Means, R. K. (1975). *Historical perspectives on school health.* Thorofare, NJ: Charles B. Slack.

Moore, H. H. (1923). *Public health in the United States.* New York: Harper & Brothers.

Pickett, G., & Hanlon, J. J. (1990). *Public health administration and practice* (9th ed.). St. Louis: Times Mirror/Mosby.

Ravenel, M. P. (Ed.). (1970). *A half century of public health.* New York: Arno Press & The New York Times.

Rogers, J. F. (1936). *Training of elementary teachers for school health work.* U.S. Department of the Interior, Office of Education, Pamphlet No. 67. Washington, DC: U.S. Government Printing Office.

Rosen, G. (1958). *A history of public health.* New York: MD Publications.

Rubinson, L., & Alles, W. F. (1984). *Health education foundations for the future.* St. Louis: Times Mirror/Mosby.

Schouten, J. (1967). *The rod and serpent of Asclepius.* Amsterdam: Elsevier.

Shattuck, L. (1850). *Report of the Sanitary Commission of Massachusetts.* Boston: Dutton and Wentworth.

Sliepcevich, E. M. (1964). *School health education study: A summary report.* Washington, D.C.: SHES.

Turner, C. E., Sellery, C. M., & Smith, S. A. (1957). *School health and health education* (3rd ed.). St. Louis: Mosby.

U.S. Department of Health and Human Services (USDHHS). (1980). *Promoting health/preventing disease: Objectives for the nation.* Washington, DC: U.S. Government Printing Office.

U.S. Department of Health and Human Services. (USDHHS) (1990). *Healthy people 2000: National health promotion and disease prevention objectives* (DHHS Publication No. PHS 90–50212). Washington, DC: U.S. Government Printing Office.

U.S. Department of Health and Human Services. (USDHHS) (1999). Changes in the Public Health System. *Morbidity and Mortality Weekly Report, 48*(50), 1141.

U.S. Department of Health and Human Services (USDHHS). (2000a). *Healthy People 2000 Fact Sheet.* Retrieved March 1, 2004 from: http://odphp.osophs.dhhs.gov/pubs/hp2000/hp2kfact.htm

U.S. Department of Health and Human Services (USDHHS). (2000). *Healthy People 2010* (Conference Edition in Two Volumes). Washington, DC: U.S. Government Printing Office.

U.S. Department of Health, Education, and Welfare (USDHEW). (1976). Health in America: 1776–1976. (DHEW Publication No. (HRA) 76-616). Washington, DC: U.S. Government Printing Office.

U.S. Public Health Service. (1979). *Healthy people: The surgeon general's report on health promotion and disease prevention.* Washington, DC: U.S. Government Printing Office.

Voices From the Past. (2004). Today's health problems and health education. American Journal of Public Health. *94*(3), 368–369.

Winslow, C. A. (1944). *The conquest of epidemic disease.* Princeton, NJ: Princeton University Press.

Ziegler, P. (1969). *The Black Death.* New York: Harper & Row.

CHAPTER 3

Philosophical Foundations

Chapter Objectives

After reading this chapter and answering the questions at the end, you should be able to:

1. Define the terms *philosophy, humanism, wellness, holistic,* and *symmetry* and explain the differences between them.
2. Discuss the importance of having a personal philosophy about life.
3. Compare and contrast the advantages and disadvantages of having a life philosophy and an occupational philosophy that are similar.
4. Formulate a statement that describes your personal philosophy of life and identify the influences that account for your philosophy.
5. Identify and explain the differences between
   a. behavior change philosophy
   b. cognitive-based philosophy
   c. decision-making philosophy
   d. freeing/functioning philosophy
   e. social change philosophy
   f. eclectic health education philosophy.
6. Explain how a health educator might use each of the five health education philosophies to address a situation in a scenario.
7. Create and defend your own philosophy of health education.

Key Terms

behavior change philosophy
cognitive-based philosophy
decision-making philosophy
eclectic health education
   philosophy

freeing/functioning
   philosophy
holistic philosophy
humanism
philosophy

philosophy of symmetry
social change philosophy
wellness

When considering the meaning of the phrase "health education philosophy," it seems almost imperative to begin by asking questions. This chapter will explore answers to questions such as:

- What is a philosophy?
- Why does a person need a philosophy?
- What are some of the philosophies or philosophical principles associated with the notion of "health"?
- What philosophical viewpoints related to health education do some of today's leading health educators hold?
- How is a philosophy developed?
- What are the predominant philosophies used in the practice of health education today?
- How will adopting any one of the health education philosophies impact the way health educators might approach their job?

The purpose of discussing the development of a health education philosophy is not to provide a treatise on "the nature of the world," so to speak, but to emphasize the importance of a guiding philosophy to the practice of any profession. Although the term *philosophy* seems to imply to many an almost ethereal, esoteric dimension, in actuality, development of a well-considered philosophy provides the underpinnings that support the bridge between theory and practice.

What Is a Philosophy?

The word *philosophy* comes from Greek and literally means "the love of wisdom" or "the love of learning." The term **philosophy** in the context of this chapter means a statement summarizing the attitudes, principles, beliefs, values, and concepts held by an individual or a group. In an academic setting, a philosopher studies the topics of ethics, logic, politics, metaphysics, theology, and/or aesthetics. It is certainly not imperative that a person be an academic philosopher to have a philosophy. All of us have convictions, ideas, values, experiences, and attitudes about one or more of the areas listed above as they apply to life. These are the building blocks (sometimes known as principles) that make up any philosophy. Therefore, the probability is high that you have already developed certain philosophical viewpoints or notions about what is real and true in the world as you know it. The manner in which you consistently act toward other people is often a reflection of your philosophy concerning the importance of people in general. The fact that you are studying to become a health educator also says something about your philosophical leanings in terms of a career. For example, the profession of health education is considered a helping profession. Those who work in the profession should value helping others.

In today's society there are many examples of the use of a philosophical stance. Corporations, for example, create slogans espousing their purported philosophy (of course, they are also trying to sell a product or service at the same time). Many of

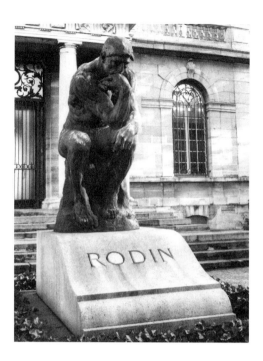

Rodin's sculpture, *The Thinker*, illustrates
the philosopher in all of us. (Art Resource)

us recognize certain companies by phrases such as "Always low prices. Always."
(WalMart), or "When you care enough to send the very best" (Hallmark Cards). The
use of caring slogans and catchy phrases is meant to convey to the public that the
company is in business solely because it is interested in the welfare of people every-
where and is responsive to their needs. If the company's actions match the slogan,
the public is more likely to perceive the slogan as a true representation of the corporate philosophy.

Additionally, many nonprofit and for-profit agencies and companies often
have mission statements. A mission statement is meant to convey a philosophy and
direction that forms a framework for all actions taken by that organization. For example, the mission statement for the Central District Health Department in Boise,
Idaho, is as follows:

> To prevent disease, disability, and premature death; to promote healthy lifestyles;
> and to protect the health and quality of the environment.

After reading this statement there is little doubt that the overriding philosophy
in this department is one of promoting prevention wherever and whenever possible. For individuals who have a philosophy that emphasizes prevention and early
intervention, this is likely to be a place where they might find employment that is
personally rewarding and professionally fulfilling.

Just as often, insight into a person's philosophy can be gained by hearing, reading, or analyzing quotes or sayings by that person. For example, the following quote
attributed to Scottish poet Robert Burns is most certainly a reflection of his life philosophy: "The purpose of life, is a life of purpose." After reading his words, it is

evident that he valued a life's work that was well considered and of benefit not only to him, but to others. As Bedworth and Bedworth (1992) state, "Philosophy is a wisdom of the nature of things—a comprehension of nature and of reality, a body of knowledge that defines the perimeters of life and living" (p. 10).

The thoughts stated above are well summarized by Loren Bensley (1993), one of the leading health educators of our time, who wrote,

> Philosophy can be defined as a state of mind based on your values and beliefs. This in turn is based on a variety of factors which include culture, religion, education, morals, environment, experiences, and family. It is also determined by people who have influenced you, how you feel about yourself and others, your spirit, your optimism or pessimism, your independence and your family. It is a synthesis of all learning that makes you who you are and what you believe. In other words, a philosophy reflects your values and beliefs which determine your mission and purpose for being, or basic theory, or viewpoint based on logical reasoning. (p. 2)

As can be seen, a philosophy does not have to be abstract. Pondering the reason for being gives people a chance to integrate their past, present, and future into a coherent whole that guides them through life.

Why Does One Need a Philosophy?

The answer to the question "Why does one need a philosophy?" is both simple and complex. Each of us already has a way we look at the world, what is true for us— our philosophy. This image helps shape the way we experience our surroundings and act toward others in our environment. In other words, people's philosophies help form the basis of reality for them.

Of course, some philosophical change is probably inevitable. New experiences, new insights, and new learnings create the possibility that a retooling of some of the tenets comprising the philosophy might occur. This is a normal part of growth. Most people's philosophical views are altered somewhat as they study and experience the world in different ways.

Usually a person's philosophy (e.g., determining how to treat others, what actions are right or wrong, and what is important in life) needs to be synchronous in all aspects of life. This means that a person's philosophical viewpoint holds at home, at school, in the workplace, and at play. If an incongruency develops between a person's philosophy and the philosophy of the leaders in the workplace, problems can occur.

As an example, consider the career of a community health educator working in HIV/AIDS prevention education who is employed by a state department of education. Assume that this individual has a philosophical view that all human life is sacred and education is the best source of prevention. Also assume that the person's work both on and off the job reflects a consistency and a commitment to those ideals. In other words, the person's actions are synonymous with the aforementioned philosophy. As long as the administration in the state department of education, and family and friends remain supportive of the role and philosophy of the HIV/AIDS educator, chances are that all will be well with this person. If, however, leadership in the state department changes and the new superintendent is not at all

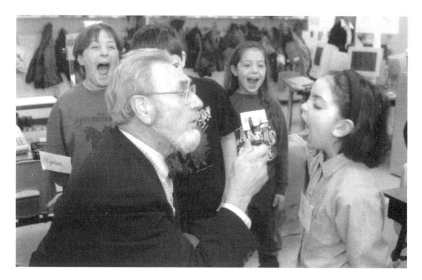

Former Surgeon General C. Everett Koop remains a staunch advocate for the value of health education as the key to prevention. (Herbert Medora, Valley News/AP/Wide World)

amenable to the idea that individuals infected with HIV are worth saving (because they chose their behaviors) or refuses to allow the term *condom* to be mentioned as a secondary source of prevention, the health educator may have a difficult time remaining in that environment. The reason is because this educator is now not allowed to act according to her beliefs, ideals, and knowledge. There is a disharmony between the philosophical stance and the ability to act in concert with that stance.

Certainly, there are exceptions to this rule. Health educators might hold philosophies on how they might personally live, yet they might be called on to educate those who have made choices that are in opposition to their belief system. This situation begins to cross the bounds of a general philosophy and get into ethics (right behavior—see Chapter 5). Although a possible moral-philosophical conflict seems apparent in this situation, health educators need to keep in mind that their primary concern is to protect and enhance the health of those within their jurisdiction. Health is not a moral issue. The health of any one of us affects the health of all of us in some manner (legally, monetarily, physically, or emotionally). At the very least, the health educator should refer this situation to another trained individual who can fulfill the obligation to the public.

Former Surgeon General C. Everett Koop was confronted with the same dilemma when he was in office. Although he was a strong conservative Christian leader and against the use of drugs or the initiation of sex before marriage, he championed the cause of HIV/AIDS education by stressing that the epidemic was a health problem needing a health-based prevention message. Through the power of his office, he insisted that HIV/AIDS prevention education include the merits of abstinence, the dissemination of needles to inner-city addicts, and the increased availability of condoms to individuals who choose to be sexually active or promiscuous.

A further example that illustrates the impact of a philosophy comes from Judy Drolet (1993), health education professor at Southern Illinois University. She comments that her philosophy of health education has served to guide her "present commitments and choices in practice, research, and programs" (p. 31). The emphasis she places on the areas of teaching, research, and service is a direct reflection of the personal and professional philosophical foundation she formed over the years. A well-reasoned philosophy often plays an important role in the choice of a career path. A recent study identifying factors that influence career choices validates that statement. Tamayose et al. (2004) surveyed public health students enrolled at a west coast university to determine what major influences led them to pursue careers in public health. Researchers found that the top two items mentioned overwhelmingly by the students were "enjoyment of the profession/commitment to health improvement" and "provide a health/community service to others." Both of these statements reflect a common philosophical thread that permeates the thinking of a majority of individuals currently practicing in the field of health education and health promotion with whom we have come in contact.

In summary, the formation of a philosophy is one of the key determining factors behind the choice of an occupation, a spouse, a religious conviction, and friends. A firm philosophical foundation serves as a beacon that lights the way and provides guidance for many of the major decisions in life.

Principles and Philosophies Associated with Health

In Chapter 1, the meaning of the term *health* was discussed. Recall that, while the term *health* is elusive to define, almost all definitions include the idea of a multidimensional construct that most people value, particularly when health deteriorates. Over the past thirty to fifty years, educators have identified several philosophies or philosophical principles that tend to be associated with the establishment and maintenance of health. These philosophies provide a set of guiding principles that help create a framework to better understand the depth of the term *health.*

Rash (1985) mentions that, while health is often not an end in itself, good health does bring a richness and enjoyment to life that will make service to others more possible. He feels that those who seek to enhance the health of others through education should espouse a **philosophy of symmetry;** that is, health has physical, emotional, spiritual, and social components, and each is just as important as the others. Health educators should seek to motivate their students or clients toward a symmetry (balance) among these components.

Oberteufer (1953) rejected the notions of a dualistic (human = mind + body) or a triune (human = mind + body + spirit) nature for humanity. Instead, he embraced the ideal of a **holistic philosophy** of health when he stated, "The mind and body disappear as recognizable realities and in their stead comes the acknowledgment of a whole being ... man is essentially a unified integrated organism" (p. 105). Thomas (1984) is convinced that the holistic view of health produces health professionals who are more passionate about creating a society in which the promotion of good health is seen as a positive goal.

Bedworth and Bedworth (1992) propose that **humanism,** one of the underlying theories of education, is worthy of consideration for each potential health

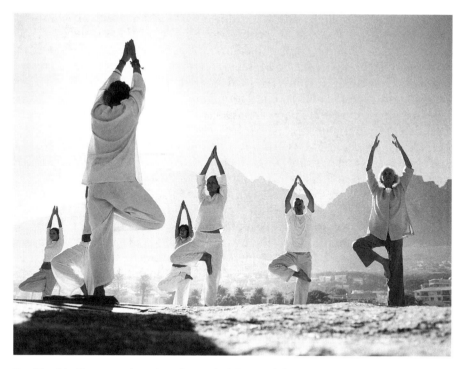

Total health allows people to function at their best. (Philip North-Coombes/Getty Images)

educator to include in formulating a philosophy of health. They note that humanism is characterized by a concern for humanity. Humanism also "promotes the basic premise of the worth of human life and the ability of individuals to achieve … self fulfillment" (p. 5).

Finally, Greenberg (1992), Donatelle (2005), Edlin and Golanty (2004), and Hales (2004), among others, have elevated the construct of wellness to the level of a philosophy. **Wellness,** always a positive quality (as opposed to illness being always a negative) is visualized as the integration of the spiritual, intellectual, physical, emotional, environmental, and social dimensions of health to form a whole "healthy person." Those who subscribe to this philosophy believe that all people can achieve some measure of wellness, no matter what limitations they have, and that achieving optimal health is an appropriate journey for everyone. The optimum state of wellness occurs when people have developed all six of the dimensions of health to the maximum of their ability. (See Figure 3.1.)

The philosophies previously mentioned are not meant to be all inclusive. The purpose for discussing them is to help provide a framework to further assist the reader in developing a philosophy about health and, ultimately, health education.

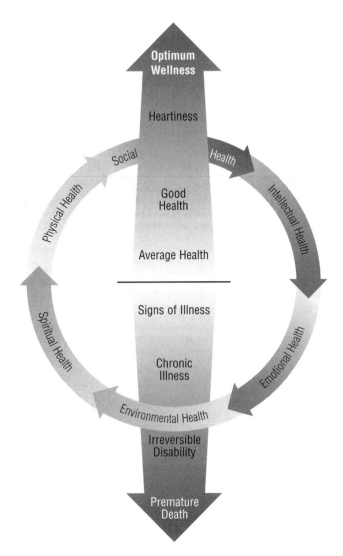

Figure 3.1   The Dimensions of Health and Wellness Continuum

Leading Philosophical Viewpoints

The December 1993 edition of *The Eta Sigma Gamma Monograph Series* was entitled "Reflections: The Philosophies of Health Educators of the 1990's." In order to assist you in formulating your own health education philosophy, we believe it is instructive to present a representative sample of the philosophies expressed in this volume. As has been previously mentioned, one of the ways a philosophical approach is developed is through the influence of role models, or mentors. The viewpoints that follow may help stimulate your thoughts and provide guidance as you consider a career in health education.

Loren Bensley (1993)

I believe health education offers an individual an invitation to be and to become—to affirm the self and become committed to the development of individual potential through decision making and action. I am committed to the philosophy of existentialism (the existential health educator sees his/her function as one of awakening learners to their own capacities and of providing opportunities for them to be responsible for their own learning opportunities and/or ignorance—[Shirreffs, 1976] as an approach to health education [p. 3]). . . . I also believe the ultimate goal of health education is to provide learning experiences from which one can develop skills and knowledge to make better informed decisions which will maintain or better their health, or the health of others (p. 4).

Joyce Fetro (1993)

I believe health education is an "ongoing process"—meaning that something is "going on." It implies continuous movement. The content and process of health education should change as individuals and current health issues change. To me, health education is an invitation to a smorgasbord. Health educators make the curriculum and program selections, arrange them in a way that is most meaningful, and appealing to their students, and replenish them when necessary (p. 59). . . . Critical to the health education feast is a forum that promotes openness and acceptance of individual differences (p. 63). . . .

Fetro concludes with this quote from Rosenstock (1960), "We must keep constantly in mind that an individual's behavior is determined by his motives and his beliefs, regardless of whether the motives and beliefs correspond to our notion of reality and what is good for him."

Marian Hamburg (1993)

Eta Sigma Gamma's *invitation to contribute has given me the chance to expound on a few of my beliefs about health education.*

1. You can't plan everything. Unexpected opportunities appear and it is important to be ready to take advantage of them (p. 68).
2. I believe in mentorship. Its power incorporated into health education programming has enormous strength for influencing positive health behaviors (p. 70).
3. I believe that effective health education programming requires appropriate inter-sectoral cooperation, and that health educators, regardless of the source of their professional preparation, must be its facilitators. School-community can be one world (p. 71).
4. I believe that we need to put more of our resources into joint efforts and coalition building. Much of health education's future as a profession depends upon the support that health educators, regardless of their specialized training, provide for the maintenance and expansion of certification (p. 73).
5. It is not surprising to me that the concept of networking has become an important basis for health education practice. We bring together people with common problems to seek solutions through the sharing of feelings and information (p. 73).

John Seffrin (1993)

I believe the most fundamental outcome of health education is the enabling of individuals to achieve a level of personal freedom not very likely to be obtained otherwise. Freedom means being able to avoid any unnecessary encumbrance on one's ability to make an enlightened choice (p. 110). . . . We need to be resourceful and open to change. In doing so, however, we need to change in ways that do not violate certain basic principles:

1. appreciation for each individual's uniqueness;
2. respect for ethnic and cultural diversity;
3. protection for individual and group autonomy;
4. promotion and preservation of free choice; and
5. intervention strategies based on good science (p. 114).

Philosophies are as individual as the people themselves, yet some common themes (development of individual potential, learning experiences that help in decision making, free choice, and enhancement of individual uniqueness) seem to emerge and hold true regardless of the health educator. Let us now examine how these philosophies are actually applied in the practice of health education.

Developing a Philosophy

Now that it is clear that a philosophy is not some abstraction that is used only by individuals such as the Dalai Lama or Gandhi, let us explore the ways in which a philosophy is formed. In previous sections, it was noted that most practicing professionals and many organizations have developed certain philosophical stances that serve as a road map and guide for living and working in the world. What provides the basis for forming a philosophy?

Assume you are searching through the Web sites of various health education programs, trying to determine which one might be best for you. In your search, you come across the Web site for the health education program at the University of Wisconsin at La Crosse (see the Weblinks section at the end of the chapter for URL references). One of the prominent features of the site is a statement of the philosophy of health education:

> "The philosophy of health education is not directed at a high level of health for health's sake, but rather to help each individual view health as a way of life that will help attain individual goals and utilize one's highest potential to the betterment of self, family, and community."

This statement is followed by a listing of values that form the underpinnings of its contents:

- Integrity of the total person
- Academic excellence
- Innovation and creativity
- Interdisciplinary professional preparation
- Relevance of academic endeavors to social needs

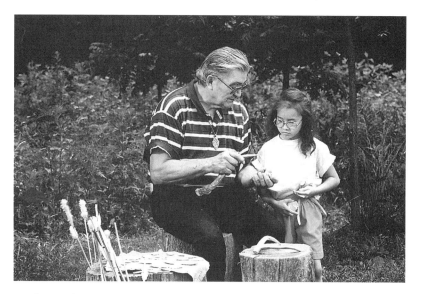

Family members, friends, mentors, and role models help shape our philosophy. (Lawrence Migdale/Stock, Boston)

The process of developing this philosophy statement most likely involved at least several meetings of faculty, staff, students, community group representatives, and administrators. During the meetings, the group discussed and then listed (and/or examined) their core beliefs or principles. These are usually formulated from personal experiences, reading and study, guidance from a trusted family member, health education peer, or mentor, and reflection on "the attributes that make a sound health educator." The final statement incorporates the essence of the core beliefs resulting from their deliberations—the philosophy.

In drafting your own philosophy statement, you should employ the same process. Think about what a health educator does and what the result of his or her work should be. Construct lists of your thoughts, under headings such as: personal values and beliefs, what "health" means to you, attributes of people you admire and trust, results of health studies and readings that you find meaningful, and outcomes you would like to see from the process of health education (e.g., better decision making, more community involvement, promotion of positive behaviors). From your lists, some common themes will emerge and the identification of these themes is a key to drafting your own health education philosophy statement. Exploring why you value the topics represented within these themes should enable you to compose your philosophy statement, or an ultimate product that will reflect a way of thinking, acting, and viewing the world that works for you.

Please note, however, that using this approach to formulate a philosophy is not a guarantee that the philosophy will remain stable. As a matter of fact, there is a strong likelihood that some changes will occur because of new learnings, activities, and experiences (e.g., working in a different culture, experiencing the premature death of a child or spouse, losing a job as a result of downsizing).

A philosophy results from the sum of knowledge, experience, and principles from which it was formed.

As a further aid to formulating a philosophy statement about health and health education, we would like to conclude this section with two short vignettes illustrating several concepts or principles that need to be considered when formulating a philosophy statement about life, health, and health education practice. The first comes from Mongolia.

> A farmer had a teenage son who caused trouble from time to time. The neighbors constantly criticized the farmer for having such a son. One day the farmer went to town and purchased a wild horse in the hope that he could tame it and use it for transportation to and from town. That evening the son sneaked out and attempted to get on the horse. It escaped. On learning of the circumstances surrounding the horse's escape, the neighbors berated the farmer for his son and the bad luck he caused. The farmer, however, responded that maybe the horse's escape was bad; maybe it wasn't. The next day, to everyone's amazement, the horse reappeared with fifteen other wild horses. The farmer and the neighbors could not believe the good fortune.
>
> That night the son tried to ride one of the wild horses, was thrown off, and broke his leg. The neighbors were quick to seize the opportunity to point out this misfortune as well. Again, the farmer responded that maybe the son's breaking his leg was bad, but maybe it wasn't. The next day the Mongols declared war on a country far away, and soldiers came to the village and conscripted every able-bodied son from every family. Of course, because of his broken leg the farmer's son was not taken. He grew to live a long, healthful, and prosperous life and became a mayor of the village.

How things turn out is many times a matter of how they are perceived. A personal philosophy is often a reflection of the individual's perspective of the world and how and why it seems to work that way.

The second story comes from the United States.

> One Saturday in late spring a family decided to visit the local zoo. As they entered, it was noted that the feature attraction for that day was a flea circus. Now, the father, being a skeptic, had heard of flea circuses before but thought them to be fictional. Approaching the area where the flea circus was supposedly housed, he was amazed to find a large piece of plywood complete with fleas jumping around. Nearby was a young woman who wore a suit with the tag "flea trainer" conspicuously inscribed on it. The father went up to the woman and asked her (tongue in cheek) how she was able to train the fleas. She responded that training them was actually quite easy. She went on to explain that a flea can jump higher for its size than any living creature. Her method involved placing the fleas in a three-inch-high box with a lid on it. At first the fleas jump and hit the lid. After a few minutes, however, they learn to jump just short of the top. When she determines that they have reached that level of training (she can no longer hear them hitting the inside of the box lid), she removes the lid and places them on the plywood. Although they have not lost any of their ability to jump, they never again go any higher than the height of the box lid.

Too many times, in determining abilities, people set their sights and dreams too low. A personal philosophy needs to incorporate the realization that life sometimes dishes out bumps and bruises. The awareness of this fact helps prevent any of us from becoming too limiting in the assessment of our place in the world.

Remember, the formation of a philosophy, whether personal or occupational, requires several steps. First, individuals need to answer the following questions in reference to themselves: What is important? What is most valued? What ideals are held? Second, they need to identify ways the answers to the first questions influence the way they believe and act. Third, after carefully considering and writing down the answers to these questions, a philosophy statement can be formulated. The statement (usually a paragraph or two in length—250 words) reflects and identifies those factors, principles, ideals, and influences that help shape reality for those individuals.

As previously mentioned, these steps can be used to formulate any type of philosophy statement. However, for those who are studying health education, there is one more important question to answer: Is this philosophy statement consistent with being a health educator? If the answer is yes, then for that person health education is a profession worthy of further consideration.

Predominant Health Education Philosophies

Butler (1997) accurately points out that, even though there are several definitions for *health education,* there are recurring themes in many of the definitions that allow for a general agreement as to the meaning of the phrase "health education." He notes, however, that the methods used to accomplish health education are less clear. The manner in which a person chooses to conduct health education can be demonstrated to be a direct reflection of that person's philosophy of health education. With that in mind, have any predominant philosophies of health education emerged? If so, what are they?

Welle, Russell, and Kittleson (1995) conducted a study to determine the philosophies favored by health educators. As part of the background for their study, they conducted a literature review and identified five dominant philosophies of health education that have emerged during the last 50–60 years. The philosophies identified were behavior change, cognitive-based, decision-making, freeing/functioning, and social change:

1. The **behavior change philosophy** involves a health educator using behavioral contracts, goal setting, and self-monitoring to try to foster a modification in an unhealthy habit in an individual with whom he is working. The nature of this approach allows for the establishment of easily measurable objectives, thus enhancing the ability to evaluate outcomes. (Example: setting up a contract to increase the number of hours of study each week)

2. A health educator who uses a **cognitive-based philosophy** focuses on the acquisition of content and factual information. The goal is to increase the knowledge of the individuals or groups so that they are better armed to make decisions about their health. (Example: simply posting statistics about the number of people killed or injured in automobile accidents who were not wearing seat belts)

3. In using the **decision-making philosophy,** a health educator presents simulated problems, case studies, or scenarios to students or clients. Each problem, case, or scenario requires decisions to be made in seeking a "best approach or answer." By creating and analyzing potential solutions, the students develop skills needed to address many health-related decisions they might face. An advantage of this approach is the emphasis on critical thinking and lifelong learning. (Example: using a variety of case study examples of the Atkin's Diet to see competing perspectives of effectiveness)

4. The **freeing/functioning philosophy** was proposed by Greenberg (1978) as a reaction to traditional approaches of health education that he felt ran the risk of blaming victims for practicing health behaviors that were often either out of their control or not seen as in their best interests. The health educator who uses this philosophical approach has the ultimate goal of freeing people to make the best health decisions possible based on their needs and interests—not necessarily the interests of society. Some health educators classify this as a subset of the decision-making philosophy discussed above. (Example: lessons on the responsible use of alcohol)

5. The **social change philosophy** emphasizes the role of health education in creating social, economic, and political change that benefits the health of individuals and groups. Health educators espousing this philosophy are often at the forefront of the adoption of policies or laws that will enhance the health of all. (Example: no smoking allowed in restaurants, or new housing developments with pedestrian-friendly areas such as sidewalks and parks)

The previously listed philosophies of health education are the products of over fifty years of study, experimentation, and dialogue within the profession. The research conducted by Welle, Russell, and Kittleson (1995) alluded to earlier found that the philosophy most preferred by both health education practitioners and academicians was decision making. Both groups listed behavior change as a second choice, and both agreed that their least favorite was cognitive based. The fact that health educators who are employed in the academic setting and those who are employed as practitioners in the field agreed on these choices as predominant philosophies speaks well for the interface between preparation programs and practice.

Another interesting finding from the study occurred when, as a part of the survey, the health educators were given health education vignettes to address or solve. In many cases, the respondents changed the philosophical approach they used depending on the setting (school, community, worksite, medical). The responding health educators had earlier identified a specific health education philosophy they favored. These results indicate that health educators are adaptable and resourceful, and they will use any health education approach that seems appropriate to the situation. The possibility exists that, in practice, health educators use an **eclectic health education philosophy.**

The results are not surprising, because in any list of philosophies there is always the possibility of one philosophy overlapping with another, so in practice not all is as clean as it might seem. Atkinson (1999) calls for the establishment of a unified, multidimensional philosophy. Perhaps a multidimensional philosophy already exists under the rubric of an eclectic philosophy. The next section will explore how adoption of any or all of these philosophies might impact the way a person practices health education.

Impacting the Delivery of Health Education

This section will use scenarios to help focus on the methods health educators might use, depending on their philosophical stance. The decision to use any philosophy involves understanding and accepting the foundation that helped create the philosophy in the first place. To this end, Welle, Russell, and Kittleson (1995) state,

> Health educators must remember that every single educational choice carries with it a philosophical principle or belief. Educational choices carry important philosophical assumptions about the purpose of health education, the teacher, and also the learner. Thus, health educators should take the time necessary for individual philosophical inquiry, in order to be able to clearly articulate what principles guide them professionally. . . . Different settings may produce the need for different philosophies. Every health educator should be aware of which elements of their individual philosophies they are willing to compromise. (p. 331)

At the outset, it is important to remember that one of the overriding goals of any health education intervention is the betterment of health for the person or the group involved. All of the philosophies have that goal. They differ in how to approach that objective.

Consider the case of Amarosa, a forty-year-old mother of two, who smokes, does not exercise regularly, and has a family history of heart disease. Amarosa is enrolled in a required health education course at a local university. She is going back to school to become an elementary school teacher. Because a health appraisal is a required part of the class, she has come in to visit the health education office. Three health educators (Felipe, Carla, and Li Ming) are employed in the center. Each one has a different philosophy of health education. How will their approaches differ? Here is a possible intervention scenario.

Felipe has adopted the philosophy of behavior change. As a proponent of this approach, he believes that all people are capable of adapting their health behavior if they can be shown the steps to success. He would use a behavior change contract method to get Amarosa to try to eliminate one or two of her negative health behaviors. As a part of this process, some preliminary analysis would be done in an attempt to identify the triggers that cause her to practice the negative health behaviors. He would help her identify short-term and long-term goals. Together they would establish objectives to reach those goals, and strategies to reach the objectives. He would also try to ensure that she receives some appropriate reward for every objective and goal she accomplishes.

Carla, on the other hand, is an advocate of the health education philosophy known as decision making. This means that she believes in equipping her clients with problem-solving and coping skills, so that they make the best possible health choices. Initially, she might sit down with Amarosa and hypothesize some situations that would necessitate Amarosa thinking through the rationale behind the negative health behaviors she practices. Carla also would most likely try to get Amarosa to see that some of her behaviors affect more people than just herself. The goals are to get Amarosa to see that some of her health behaviors need to be changed and to help her identify the reasons that changing them would make her life better.

Finally, Li Ming advocates a freeing/functioning philosophy of health education. She feels that, too often, health educators fail to find out the needs and desires of the client. They simply "barge in" and either overtly or covertly blame the client for any negative health behaviors. Li Ming would advocate change only if the behavior were infringing on the rights of others. In the beginning, Li Ming would confer with Amarosa and find out "how her life was going." She would ask Amarosa to identify any behaviors she wanted to change, making certain that Amarosa had all of the information necessary to make an informed decision. Although Li Ming might believe that Amarosa should stop smoking and start exercising, she would help Amarosa change only those behaviors Amarosa wanted to change.

One sidelight needs to be mentioned at this time. The fact that Amarosa was required to take a health education course in her teacher preparation program and that the instructor required a health assessment illustrates at a microlevel the social change philosophy at work. If health were not a state requirement (legislation) in the first place, she might not have considered changing any of her negative health behaviors.

Amarosa's situation demonstrates a point made earlier—in practice, there often is a natural mixing of some of the philosophies. For example, all of the approaches mentioned used portions of the cognitive-based health education philosophy. To reiterate, this philosophy is based on the premise that persons need to be provided with the most current information that impacts their health behaviors, and the acquisition of that information should create a dissonance and cause change.

The fifth philosophy, social change, is probably not as well suited to addressing the health behaviors of individuals one on one. Proponents stress changes in social, economic, and political arenas to impact the health of populations. Of course, populations are made up of individuals, so changing the environment of an inner-city neighborhood to be healthier (for example, creating jobs, assuring adequate and safe housing and safe schools, providing health care coverage for all) ultimately impacts the health of people at the individual level as well.

SUMMARY

The term *philosophy* means a statement summarizing the attitudes, principles, beliefs, and concepts held by an individual or a group. Forming both a personal and an occupational philosophy requires reflection and the ability to identify those factors, principles, ideals, and influences that help shape your reality. The decision to use any philosophy involves understanding and accepting the foundation that helped create the philosophy in the first place. A sound philosophical foundation serves as a guidepost for many of the major decisions in life.

The five predominant philosophies of health education that were identified in the chapter are behavior change, cognitive based, decision making, freeing/functioning, and social change. Health educators might disagree on which philosophy works best. They might even use an eclectic or multidimensional philosophical approach, depending on the setting or situation. However, it is important to remember that one of the overriding goals of any health education intervention is the betterment of health for the person or group involved. All of the philosophies have that goal. They simply differ in how to reach it.

REVIEW QUESTIONS

1. Define each of the following and explain their relationship to one another.
   - Philosophy
   - Humanism
   - Wellness
   - Holistic
   - Symmetry
2. Why is it important to have a personal philosophy about life?
3. Compare and contrast the value of having a personal life philosophy and an occupational life philosophy that are similar.
4. Define and explain the differences between:
   - Behavior change philosophy
   - Cognitive-based philosophy
   - Decision-making philosophy
   - Freeing/functioning philosophy
   - Social change philosophy
   - Eclectic health education philosophy
5. Explain how a person might use each of the five health education philosophies to address a societal problem that can be addressed by health education (e.g., smoking, seat belt use, air pollution).

CRITICAL THINKING QUESTIONS

1. Of the five basic health education philosophies identified by Welle, Russell, and Kittleson (1995), why do you think that the least favorite among health educators was the cognitive philosophy? Why do you think decision making was viewed as most popular?
2. What is the purpose of health education? How might the formulation of a purpose statement be reflected in your philosophy of health education?
3. You have been hired by a local pharmacy to provide health education services to customers and employees. Shortly after you begin work, however, you discover that much of your job is marketing nutritional supplements and nonpharmaceutical health-related services provided by the pharmacy and not the health education you had envisioned. How might this supposed conflict of interest have been avoided?
4. Assume you are a proponent of the social change health education philosophy. What advantage does this philosophy have for the health educator that might be a disadvantage for the consumer of health services and education? Defend your answer.

5. A recent article by Bruess (2003) in the *American Journal of Health Education* discusses the notion of "role modeling" for health educators. The reference for the article can be found at the end of this chapter. After reading the article, summarize Dr. Bruess's main points, and use your answer to determine which philosophical viewpoint(s) a health educator must hold to feel as Dr. Bruess does on the issue of role modeling. Finally, assess how you feel about the issue. Do you agree or disagree with him? Provide a rationale for your answer.

Activities

1. Reread the story of the Mongolian farmer. How would you describe the farmer's philosophy of life? What values or ideals of the farmer helped form the basis of his philosophy? What life experiences do you think he had that helped shape his philosophy?

2. After reexamining the philosophies of health, write a paragraph that could be used to explain your philosophy of health to a friend or colleague.

3. Interview a school or community health educator in your city. Ask what his or her philosophy of health education is. Then ask about the influences that helped the educator form his or her philosophy. Summarize the interview in a one-page paper.

4. Use any three of the five philosophical approaches to health education discussed in the chapter and address the following situation:

   In the past week in your community, two teenagers have been killed in separate incidents while riding bicycles. In neither case was the person wearing a helmet. A local citizens group has asked you and two of your health education colleagues to attend a meeting concerning what to do about this issue.

Weblinks

1. **http://perth.uwlax.edu/academicprograms/html/healthed.htm**

   Health Education Program in the Department of Health, Physical Education, and Recreation at the University of Wisconsin, La Crosse

   This site provides a fine example of a philosophy of health education and the supporting principles or values that serve as foundations for that philosophy.

2. **http://the.dublinschools.net/curriculum/health%20course%20of%20study /health%20GCOS.pdf**

   School District of Dublin, Ohio

   This Web site of their health course lists the district's mission statement and statement of philosophy of health education and shows how they link to the health education curriculum.

3. **http://homepages.wmich.edu/~cummings/Philosophy_State.html**

   Western Michigan University (College of Education)

   This site gives some guidance in how to proceed in writing a philosophy statement. Although the site is designed for students writing a "philosophy of education" statement, the approach is sound and relevant and augments the discussion in this chapter.

CASE STUDY

You are entering the final semester of the senior year of study with a major in community health education. In anticipation of program completion and graduation, you are beginning to look for possible job openings. After perusing the position announcements in professional journals, visiting the state job availability center, and viewing some health-related job listing Web sites, you find three positions that are of interest to you.

After authoring a resume and filling out the requisite application forms, you wait for word as to whether or not you are chosen for an interview. Two weeks later you receive letters from the managers of two of the jobs, requesting that you call and set up an appointment for an interview. Both letters outline possible questions that you might be asked. You notice that one of the questions listed involves statements relating to personal and professional philosophy. The inclusion of philosophy to the list of question possibilities surprises you because you really haven't thought much about philosophy since your introductory course in health education nearly four years ago.

Digging out your old notes, you begin to formulate both personal and professional philosophy statements. You begin wondering if it is necessary to have a congruence between the personal and professional philosophies. In addition, is it important that the business philosophy or mission statements of the places to which you are applying match your personal or professional philosophy? What concerns would you have if your employer's management had a vastly different philosophy from yours? Just what are the considerations inherent in creating a philosophy? Create an outline of the major points of your philosophy and an outline of what you would like to see in the mission statement or philosophy of a business where you were employed. Compare and contrast these outlines.

REFERENCES

Atkinson, D. (1999). United direction 2000? *Journal of School Health, 69*(8), 300.

Bedworth, D. A., & Bedworth, A. E. (1992). *The profession and practice of health education.* Dubuque, IA: Wm. C. Brown.

Bensley, L. B. (1993). This I believe: A philosophy of health education. *The Eta Sigma Gamma Monograph Series, 11*(2),1–7.

Bruess, C. E. (2003). The importance of health educators as role models. *American Journal of Health Education, 34*(4), 237–239.

Butler, J. T. (1997). *The principles and practices of health education and health promotion.* Englewood, CO: Morton.

Donatelle, R. J. (2005). *Health: The basics* (6th ed.). San Francisco: Benjamin Cummings.

Drolet, J. C. (1993). Pondering a professional philosophy. *The Eta Sigma Gamma Monograph Series, 11*(2), 26–38.

Edlin, G., & Golanty, E. (2004). *Health and wellness* (8th ed.). Sudbury, MA: Jones and Bartlett.

Fetro, J. S. (1993). Health education: A smorgasbord of life. *The Eta Sigma Gamma Monograph Series, 11*(2), 56–66.

Greenberg, J. S. (1978). Health education as freeing. *Health Education, 9*(2), 20–21.

Greenberg, J. S. (1992). *Health education: Learner centered instructional strategies* (2nd ed.). Dubuque, IA: William C. Brown.

Hales, D. (2004). *An invitation to health* (3rd ed). Belmont, CA: Thomson-Wadsworth.

Hamburg, M. V. (1993). Would I do it all over! *The Eta Sigma Gamma Monograph Series, 11*(2), 67–74.

Hills, M. D., & Lindsey, E. (1994). Health promotion: A viable curriculum framework for nursing education. *Nursing Outlook, 42*(4), 158–162.

Oberteufer, D. (1953). Philosophy and principles of school health education. *The Journal of School Health, 23*(4), 103–109.

O'Rourke, T. (1989). Reflections on the directions in health education: Implications for policy and practice. *Health Education, 28*(6), 4–14.

Pigg, R. M. (1993). Three essential questions in defining a personal philosophy. *The Eta Sigma Gamma Monograph Series, 11*(2), 94–101.

Rash, J. K. (1985). Philosophical bases for health education. *Health Education, 16*(3), 48–49.

Rosenstock, I. M. (1960). *Decision-making by individuals.* Paper presented at the Annual Meeting of the Society for Public Health Educators, October 29, San Francisco, CA.

Seffrin, J. R. (1993). Health education and the pursuit of personal freedom. *The Eta Sigma Gamma Monograph Series, 11*(2), 109–118.

Shirreffs, J. (Spring, 1976). A philosophical approach to health education. *The Eta Sigma Gamman,* 21–23.

Tamayose, T. S. et al. (2004). Important factors when choosing a career in public health. *Californian Journal of Health Promotion 2(1),* 65–73.

Thomas, S. B. (1984). The holistic philosophy and perspective of selected health educators. *Health Education, 15*(1), 15–20.

Welle, H. M., Russell, R. D., & Kittleson, M. J. (1995). Philosophical trends in health education: Implications for the 21st century. *Journal of Health Education, 26*(6), 326–333.

CHAPTER 4

Theoretical Foundations

Chapter Objectives

After reading this chapter and answering the questions at the end, you should be able to:

1. Define and explain the difference among *theory, concept, construct, variable,* and *model.*

2. Explain the importance of theory to health education and promotion.

3. Distinguish between theories/models of implementation (planning models) and change process theories.

4. Identify the planning models and their components used in health education/health promotion and briefly explain each:

   a. PRECEDE-PROCEED

   b. Multilevel Approach To Community Health (MATCH)

   c. CDCynergy

   d. Social Marketing Assessment and Response Tool (SMART)

   e. Mobilizing for Action through Planning and Partnerships (MAPP)

   f. Generalized Model for Program Planning (GMPP)

5. Identify the theories and models focusing on behavior (change process theories) and their components used in health education/promotion and briefly explain each:

   a. health belief model

   b theory of planned behavior

   c. transtheoretical model

   d. precaution adoption process model

   e. social cognitive theory

   f. theory of diffusion

6. Explain the difference between continuum theories and stage theories.

Key Terms

action stage

administrative and policy
  assessment

attitude toward the behavior

behavioral assessment

behavioral capability

CDCynergy

change process theories

concepts

construct

contemplation stage

continuum theory

cue to action

early adopters

early majority

ecological perspective

educational and ecological
  assessment

emotional-coping response

enabling factor

environmental assessment

epidemiological assessment

expectancies

expectations

impact evaluation

implementation

innovators

laggards

late majority

likelihood of taking action

locus of control

maintenance stage

MAPP

MATCH

model

outcome evaluation

perceived barriers

perceived behavioral control

perceived benefits

perceived
  seriousness/severity

perceived susceptibility

perceived threat

PRECEDE-PROCEED

precontemplation stage

predisposing factor

preparation stage

process evaluation

reciprocal determinism

reduction of threat

reinforcement

reinforcing factor

self-control (self-regulation)

self-efficacy

SMART

social assessment

social marketing

stage theories

subjective norm

termination

theories/models of
  implementation

theory

variable

As noted in Chapter 1, health education/health promotion is a multidisciplinary field of practice that has evolved from the theory and practice of a number of other biological, behavioral, sociological, and health science disciplines. As the profession has grown, the theoretical base on which it was formed has become more apparent. In this chapter, we will introduce the definitions of *theory, concept, construct, variable,* and *model;* explain why it is important to use theory in health education/promotion; provide an overview of the different theories and models that will be used in your future work; and leave you with a word of caution about the application of theories and models.

Definitions

In order to be able to understand the theoretical foundations presented in this chapter, it is important to be familiar with some key related words. Let us begin with theory. One of the most frequently quoted definitions of **theory** is one in which Glanz, Lewis, and Rimer (2002) modified an earlier definition written by Kerlinger (1986). It states, "A *theory* is a set of interrelated concepts, definitions, and propositions that presents a *systematic* view of events or situations by specifying relations among variables in order to *explain* and *predict* the events of the situations" (p. 25). Stated a little differently, "a theory is a systematic arrangement of fundamental principles that provide a basis for explaining certain happenings of life" (McKenzie, Neiger, & Smeltzer, 2005, p. 144). Thus, "the role of theory is to untangle and simplify for human comprehension the complexities of nature" (Green et al., 1994, p. 398). As applied to the profession of health education, a theory is a general explanation of why people act or do not act to maintain and/or promote the health of themselves, their families, organizations, and communities. The primary elements of theories are known as **concepts** (Glanz et al., 2002). When a concept has been developed, created, or adopted for use with a specific theory, it is referred to as a **construct** (Kerlinger, 1986). In other words, constructs are synthesized thoughts or key concepts of specific theories. The operational (practical use) form of a construct is known as a **variable.** Variables "specify how a construct is to be measured in a specific situation" (Glanz et al., 2002, p. 27).

"A **model** is a subclass of a theory" (McKenzie et al., 2005, p. 144). "Models draw on a number of theories to help people understand a specific problem in a particular setting or context" (Glanz et al., 2002, p. 27). Models provide health educators with a framework on which to create plans for programs. Unlike theories, models do "not attempt to explain the processes underlying learning, but only to represent them" (Chaplin & Krawiec, 1979, p. 68).

Now consider how these terms are used in practical application. A personal belief is a *concept* that has been shown to relate to various health behaviors. Using a *theory* that includes the concept of personal beliefs helps explain why people fear being trapped in a burning vehicle if they use their safety belts. This personal belief of fear acts as a perceived barrier to safety belt use. Perceived barrier is a part of a specific theory and is referred to here as a *construct.* If a health educator develops a program around a theory to help people overcome this barrier and wear their safety belts, then safety belt use is the *variable* being studied. The health educator realizes that this theory, which emphasizes personal beliefs, will not explain all the reasons that people do not wear safety belts. Thus, other theories, which emphasize other concepts (i.e., knowledge, environment, incentives, comfort, convenience, etc.) need to be considered.

Eventually, all of these theories may be combined into a *model* that will explain, at least in part, why people wear safety belts. If a model were a perfect model, it would predict with 100 percent accuracy who would wear safety belts. Unfortunately, behavior is very complex and there are no perfect models in health education. It is therefore important for health educators to keep revising their models to improve their understanding of health behavior.

The Importance of Using Theory in Health Education/Promotion

Theory is important to the profession because it helps guide the practice of health educators. It can help during the various stages of planning, implementing, and evaluating a program (Glanz & Rimer, 1995). "Behavioral and social science theory provides a platform for understanding why people engage in health-risk or health-compromising behavior and why (as well as how) they adopt health-protective behavior" (Crosby, Kegler, & DiClemente, 2002, p. 1). Using the most appropriate theory and practice strategies for a given situation greatly enhances the chances for effective health education/promotion practice (Glanz et al., 2002). Though not all health education/health promotion programs are successful, those that are based on sound theory are more likely to succeed than those that are not.

An Overview of the Theories and Models Used in Health Education/Promotion

The remaining portions of this chapter present many of the theories and models that are often used in the discipline of health education/promotion. There are a number of ways that the theories and models could be organized and presented in this chapter. We will present the theories and models in two groups. The first are those used in planning, implementing, and evaluating health education/promotion programs. Some have referred to these as the **theories/models of implementation.** To lessen the confusion of terminology, we will refer to them as planning models. The second group includes the theories and models that focus on behavior change. McLeroy and colleagues (1992) have referred to these theories as change process theories. **Change process theories** "specify the relationships among causal processes operating both within and across levels of analysis" (McLeroy et al., 1992, p. 3). In other words, change process theories help explain, through their constructs, how change takes place. For example, the change of getting a nonexerciser to exercise can be explained in part by change process theories.

Planning Models (Theories/Models of Implementation)

Good health promotion programs are not created by chance. They are the result of much hard work and are organized around a well-thought-out and well-conceived model. Models for planning provide health educators with a frame on which to develop a plan. A number of models have been developed over the years. Although many of the models have common elements, those elements may have different labels. In fact, "the underlying principles that guide the development of the various models are similar; however, there are important differences in sequence, emphasis, and the conceptualization of the major components that make certain models more appealing than others to individual practitioners" (Simons-Morton, Greene, & Gottlieb, 1995, pp. 126–127).

There is not space in this textbook to present all of the planning models that have been used for health education/promotion programs. We have selected six models that have been used successfully and represent a wide range of planning approaches. Box 4.1 lists other planning models that may be just as good from a theoretical perspective but are not currently used as much as the six we present. Please note that the presentation of the models here is just to familiarize you with the names and components of the major planning models. It is assumed that you will obtain a working knowledge of the models in your upper-level health education classses. For more detailed explanations of the models, see the original publications of the models.

> ### Box 4.1 Other Planning Models
>
> - Comprehensive Health Education Model, Sullivan (1973)
> - Model for Health Education Planning, Ross & Mico (1980)
> - Model for Health Education Planning and Resource Development, Bates & Winder (1984)
> - Planned Approach To Community Health (PATCH), CDC (no date)
> - Generic Health/Fitness Delivery System, Patton et al. (1986)
>
> - Assessment Protocol for Excellence in Public Health (APEX/PH), NACHO (1991)
> - Health Plan-It, CDC (2000)
> - The Health Communication Model, NCI (2002)
> - The Planning, Program Development, and Evaluation Model, Timmreck (2003)

PRECEDE-PROCEED.   Currently, the best known and most often used theory of implementation is the **PRECEDE-PROCEED** model. "PRECEDE is an acronym for *p*redisposing, *r*einforcing, and *e*nabling *c*onstructs in *e*ducational/*e*cological *d*iagnosis and *e*valuation" (Green & Kreuter, 1999, p. 34). "PROCEED stands for *p*olicy, *r*egulatory, and *o*rganizational *c*onstructs in *e*ducational and *e*nvironmental *d*evelopment" (Green & Kreuter, 1999, p. 34). The PRECEDE-PROCEED model was developed over a period of fifteen to twenty years, with the PRECEDE framework being conceived in the early 1970s (Green, 1974) and evolving into a planning model in the late 1970s (Green, 1975, 1976; Green, Levine, & Deeds, 1975; Green et al., 1978; Green et al., 1980). The PROCEED portion was developed in the early to mid-1980s (Green, 1979, 1980, 1981a, 1981b, 1982, 1983a, 1983b, 1984a, 1984b, 1984c, 1984d, 1986a, 1986b, 1986c, 1986d, 1986e, 1987a, 1987b; Green & Allen, 1980; Green & McAlister, 1984; Green, Mullen, & Friedman, 1986; Green, Wilson, & Lovato, 1986; Green, Wilson, & Bauer, 1983). It "is essentially an elaboration and extension of the administrative diagnosis step of PRECEDE, which was the final and least developed link in the PRECEDE framework" (Green & Kreuter, 1991, p. 25).

As is noted in Figure 4.1, PRECEDE-PROCEED is comprised of nine phases. The first five phases, which make up the PRECEDE portion of the model, deal with assessment. The last four phases, the PROCEED portion, are implementation and evaluation (process, impact, and outcome) phases, with emphasis on the latter to improve the former (Glanz & Rimer, 1995). At first glance, the PRECEDE-PROCEED model appears overly complicated, but on close examination you will find that there is a very logical sequence to the nine phases that outlines the health promotion planning process. "The underlying approach of this model is to begin by identifying the desired outcome, to determine what causes it, and finally to design an intervention aimed at reaching the desired outcome. In other words, PRECEDE-PROCEED begins with the final consequences and works backwards to the causes" (McKenzie et al., 2005, p. 18). Table 4.1 provides an overview of the nine phases of the model.

PRECEDE

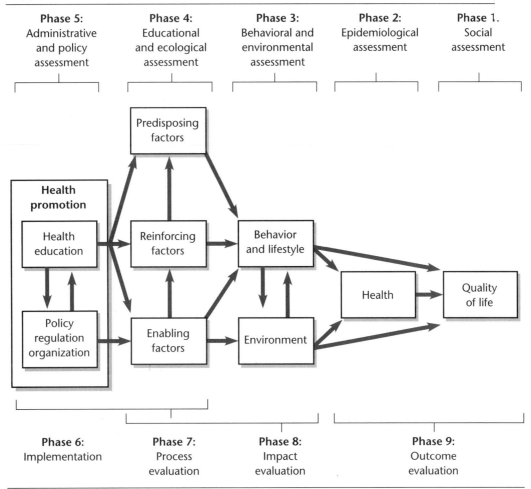

Figure 4.1   PRECEDE-PROCEED Model for Health Promotion, Planning, and Evaluation

Source: Adapted from Green, L. W., and M. W. Kreuter. 1999. *Health promotion planning: An educational and ecological approach* (3rd ed.). San Francisco: Mayfield.

MATCH.   **MATCH** is an acronym for Multilevel Approach To Community Health. This planning model (see Figure 4.2 on page 103) was developed in the late 1980s (Simons-Morton, Simons-Morton, Parcel, & Bunker, 1988). Like the PRECEDE-PROCEED model, MATCH has also been used in a variety of settings, including in the development of several intervention handbooks created by the Centers for Disease Control and Prevention (Simons-Morton et al., 1995). MATCH is an ecological planning perspective that recognizes that intervention activities can and should be aimed at a variety of objectives and individuals (B. Simons-Morton, personal communication, October 10, 1999). This is

Table 4.1   The Nine Phases of the PRECEDE-PROCEED Model

Phase 1.	**Social assessment** is "the assessment in both objective and subjective terms of high-priority problems or aspirations for the common good, defined for a population by economic and social indicators and by individuals in terms of their quality of life."
Phase 2.	**Epidemiological assessment** is "the delineation of the extent, distribution, and causes of a health problem in a defined population."
Phase 3.	**Behavioral assessment** is the "delineation of the specific health-related actions that will most likely cause a health outcome," and **environmental assessment** is "a systematic assessment of factors in the social and physical environment that interact with behavior to produce health effects or quality-of-life outcomes. Also referred to as **ecological assessment.**"
Phase 4.	**Educational assessment** is "the delineation of factors that predispose, enable, and reinforce a specific behavior or that through behavior affect environmental changes," and **ecological assessment** (see environmental assessment, above). **Predisposing factor** is "any characteristic of a person or population that motivates behavior prior to the occurrence of the behavior"; **enabling factor** is "any characteristic of the environment that facilitates action and any skill or resource required to attain a specific behavior"; **reinforcing factor** is "any reward or punishment following or anticipated as a consequence of a behavior, serving to strengthen the motivation for or against the behavior."
Phase 5.	**Administrative and policy assessment** is "an analysis of the policies, resources, and circumstances prevailing in an organization to facilitate or hinder the development of the health promotion program."
Phase 6.	**Implementation** is "the act of converting program objectives into actions through policy changes, regulation, and organization."
Phase 7.	**Process evaluation** is "the assessment of policies, materials, personnel, performance, quality of practice or services, and other inputs and implementation experiences."
Phase 8.	**Impact evaluation** is "the assessment of program effects on intermediate objectives including changes in predisposing, enabling, and reinforcing factors, as well as behavioral and environmental changes."
Phase 9.	**Outcome evaluation** is an "assessment of the effects of a program on its ultimate objectives, including changes in health and social benefits or quality of life."

Source: Green, L. W., and M. W. Kreuter. 1999: pp. 503–509. *Health promotion planning: An educational and ecological approach* (3rd ed.). Mountain View: Mayfield.

represented in Figure 4.2 by the various levels of influence. The MATCH framework is recognized for emphasizing program implementation (Simons-Morton et al., 1995). "MATCH is designed to be applied when behavioral and environmental risk and protective factors for disease or injury are generally known and when general priorities for action have been determined, thus providing a convenient way to turn the corner from needs assessment and priority setting to the development of effective programs" (Simons-Morton et al., 1995, p. 155).

Table 4.2 on page 104 presents the phases and steps of MATCH along with an explanation of each.

CDCynergy.   **CDCynergy**, or **Cynergy** for short, is a health communication planning model developed by the Office of Communication at the Centers for Disease Control and Prevention (CDC) in 1997 and first issued in July 1998 (Parvanta & Freimuth, 2000). Cynergy was developed primarily for the public health

Box 4.2 *Practitioner's Perspective: Planning Models*

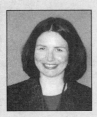

NAME: Maggie Mann

MAJOR: Community Health Education

DEGREE/INSTITUTION: B.S., University of Nebraska, Lincoln, 1992

CURRENT POSITION/TITLE: Health Promotion Director

EMPLOYER: Southeastern District Health Department, Pocatello, ID

How I obtained my job: I had just begun participating in a community coalition on adolescent pregnancy prevention, which was facilitated by the Southeastern District Health Department (SDHD). One of the members, an employee of SDHD, told me about an opening for the position I currently hold. Though SDHD is not a state of Idaho agency, it does utilize some of the systems operated by the state, such as the Idaho Personnel Commission. For this reason, all SDHD employees must test through a "register" process. The register is only open for testing for brief periods during the year, usually when a position opens up. I took the test, which consisted of a series of questions related to my education, experience, and knowledge base. The test is then submitted to the Idaho Personnel Commission, which scores each test, then routes a list of eligible candidates back to the requesting agency. After being placed on the register, I had an opportunity to interview with the SDHD Director. I was offered the position and accepted.

Using planning models in health education: Planning models, such as the stages of change model or the health belief model, are used on a regular basis to assess the need for programs, and to strategize and make decisions as to where programs are headed (e.g., defining goals and objectives). In addition, some models are used as a "check and balance" for what programs are actually accomplishing (e.g., the logic model).

Examples of utilizing planning models in the practice setting: Virtually all health promotion programs of the public health districts in Idaho now begin with the use of a model to help identify program goals, program outcomes for the short and long term, and methods to assess whether the outcomes have been attained. This process is similar to phases of the PRECEDE-PROCEED model. Planning in this manner is helpful in that it forces us to identify what our ultimate outcome should be from the very start of program planning. We then work backward to identify what strategies can help us to achieve that outcome, what resources are needed, and how to evaluate progress.

A different example would be use of the stages of change model with tobacco cessation clients. We use this model to assess readiness to quit, and we then tailor interventions and messages to match the stage that corresponds to the place where the clients are.

Recommendations for those preparing to be health educators: In public health, communicating the value and critical nature of what we do on a daily basis has been problematic; this is true at national, state, and local levels. Two primary reasons contribute to this difficulty. First, when public health is doing its job, it's largely invisible and difficult for people to recognize. Second, many public health initiatives are grounded in primary prevention, and it is close to

(Box 4.2 continues)

(Box 4.2 *continued*)

impossible to gauge effectiveness of primary prevention in the short term. Therefore, a significant challenge for public practitioners is the ability to market public health in such a way that decision makers value public health efforts enough to fund initiatives and public health infrastructure. For this reason, I would strongly recommend that health educators pursue a line of coursework that includes classes in marketing and business strategy. An important part of marketing is media advocacy. I would also suggest that health educators and health promotion specialists who are interested in working in the public health arena learn as much as they can about this complex venue.

Finally, because of limited resources, public health practitioners must forge strong collaborative partnerships with agencies and organizations that have not traditionally been public health partners. For this reason, communication skills, especially negotiation and group facilitation, are essential.

professionals at CDC who have responsibilities for health communication. However, because of widespread interest in the model, CDC made it available to other health professionals who found the model useful in a variety of health promotion settings. Although Cynergy is considered to be in the public domain (meaning restrictions are not placed on general use or copying), CDC currently requires training before releasing a copy of the CD-ROM. At the time this textbook was being prepared there were plans to make the next version of Cynergy Web based.

The basic edition of Cynergy presents a general methodology for health communication planning, a step-by-step guide, a reference library, and links to templates that allow tailored plans to be created (CDC, 2003). Cynergy uses six phases involving multiple steps to help planners acquire a thorough understanding of a health problem and whom it affects; explore a wide range of possible intervention strategies for influencing the problem; systematically select the intervention strategies that show the most promise; understand the role communication can play in planning, implementing, and evaluating selected strategies; and develop a comprehensive communication plan (2003). Table 4.3 on page 105 displays the six sequential yet interrelated phases, which are designed to build upon the previous phases and prepare program planners for subsequent phases. Completion of these phases will lead to a strategic communication plan that is both science and audience based.

In addition to the basic edition of Cynergy, CDC and its partners have produced content-specific editions of Cynergy to meet the specific needs of health educators addressing various health problems (McKenzie et al., 2005). There are content-specific editions for: American Indian/Alaska Native Diabetes, Cardiovascular Disease, Diabetes, Emergency Risk Communication, Immunizations, Micronutrients, Social Marketing, STD Prevention, and Tobacco Prevention and Control. Several other content-specific editions were being developed at the time this book was written.

(*Text continues on page 106*)

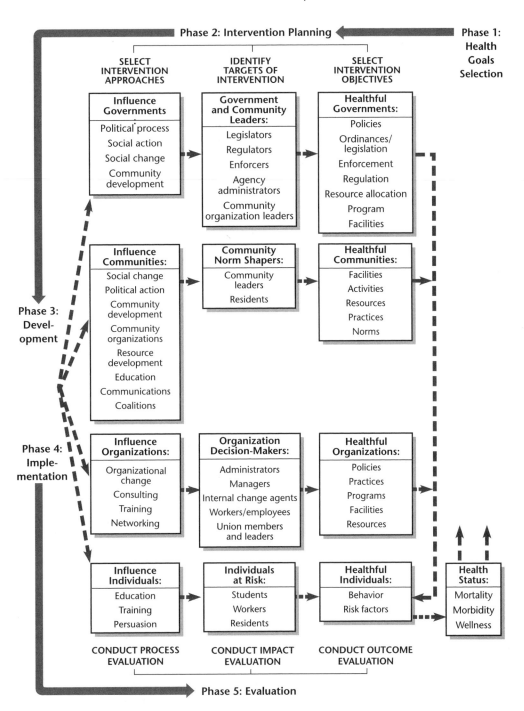

Figure 4.2   MATCH: Multilevel Approach to Community Health

Source: From Simons-Morton, B. G., W. H. Greene, and N. H. Gottlieb. 1995. *Introduction to health education and health promotion* (2nd ed.). Long Grove, IL: Waveland Press, Inc. All rights reserved. Reprinted by permission of Waveland Press, Inc.

Table 4.2   MATCH Phases and Steps

PHASE I: GOALS SELECTION

Step 1: Select health status goals
Step 2: Select high-priority population(s)
Step 3: Identify health behavior goals
Step 4: Identify environmental factor goals

Explanation of Phase I: Planners select health status goals based upon several different factors including the prevalence of the health problem, the relative importance of the health problem, the changeability of the problem, and other considerations unique to the program. Also, planners need to select the high-priority populations, identify the health behaviors most associated with the health status goals in order to create health behavior goals, and identify the environmental factors such as access, availability of resources, enabling practices, and barriers so that environmental goals can be created.

PHASE II: INTERVENTION PLANNING

Step 1: Identify the targets of the intervention
Step 2: Select intervention objectives
Step 3: Identify mediators of the intervention objectives
Step 4: Select intervention approaches

Explanation of Phase II: This phase begins with the matching of objectives with the intervention targets and intervention actions. Targets of the intervention actions are those individuals that exert influence or control over the personal or environmental conditions that are related to the target health and behavior goals. After identifying the TIAs, they are matched with the health behavioral and environmental factors identified in Phase I. Once this match is made, planners select an intervention action(s) to be used. Intervention actions commonly used by health educators include teaching, training, counseling, policy advocacy, consulting, community organization, social marketing, and social action.

PHASE III: PROGRAM DEVELOPMENT

Step 1: Create program units or components
Step 2: Select or develop curricula and create intervention guides

Step 3: Develop session plans
Step 4: Create or acquire instructional materials, products, and resources

Explanation of Phase III: After the creation of the program components, planners either select from already developed curricula or develop their own guides. This would include the development of individual session or lesson plans, and the acquisition or creation of instructional materials, products, and resources.

PHASE IV: IMPLEMENTATION PREPARATIONS

Step 1: Facilitate adoption, implementation, and maintenance
Step 2: Select and train implementers

Explanation of Phase IV: Planners prepare for implementation and conduct the interventions. To achieve effective implementation planners must (a) develop a specific proposal and advocate for the adoption of change, (b) develop the need, readiness, and environmental supports for change, (c) provide evidence that the intervention works, (d) identify and select change agents and opinion leaders and sell them on the need for change, and (e) establish good working relationships with the decision makers. In addition, depending on who will implement the program, there may be a need to select, train, support, and monitor those who do the implementation.

PHASE V: EVALUATION

Step 1: Conduct process evaluation
Step 2: Measure impact
Step 3: Monitor outcomes

Explanation of Phase V: Planners carry out three different types of evaluation—process (utility, extent, quality, and effects of implementation on immediate learning outcomes), impact (assessing target mediators such as knowledge, attitudes and practices), and outcome (long-term effects of the program, usually health behaviors or environmental factors).

Table 4.3   *CDCynergy Lite* (This is an abridged version of the CDCynergy health communication model.)

PHASE 1: DESCRIBE PROBLEM
- Identify and define health problems that may be addressed by your program interventions.
- Examine and/or conduct necessary research to describe the problems.
- Assess factors and variables that can affect the project's direction, including strengths, weaknesses, opportunities, and threats (SWOT).

PHASE 2: ANALYZE PROBLEM
- List causes of each problem you plan to address.
- Develop goals for each problem.
- Consider strengths, weaknesses, opportunities, threats, and ethics of health 1) engineering, 2) communication/education, 3) policy/enforcement, and 4) community service intervention options.
- Select the types of intervention(s) that should be used to address the problem(s).

PHASE 3: PLAN INTERVENTION
- Decide whether communication is needed as a dominant intervention and/or as support for other intervention(s).
  - If communication is used as a dominant intervention, list possible audiences.
  - If communication is to be used to support Community Services, Engineering, and/or Policy/Enforcement interventions, list possible audiences to be reached in support of each selected intervention.
- Conduct necessary audience research to segment intended audiences.
- Select audience segment(s) and write communication objectives for each audience segment.
- Write a creative brief to provide guidance in selecting appropriate concepts/messages, settings, activities, and materials.

PHASE 4: DEVELOP INTERVENTION
- Develop and test concepts, messages, settings, channel-specific activities, and materials with intended audiences.
- Finalize and briefly summarize a communication implementation plan. The plan should include:
  - Background and justification, including SWOT and ethics analyses
  - Audiences
  - Communication objectives
  - Messages
  - Settings and channels for conveying your messages
  - Activities (including tactics, materials, and other methods)
  - Available partners and resources
  - Tasks and timeline (including persons responsible for each task, date for completion of each task, resources required to deliver each task, and points at which progress will be checked)
  - Internal and external communication plan
  - Budget
- Produce materials for dissemination.

PHASE 5: PLAN EVALUATION
- Determine stakeholder information needs.
  - Decide which types of evaluation (e.g., implementation, reach, effects) are needed to satisfy stakeholder information needs.
  - Identify sources of information and select data collection methods.
  - Formulate an evaluation design that illustrates how methods will be applied to gather credible information.
  - Develop a data analysis and reporting plan.
    - Finalize and briefly summarize an evaluation implementation plan. The plan should include:
    - Stakeholder questions

(Table 4.3 *continues*)

(Table 4.3 *continued*)

- Intervention standards
- Evaluation methods and design
- Data analysis and reporting
- Tasks and timeline (including persons responsible for each task, date for completion of each task, resources required to deliver each task, and points at which progress will be checked)
- Internal and external communication plan
- Budget

PHASE 6: IMPLEMENT PLAN

- Integrate, execute, and manage communication and evaluation plans.
- Document feedback and lessons learned.
- Modify program components based on feedback.
- Disseminate lessons learned and evaluation findings.

Source: Centers for Disease Control and Prevention (CDC), U.S. Department of Health and Human Services (USDHHS). 2003. *CDCynergy 3.0: Your Guide to Effective Health Communication (CD-ROM Version 3.0)*. Atlanta, GA: Author.

SMART. **Social marketing** has been defined as "a process for influencing human behavior on a large scale, using marketing principles for the purpose of societal benefit rather than commercial profit" (Smith, 1999 as cited in Smith, 2000, p. 11). This process offers benefits the audience wants, reduces barriers the audience faces, and uses persuasion to influence intentions to act favorably (Albrecht, 1997). The concept of social marketing is more than thirty years old, but its application to health promotion/education is much more recent (McDermott, 2000). Even though the use of social marketing is relatively new in health promotion/education, several different authors (Andreasen, 1995; Bryant, 1998; Walsh, Rudd, Moeykens, & Moloney, 1993) have presented planning processes, models, or frameworks based upon social marketing. The Social Marketing Assessment and Response Tool (**SMART**) is a social marketing planning framework developed by Neiger (1998). It is presented here because it provides a composite of other social marketing models, and because it has been used from start to finish on multiple occasions in several social marketing interventions (Neiger & Thackeray, 2002). This model also provides an excellent overview of social marketing in general (McKenzie et al., 2005).

SMART is composed of seven phases (see Table 4.4). "Like other social marketing planning frameworks, the central focus of SMART is consumers. The heart of this model, composed of Phases 2 through 4, pertains to acquiring a broad understanding of the consumers who will be the recipients of a program and its interventions. These three phases seek to understand consumers before interventions are even developed or implemented. Social marketing represents an honest attempt to respond directly to consumer feedback" (McKenzie et al., 2005, pp. 36–37).

MAPP. **MAPP** is an acronym for Mobilizing for Action through Planning and Partnerships. It is a relatively new planning model created by the National Association of County and City Health Officials (NACCHO) to assist local public health agencies (LPHAs) at the city or county level with planning. This model blends

Table 4.4   The SMART Model

PHASE 1: PRELIMINARY PLANNING
- Identify a health problem and name it in terms of behavior.
- Develop general goals.
- Outline preliminary plans for evaluation.
- Project program costs

PHASE 2: CONSUMER ANALYSIS
- Segment and identify the priority population.
- Identify formative research methods.
- Identify consumer wants, needs, and preferences.
- Develop preliminary ideas for preferred interventions and communication strategies.

PHASE 3: MARKET ANALYSIS
- Establish and define the market mix (4Ps).
- Assess the market to identify competitors (behaviors, messages, programs, etc.), allies (support systems, resources, etc.), and partners.

PHASE 4: CHANNEL ANALYSIS
- Identify appropriate communication channels.
- Assess options for program distribution. Determine how channels should be used.
- Assess options for program distribution.
- Identify communication roles for program partners.

PHASE 5: DEVELOP INTERVENTIONS, MATERIALS, AND PRETEST
- Develop program interventions and materials using information collected in consumer, market, and channel analyses.
- Interpret the marketing mix into a strategy that represents exchange and societal good.
- Pretest and refine the program.

PHASE 6: IMPLEMENTATION
- Communicate with partners and clarify involvement.
- Activate communication and distribution strategies.
- Document procedures and compare progress to timelines.
- Refine the program.

PHASE 7: EVALUATION
- Assess the degree to which the priority population is receiving the program.
- Assess the immediate impact on the priority population and refine the program as necessary.
- Ensure that program delivery is consistent with established protocol.
- Analyze changes in the priority population.

Source: Adapted from Walsh, R. E., et al., 1993. Social marketing for public health. *Health Affairs 12*: 104–119, by Neiger, B. L. (1998). *Social marketing: Making public health sense.* Paper presented at the annual meeting of the Utah Public Health Association, Provo, UT.

many of the strengths of the four planning models already presented in this chapter. The MAPP approach is designed to improve health and quality of life by mobilizing partnerships and taking strategic action (NACCHO, 2001).

MAPP is comprised of multiple steps within six phases (see Figure 4.3). In the first phase of MAPP, Organizing for Success and Partnership Development, planners assess whether or not the MAPP process is timely, appropriate, and even possible. This involves assessing resources including funding, personnel, and general interest of

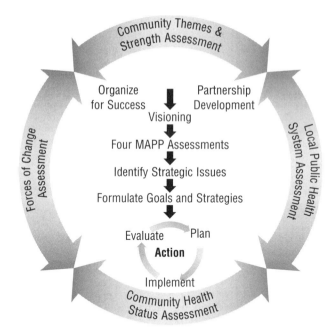

Figure 4.3   Mobilizing for Action through Planning and Partnerships (MAPP) Model

Source: National Association of County and City Health Officials (NACCHO). (2000). *Mobilizing for action through planning and partnerships (MAPP).* Retrieved February 19, 2004, from http://mapp.naccho.org/view_model.asp?image+MAPP+model

community members. If resources are not in place, the process is delayed. If resources are sufficient, the following work groups are created: (1) a core support team, which prepares most, if not all, of the material needed for the process; (2) the MAPP Committee, composed of key sponsors from the community who provide legitimacy and resources, and stakeholders who guide and oversee the process; and (3) the community itself, which provides input, representation, and decision making.

In Phase 2, Visioning, the community is guided through a process that results in a shared vision—what the ideal future looks like—and common values—principles and beliefs that will guide the remainder of the planning process (NACCHO, 2001). This phase is usually handled by a facilitator and involves anywhere from 50–100 participants, including the advisory committee, the MAPP committee, and key community leaders.

The strength and defining characteristic of MAPP are found in Phase 3, the Four MAPP Assessments. "The four assessments include: (1) the community themes and strengths assessment (community or consumer opinion); (2) the local public health assessment (general capacity of the local health department); (3) the community health status assessment (measurement of the health of the community by use of epidemiological data); and (4) the forces of change assessment (forces such as legislation, technology, and other environmental or social phenomena that do or will

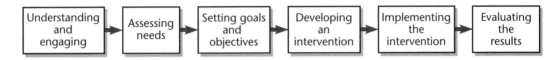

Figure 4.4   Generalized Model for Program Planning

Source: From McKenzie, J. F., B. L. Neiger, and J. L. Smeltzer. 2005. *Planning implementing, and evaluating health promotion programs: A primer.* Copyright © 2005 by Benjamin Cummings. Reprinted by permission.

impact the community)" (McKenzie et al., 2005, pp. 42–43). The four assessments help identify the gaps that exist between current status in the community and the vision identified in Phase 2, as well as strategic direction for goals and strategies (NACCHO, 2001).

In Phase 4, Identify Strategic Issues, a prioritized list of the issues facing the health of the community is developed. "Only issues that jeopardize the vision and values of the community are considered. An important task in this phase is consideration of what would happen if certain issues are not addressed, understanding why an issue is strategic, consolidating overlapping issues and identifying a prioritized list" (McKenzie et al., 2005, p. 43).

In Phase 5, Formulate Goals and Strategies, the goals and strategies to reach the vision are created. Finally, Phase 6, The Action Cycle, is similar to implementation and evaluation phases in other planning models. In this phase, implementation details are considered, evaluation plans are developed, and plans for disseminating results are made (NACCHO, 2001).

A Generalized Model for Program Planning (GMPP).   As can be noted in the models presented so far, there are a variety of approaches and frameworks on which to develop a program. Each model seems to have its own characteristics, whether it is the terminology used (e.g., predisposing, enabling, and reinforcing or analyze problem or consumer analysis), the number of components (e.g., nine phases versus six steps), or the progression through the phases or steps (e.g., circular, linear, or starting with the desired end and working backward). In other words, there are a number of ways to get from point A to point B. However, on closer examination in each of the models previously presented, you will see that each revolves around the six primary tasks incorporated in the Generalized Model for Program Development (McKenzie et al., 2005). The six tasks are:

1. Understanding the community and engaging the priority population
2. Assessing the needs of the priority population
3. Developing appropriate goals and objectives
4. Creating an intervention that considers the peculiarities of the setting
5. Implementing the intervention
6. Evaluating the results (see Figure 4.4)

To better understand the planning process in health education and the various models presented, consider the following scenario. A health educator was hired to develop health promotion programs in a corporate setting. Her first task was to find out as much as possible about the "community" of this corporate setting and get those in the priority population involved in the program planning process. She did this by reading all the material she could find about the company, spending time talking with various individuals and subgroups in the company (i.e., new employees, longtime employees, management, clerical staff, labor representatives, etc.) to find out what they wanted from a health promotion program, and reviewing old documents of the company (i.e., health insurance records, labor agreements, written history of the company, etc.). Also as a part of this first task, she formed a program planning committee with representation from the various subgroups of the work force. With the help of the planning committee, her second task was to assess the needs of the priority population. She did this by reviewing the relevant literature, examining company health insurance claims, conducting a survey of employees, and holding focus groups with selected employees. As a result of the needs assessment, she was able to identify a target health problem. In this company, the problem was a higher than expected number of breast cancer cases in the priority population. This was due in part to (1) the limited knowledge of employees about breast cancer, (2) the limited number of employees conducting breast self-examination (BSE), and (3) the low number of employees having mammograms on a regular basis.

In task three, the health educator created specific objectives to (1) increase the employees' knowledge of breast cancer from baseline to after program participation, (2) increase the number of women receiving mammograms by 30 percent, and (3) increase the number of women reporting monthly breast self-examination by 50 percent. With these objectives in mind, the health educator developed multiple intervention activities in task four:

1. An information sheet to be distributed with employee paychecks on the importance of BSE and mammography

2. A mobile mammography van to be at the site every other month

3. Plastic BSE reminder cards that can be hung from the showerhead distributed to all female employees

4. An article in the company newsletter on the high rate of breast cancer in the company and the new program to help women reduce their risk

5. Posters and pamphlets from the American Cancer Society to be displayed in the lunchroom

In task five, all of the listed intervention activities were carried out. And, finally, in task six, the health educator completed an evaluation to determine if there was an increase in knowledge, mammograms, and monthly BSE.

As can be seen from this scenario, health education involves careful, systematic planning. The skills needed to conduct a program like the one described can be acquired in upper-division classes. For now, it is enough to see the type of work a health educator is involved in and to understand the importance of using planning models to achieve successful programs.

Theories and Models Focusing on Health Behavior Change (Change Process Theories)

As with planning models, there are a number of theories and models that health educators can use to design appropriate health education interventions to help those in the priority populations with behavior change. And, as with planning models, each of these theories and models works better in some situations than in others, depending on the level of influence at which the health education program is being planned. However, before presenting the theories and models focusing on health behavior change, we need to present the concept of level of influence.

The concept of level of influence is included in the **ecological perspective** (McLeroy et al., 1988). This perspective includes five levels of influence on health-related behaviors and conditions:

1. Intrapersonal, or individual, factors
2. Interpersonal factors
3. Institutional, or organizational, factors
4. Community factors
5. Public policy factors

The ecological perspective "recognizes that health behaviors are part of the larger social system (or ecology) of behaviors and social influences, much like a river, forest or desert is part of a larger biological system (or ecosystem), and that lasting changes in health behaviors require supportive changes in the whole system, just as the addition of a power plant, the flooding of a reservoir, or the growth of a city in a desert produce changes in the whole ecosystem" (O'Donnell, 1996, p. 244).

Figure 4.5, which was created by Eng (1997), provides a visual representation of the ecological perspective. To apply this perspective to health education, let us look at how health educators can use it in assisting people to quit smoking. Health educators can provide the smoking cessation program that gives smokers important knowledge and skills necessary to quit. This is an individual strategy depicted in the center circle of Figure 4.5. Going beyond this individual approach, the health educators can also consider the social networks (friends and family) of the individuals and try to help them to be more supportive. Family members can be provided information on how to help support the behavior change. This is the interpersonal level. Next the health educators can examine the institutions to which the individuals belong to encourage them to support the new behavior. This might include the smokers' religious community, social groups, or work environment. A strategy at this level would be to encourage worksites to be smoke free or churches to provide support and prayer groups for smokers trying to quit. Beyond this level are the communities in which the smokers reside. What are the prevailing attitudes toward smoking, and how can these attitudes be modified to help support nonsmoking behaviors? Will the community culture support a nonsmoking environment? Finally, the health educators might look beyond the local communities to the population or society as a whole. Is there support for public policy? Are people willing to push for appropriate laws limiting smoking, and can such laws be enforced?

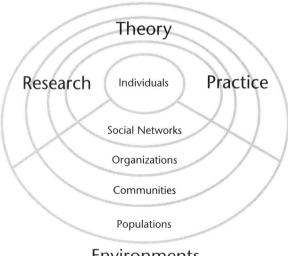

Figure 4.5 Social Ecological Framework

Source: From E. Eng, "Room with a View for a Change." Keynote address to the 1997 Annual Meeting of the National Society of Public Health Education, Indianapolis, IN. Used with permission of author.

In addition to the levels noted in Figure 4.5, there are four terms noted in bold print: *theory, practice, environments,* and *research.* Eng (1997) noted that, for the ecological perspective to be successful, the theory must be placed into practice in multiple environments, where research can be conducted to determine its effectiveness.

Having presented the concept of level of influence as it is found in the ecological perspective, we are now ready to present the theories and models focusing on behavior change. For the purpose of this presentation, we are using a modification of the ecological perspective, whereby the final three levels—institutional, community, and public policy factors—are combined into a single level called community. The modification was used earlier by Glanz and Rimer (1995). Please be aware that there are more theories and models that could be presented; however, we do not want to overwhelm you with too many at one time. We are assuming that you will have an opportunity to study these and other theories in greater detail in your upper-level major courses.

Intrapersonal (Individual) Theories. Intrapersonal theories focus on factors within individuals such as knowledge, attitudes, beliefs, self-concept, mental history, past experiences, motivation, skills, and behavior (Glanz & Rimer, 1995). Four theories that are useful in helping health educators develop interventions at the intrapersonal level are the health belief model (HBM), the theory of planned behavior (TPB), the transtheoretical model (TTM), and the precaution adoption process model (PAPM). Although all of these theories fall into the intrapersonal theories category, they can be further subdivided into either continuum theories or stage theories. The approach of **continuum theories**

is to identify variables that influence action (such as perceptions of risk and precaution effectiveness) and to combine them in a prediction equation. When applied

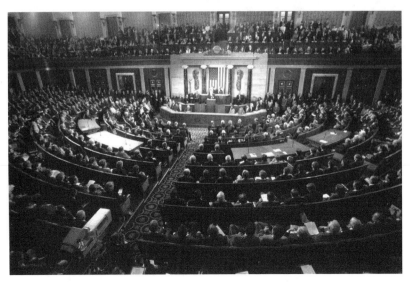

Public policy has become an important intervention strategy for health promotion. (Ron Edmonds/AP/Wide World)

to a particular individual, the value generated by the equation indicates the probability that this person will act. Thus, each person is placed along a continuum of action likelihood. Because each theory has only a single prediction equation, the way in which variables combine to influence action is expected to be the same for everyone (Weinstein, Rothman, & Sutton, 1998, p. 291).

The HBM and the TPB are examples of continuum theories that are appropriate for use at the intrapersonal level.

A **stage theory** is one that is comprised of an ordered set of categories into which people can be classified, and which identifies factors that could induce movement from one category to the next (Weinstein & Sandman, 2002b). More specifically, stage theories have four principal elements (Weinstein & Sandman, 2002a): (1) a category system to define the stages, (2) an ordering of stages, (3) people in a stage facing common barriers to change, and (4) people in different stages facing different barriers to change. Several different stage models have been proposed, but the two most commonly reported in the literature are the transtheoretical model (TTM) (Prochaska, 1979; Prochaska & DiClemente, 1983) and the precaution adoption process model (PAPM) (Weinstein, 1988; Weinstein et al., 1998).

Health Belief Model. The *health belief model* "addresses a person's perceptions of the threat of a health problem and the accompanying appraisal of a recommended behavior for preventing or managing the problem" (Glanz & Rimer, 1995, p. 17). It was developed in the 1950s by a group of psychologists to help explain why people would or would not use health services (Rosenstock, 1966). A graphic representation of this model is presented in Figure 4.6. Refer to that figure as you read this example of why a person may or may not do self-screening for cancer. While reading a weekly news magazine, the person sees an advertisement about self-screening for

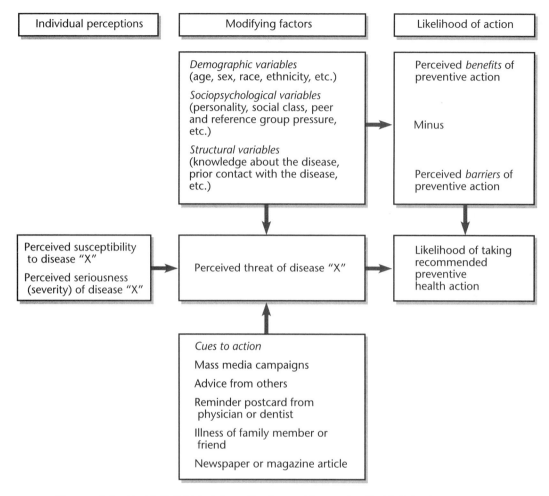

Figure 4.6   Health Belief Model as a Predictor of Preventive Health Behavior

Source: From M. H. Becker, R. H. Drachman, & J. P. Kirscht, "A New Approach to Explaining Sick-Role Behavior in Low Income Populations" in *American Journal of Public Health* 64, March 1974. Copyright © 1974 American Public Health Association.

cancer. This is a **cue to action** that gets the person thinking about his possibility of getting cancer. There may be some variables (demographic, sociopsychological, and structural) that cause the person to think about it a bit more. The person remembers his college health course, which included information about self-screenings and cancer. This person knows he is at a higher than normal risk for cancer because of family history, age, and less than desirable health behavior. Therefore, he comes to the conclusion that he is susceptible to cancer (**perceived susceptibility**). The person also believes that, if he develops cancer, it can be very serious (**perceived seriousness/severity**). Based on these factors, the person thinks that there is reason to be concerned about cancer (**perceived threat**). This person knows that self-screening can help detect cancer earlier and thus reduce the severity (**perceived**

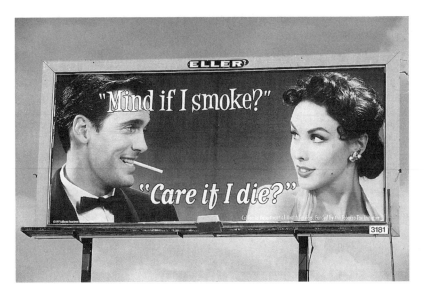

A single billboard along a highway can serve as a cue to action for many people. (Stock, Boston)

benefits). But self-screening takes time to do, and this person does not always remember to do it (**perceived barriers**). He must now analyze the difference between the benefits of self-screening and the barriers to self-screening (**reduction of threat**). For this person, the **likelihood of taking action** (self-screening) will be determined by weighing the perceived threat against the reduction of threat.

When the health belief model (HBM) was first conceived in the 1950s, **self-efficacy** (one's confidence in one's ability to perform a certain task or function) was not part of the model. But in recent years it has become a more meaningful concept in the perceived barriers construct. However, it is now believed that "for behavior change to succeed, people must (as the original HBM theorizes) feel threatened by their current behavioral patterns (perceived susceptibility and severity) and believe that change of a specific kind will result in a valued outcome at acceptable cost. They must also feel themselves competent (self-efficacious) to overcome perceived barriers to taking action (Janz, Champion, & Strecher, 2002, p. 51).

Theory of Planned Behavior.   According to the *theory of planned behavior,* individuals' intention to perform a given behavior is a function of their attitude toward performing the behavior, their beliefs about what relevant others think they should do, and their perception of the ease or difficulty of performing the behavior. The theory of planned behavior (see Figure 4.7) is an extension of the theory of reasoned action (Fishbein & Ajzen, 1975). Unlike the theory of reasoned action, the theory of planned behavior addresses behaviors in which there is both complete and incomplete volitional control. To use the example of the use of spit tobacco as a

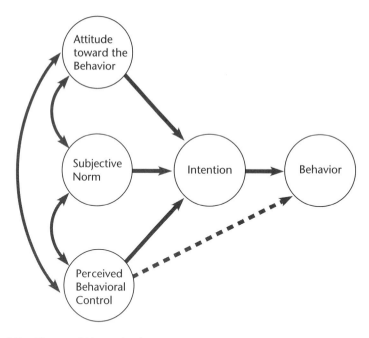

Figure 4.7   Theory of Planned Behavior

Source: From I. Ajzen, *Attitudes, Personality, and Behavior,* 1988, Dorsey Press. Copyright © 1988 Open University Press. Reprinted by permission.

behavior not fully under volitional control, the theory of planned behavior predicts that people intend to give up its use if they

1. Have a positive attitude toward quitting **(attitude toward the behavior)**
2. Think others whom they value believe it would be good for them to quit **(subjective norm)**
3. Perceive that they have control over whether or not they quit **(perceived behavioral control)**

Transtheoretical Model.   "The Transtheoretical Model is an integrative framework for understanding how individuals and populations progress toward adopting and maintaining health behavior change for optimal health. The Transtheoretical Model uses stages of change to integrate processes and principles of change from across major theories of intervention, hence the name 'Transtheoretical'" (Prochaska, Johnson, & Lee, 1998, p. 59). The core constructs of the transtheoretical model include the stages of change, the processes of change, the pros and cons of changing, and self-efficacy. Though each of the constructs is important, it is the stages of change for which this model is best known. (See Figure 4.8.) The model suggests that "people move from *precontemplation,* not intending to change, to *contemplation,* intending to change within 6 months, to *preparation,* actively planning change, to *action,* overtly making changes, and into *maintenance,* taking steps to sustain change and resist temptation to relapse" (Prochaska et al., 1994, p. 473). The model was first used in psychotherapy and was developed by Prochaska (1979) after he completed

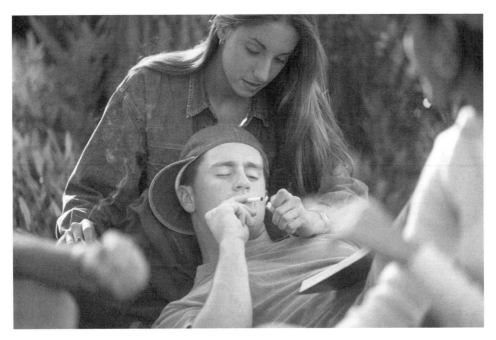

Subjective norm is an important construct to be considered when planning programs for adolescents and young adults. (Tom & DeeAnn McCarthy/The Stock Market)

a comparative analysis of a number of therapy systems and many therapy studies. Since its development, the model has been used by program planners with a variety of topics ranging from alcohol abuse to weight control.

Here is an example of applying the transtheoretical model to smoking cessation. In the **precontemplation stage,** smokers are not seriously thinking about stopping smoking in the next six months. "Many individuals in this stage are unaware or underaware of their problems" (Prochaska, DiClemente, & Norcross, 1992, p. 1103). In the **contemplation stage,** smokers know that smoking is bad for them and consider quitting, but they are not quite ready to do so. In the third stage, the **preparation stage,** the smokers have combined intention and behavioral criteria. "Individuals in this stage are intending to take action in the next month and have unsuccessfully taken action in the past year" (Prochaska et al., 1992, p. 1104). By now the smokers may have cut back on the number of cigarettes smoked, but they have not reached an effective criterion for effective action (Prochaska et al., 1992).

In the fourth stage, the **action stage,** smokers are overtly making changes in their behavior, experiences, or environment in order to stop smoking. This stage of the model reflects a consistent behavior pattern, is usually most visible, and receives the greatest external recognition (Prochaska et al., 1992). As the smokers make these changes, they are moving toward the fifth stage, maintenance.

The focus of the **maintenance stage** is to prevent relapse. Thus individuals who have quit smoking are working not to smoke again. People in this stage have changed

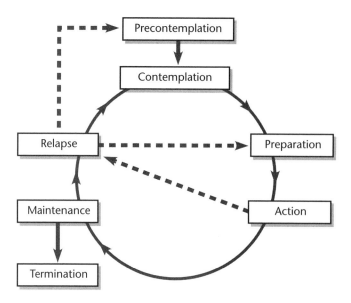

Figure 4.8   The Stages of Change

Source: From M. G. Goldstein, J. DePue, A. Kazura, and R. Niaura, "Models for Provider-Patient Interaction: Applications to Health Behavior Change," in S. A. Shumaker, E. B. Schron, J. K. Ockene, and W. L. McBee (eds.), *The Handbook of Health Behavior Change* (2nd ed.) (New York: Springer, 1998), p. 98. Springer Publishing Company, Inc., New York 10012. Used by permission.

their problem behavior for at least six months and are increasingly more confident that they can continue their changes (Prochaska et al., 1998; Redding, Rossi, Rossi, Velicer, & Prochaska, 1999). Their change has become more of a habit and their chance of relapse is lower, but it still requires some attention (Redding et al., 1999).

The final stage is **termination**. This stage is defined as the time when the individuals who have changed have zero temptation to return to their old behavior and have 100 percent self-efficacy (a lifetime of maintenance). In our example, smokers have become nonsmokers. No matter what their mood, they will not return to their old behavior (Prochaska et al., 1998). This is a stage that few people reach with certain behaviors (e.g., alcoholism).

Precaution Adoption Process Model.   The goal of the precaution adoption process model (PAPM) "is to explain how a person comes to the decision to take action, and how he or she translates that decision into action" (Weinstein & Sandman, 2002a, p. 124). Though the transtheoretical model and PAPM are both stage models and appear similar, they are applied quite differently. The PAPM is most applicable for use with the adoption of a new precaution (e.g., getting a mammogram or a hepatitis B vaccination) or the abandonment of a risky behavior that requires a deliberate action (e.g., not wearing a safety belt). It can also be used to explain why and how people make deliberate changes in habitual patterns (e.g., flossing one's teeth two times a day instead of one). It is not applicable for actions that require the gradual development of habitual patterns of behavior, such as exercise and diet (Weinstein & Sandman, 2002b).

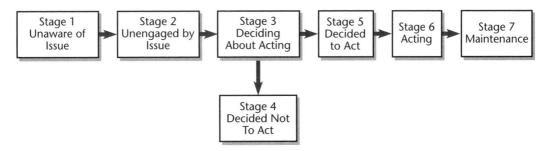

Figure 4.9   Stages of the Precaution Adoption Process Model (PAPM)

Source: Weinstein, N. D., and P. M. Sandman. 2002a. The precaution adoption process model. In K. Glanz, B. K. Rimer, and F. M. Lewis (Eds.), *Health behavior and health education: Theory, research, and practice* (3rd ed.). San Francisco: Jossey-Bass, p. 125.

Here is an example of applying the seven stages of PAPM (see Figure 4.9) to participating in a medical screening program. In Stage 1, Unaware, people are totally unaware of the need to be screened. When people first learn something about the screening, they are no longer unaware, but they are not necessarily engaged by it, either. This is Stage 2, Unengaged. In Stage 3, Deciding About Acting, people have become engaged in thinking about the screening and are considering participating. This decision-making process can result in one of two outcomes. If they decide not to participate in the screening, they are in Stage 4, Decided Not to Act, and the process is over at least for the time being. But if they decide to get screened, they are in Stage 5, Decided to Act. Once the people participate in the screening, they have initiated the behavior and are in Stage 6, Acting. And finally, if the people participate in the screening at the medically recommended intervals, they are in Stage 7, Maintenance. Note that this last stage of the PAPM is not applicable to some decision making processes such as for an action that is required only once in a lifetime, such as a vaccination that immunizes for life (Weinstein & Sandman, 2002b).

Interpersonal Theories.   The category of interpersonal theories is comprised of theories that "include factors related to individuals' experience and perceptions of their environments in combination with their personal characteristics" (Glanz & Rimer, 1995, p. 22). Included in this category are theories dealing with social learning, social power, interpersonal communication, social networks, and social support. Because of the importance of social learning to health education/promotion and because of space limitations, the only theory we will discuss is the social cognitive theory.

The social cognitive theory (SCT) (Bandura, 1986) dates back to the 1950s (Bandura, 1977; Rotter, 1954), when it was known as the social learning theory (SLT). Some still refer to it as the SLT. In brief, the SCT describes learning as a reciprocal interaction among an individual's environment, cognitive processes, and behavior (Parcel, 1983). Those who espouse the SCT believe that reinforcement contributes to learning, but it is the combination of reinforcement with an individual's expectations of the consequences of the behavior that determines the behavior. The SCT explains learning through its constructs. Those constructs that have been most

Table 4.5   Often-Used Constructs of the Social Cognitive Theory and Examples of Their Application

Construct	Definition	Example
Behavioral capability	Knowledge and skills necessary to perform a behavior	If people are going to exercise aerobically, they need to know what it is and how to do it.
Expectations	Beliefs about the likely outcomes of certain behaviors	If people enroll in a weight-loss program, they expect to lose weight.
Expectancies	Values people place on expected outcomes	How important is it to people that they become physically fit?
Locus of control	Perception of the center of control over reinforcement	Those who feel they have control over reinforcement are said to have internal locus of control. Those who perceive reinforcement under the control of an external force are said to have external locus of control.
Reciprocal determinism	Behavior changes result from an interaction between the person and the environment; change is bidirectional (Glanz & Rimer, 1995).	Lack of use of vending machines could be a result of the choices within the machine. Notes about the selections from the nonusing consumers to the machine's owners could change the selections and change the behavior of the nonusing consumers to that of users.
Reinforcement (directly, vicariously, self-management)	Responses to behaviors that increase the chances of recurrence	Giving verbal encouragement to those who have acted in a healthy manner
Self-control, or self-regulation	Gaining control over own behavior through monitoring and adjusting it	If clients want to change their eating habits, have them monitor their current eating habits for seven days.
Self-efficacy	People's confidence in their ability to perform a certain desired task or function	If people are going to engage in a regular exercise program, they must feel they can do it.
Emotional-coping response	For people to learn, they must be able to deal with the sources of anxiety that surround a behavior.	Fear is an emotion that can be involved in learning, and people would have to deal with it before they could learn a behavior.

often used in health education/promotion are presented in Table 4.5, along with an example of each.

Community Theories.   As noted earlier, this group of theories includes three categories of factors from the ecological perspective—institutional, community, and public policy. Institutional factors include such things as rules, regulations, and policies of an organization that can impact health behavior. Community factors include social networks and norms, while public policy includes legislation that can impact health behavior. Theories associated with these three factors include theories of community organizing and community building (see Chapter 1), organizational change, and the diffusion theory. It is this later theory that we will present here.

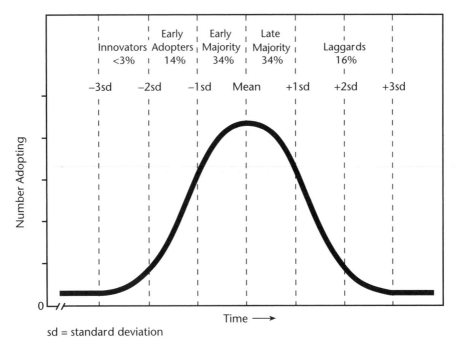

sd = standard deviation

Figure 4.10   Bell-shaped Curve and Adopter Categories

Source: Adapted with the permission of The Free Press, a Division of Simon & Schuster from *Diffusion of Innovations,* Fourth Edition by Everett M. Rogers. Copyright © 1995 by Everett M. Rogers. Copyright © 1962, 1971, 1983 by The Free Press.

The *diffusion theory* provides an explanation for the diffusion of innovations in populations. In health education/promotion, innovations come in the form of new ideas, techniques, behaviors, and programs. When people become "consumers" of an innovation, they are referred to as adopters.

Rogers (2003) has categorized adopters on the basis of when they adopt innovations. They include innovators, early adopters, early or late majority, and laggards. The rate at which people become adopters can be represented by the bell-shaped curve (see Figure 4.10). **Innovators** are the first to adopt an innovation. They are venturesome, independent, risky, and daring. They want to be the first to do something. The second group consists of the **early adopters.** These people are very interested in innovation, but they do not want to be the first involved. Early adopters are respected by others in the social system and looked at as opinion leaders. Following the early adopters is the **early majority.** This group of people may be interested in the innovation but will need some external motivation to get involved. These people, along with those in the late majority, comprise the largest groups. The **late majority** is comprised of people who are skeptical and will not adopt an innovation until most people in the social system have done so. The last group, the **laggards,** will be the last to get involved in an innovation, if they get involved at all. Let us look at an application of this theory. If the health education staff at the Walkup Health Maintenance Organization (HMO) is beginning a new series of stress management classes for the HMO members, they can expect that about 3 percent of the priority population (the innovators) will sign up and attend as soon as they hear about the series. Shortly thereafter, another 14 percent (early adopters) will probably get involved, possibly after reading about the merits of the program. At this point, the health education staff will have to get a little more aggressive in attracting the others to the program. It will take constant reminders to get the early majority involved, while buddy, peer, or mentoring programs might be needed to get the late majority involved. The laggards will probably not attend the series at all.

Some Final Thoughts about Theories and Models

Having spent a number of pages discussing the theories (and some models) commonly used in the profession, also note that there are some individuals in the profession who feel that the theories presented in this chapter, and some others not discussed (see Glanz, Rimer, & Lewis, 2002, and DiClemente, Crosby, & Kegler, 2002, for other theories and models), still are not as useful to health educators as they should or could be in helping move from theory to practice. Stated another way, these theories have limited usefulness in explaining (accounting for) the desired outcomes of health education/promotion programs. The criticism is that much of what is presented in this chapter is based on logical positivism. Logical positivism can be thought of as experimental, hypothesis-testing methodology, in which those "conducting" the experiment have a great amount of control over the process (Buchanan, 1994). It is an approach that has worked well in the natural sciences, but can it be assumed that it will work in the social sciences too? To do so, Buchanan (1992) states that it would have to be assumed

> that there is no essential difference between human behavior and the behavior of chemicals in a test tube, gases in a bubble chamber, or planets in space. Human behavior may be more complex, but in principle, it is no different from any [other] natural process. It is governed by immutable laws that are determined by very structured nature. Based on this assumption, positivists claim the methods and "language" (i.e., mathematics) of physics and chemistry are not only the best, but even more strongly, the only valid and reliable means to explain human behavior. (p. 129)

A question now facing the profession is whether the theories presently available to health educators are adequate and should continue to be used, or should there be a movement toward the development of new theories to help guide health educators' work? The need to expand the theoretical foundations of health education to go beyond logical positivism has been discussed by several authors (Buchanan, 1992, 1994; Burdine & McLeroy, 1992; Labonte & Robertson, 1996; McLeroy et al., 1992; McLeroy et al., 1993). Some of the issues raised in these articles have been discussed and countered in another work (Green et al., 1994). Space does not permit a full discussion of this debate here. Though there may not be agreement on whether health educators can build on the theories and models now in use or must replace them, both sides agree that theories and models are necessary components in guiding the work of health educators.

SUMMARY

Health education/health promotion is a multidisciplinary field of practice that has evolved from the theory and practice of a number of other biological, behavioral, sociological, and health science disciplines. The theories and models that are used in health education/promotion have also evolved from these other disciplines. This chapter presented an overview of the theoretical foundations of health education. Readers were introduced to the definitions of *theory, concept, construct, variable,* and *model.* A rationale was also provided to explain why it is important that health educators use theory in their work. Readers were then introduced to six planning models (theories/models of implementation) and six theories and models used in helping change health behavior (theories of change). The latter theories and models were presented within the five levels of the ecological perspective. The chapter concluded with a word of caution about the application of theories and models and what the future may hold for theories used by health educators.

REVIEW QUESTIONS

1. Define each of the following and explain how they relate to each other.
   • Theory
   • Concept
   • Construct
   • Variable
   • Model
2. Why is it important to use theory in the practice of health education/promotion?
3. What is the difference between planning models and the theories and models focusing on behavior change (change process theories)?
4. Name the six planning models (theories/models of implementation) presented in this chapter and list one distinguishing characteristic of each.
5. Of the six planning models (theories/models of implementation) presented in this chapter, which one is most commonly used? Name the phases of this model.
6. What six components seem to be common to the planning models (theories of implementation) presented in this chapter?
7. What are the five levels within the ecological perspective? How do they relate to the theories of change (change process theories)?
8. Identify the six theories and models presented in this chapter that focus on health behavior change (change process theories). Briefly describe each of the theories or models and name their components.
9. Explain why it might be important that health educators have a good understanding of the stage models.

CRITICAL THINKING QUESTIONS

1. This chapter presented a number of different theories and models focusing on health behavior change. If you were trying to help a friend stop smoking, at the friend's request, what behavior change theory/model would you use to develop the

intervention to help your friend? Defend why you selected this theory/model and explain how you would apply each of the constructs.

2. You have been invited by the Garber Corporation to interview for a newly created position in the company as a health educator. The position has been described as one that will focus on helping employees change their health behavior. As a part of the interview, the director of human resources asks you this question: "Of all the theories and models related to health education/promotion you studied in your college courses, which one do you think will have the greatest application to your work here at the Garber Corporation?" Defend your response.

3. You have been given an assignment by one of your college professors to conduct an in-depth study of one of the theories/models presented in this chapter. Which one would you select? Why?

ACTIVITIES

1. Interview a practicing health educator, asking about the theories and models the person has used in planning and implementing health education/promotion programs. Ask why those theories and models were used. Also, find out if the health educator has run into any problems trying to use the theories and models. Summarize the interview in a one-page paper.

2. Choosing and selecting from the components found in the theories of implementation, create your own model. Draw a diagram of your model and, in two paragraphs, explain why you have included the components you did.

3. Pick one of the theories of change. Then choose a health behavior. In a one-page paper, explain how the theory can be applied to the health behavior you chose.

WEBLINKS

1. **http://mapp.naccho.org/mapp_introduction.asp**

   National Association of County and City Health Officials

   At this Web site, the MAPP model is comprehensively diagrammed and explained. The Four MAPP Assessments are described, including how they are implemented, how to use subcommittees for each assessment, and how to make linkages between assessments.

2. **http://www.cdc.gov/communication/cdcynergy.htm**

   Communication at the Centers for Disease Control and Prevention

   This Web site provides an overview of *CDCynergy,* news and updates, information on all editions, current campaigns, practice areas, and resources.

3. **http://www.uri.edu/research/cprc/**

   Cancer Prevention Resource Center (CPRC), University of Rhode Island

   This is the Web site of the CPRC, which is the home of the transtheoretical model. Information about the model as well as measures that can be used to "stage" a person can be found at this site.

4. **http://www.cdc.gov/std/program/community/9-PGcommunity.htm**

   National Center for HIV, STD, and TB prevention, Division of Sexually Transmitted Diseases

This Web site provides an overview of the following behavior change theories: health belief model, theory of reasoned action, social (cognitive) learning theory, transtheoretical model (stages of change), diffusion of innovations, and empowerment theory/popular education.

5. **http://oc.nci.nih.gov/services/Theory_at_glance/HOME.html**

National Cancer Institute (NCI)

The Web page is part of the NCI Web site. This site presents the primer *Theory at a Glance: A Guide for Health Promotion Practice*. This volume explains why theories and models are important and how to use theory, and provides explanations of several behavior change theories, as well as a couple of program planning models.

CASE STUDY

Mike graduated a year ago with a bachelor's degree in health education. He felt extremely lucky to "beat out" fifteen interviewees for the health educator position at the Lancaster County Health Department. Though the health department has a good reputation throughout the state, Mike is the only person on the staff hired to do health education. Mike's supervisor Dan Santoro, Coordinator of Chronic and Infectious Disease for the health department, has worked for the department for about thirty years. He also holds a bachelor's degree from the same university Mike graduated from. However, Mr. Santoro received his degree in health and physical education prior to the implementation of the current community health education major. Throughout Mike's tenure with the health department, he and Mr. Santoro have had a good working relationship. However, while planning a weight-loss program for a group of teenagers in the county, Mike ran into a situation that caused him some concern. After conducting a needs assessment and writing the program goals and objectives, he could not decide which change process theory or model to use to plan his intervention. He decided to seek Mr. Santoro's advice. When he asked Mr. Santoro what theory or model he would recommend, Mr. Santoro responded, "Theory-shmeary, you don't need to use that stuff, just skip the theory part and plan the intervention. This program needs to be up and running by the end of the month." Based on this short conversation with Mr. Santoro, Mike was not sure how to proceed because during his undergraduate preparation at the university he was told to "never plan an intervention that was not based on theory." Mike does not want to upset his supervisor, but he also knows that his program should be grounded in theory. What do you see as Mike's options at this point? What do you think Mike should do next? How would you solve this dilemma?

REFERENCES

Ajzen, I. (1988). *Attitudes, personality, and behavior.* Chicago: Dorsey Press.

Albrecht, T. L. (1997). Defining social marketing: Twenty five years later. *Social Marketing Quarterly, 3,* 21–23.

Andreasen, A. (1995). *Marketing sound change: Changing behavior to promote health, social development, and the environment.* San Francisco: Jossey-Bass.

Bandura, A. (1977). *Social learning theory.* Englewood Cliffs, NJ: Prentice-Hall.

Bandura, A. (1986). *Social foundations of thought and action.* Englewood Cliffs, NJ: Prentice-Hall.

Bates, I. J., & Winder, A. E. (1984). *Introduction to health education.* Palo Alto, CA: Mayfield.

Bryant, C. (1998). *Social marketing: A tool for excellence.* Eighth annual conference on social marketing in public health. Clearwater Beach, FL.

Buchanan, D. R. (1992). An uneasy alliance: Combining qualitative and quantitative research methods. *Health Education Quarterly, 19*(3), 117–135.

Buchanan, D. R. (1994). Reflections on the relationship between theory and practice. *Health Education Research, 9*(3), 273–283.

Burdine, J. N., & McLeroy, K. R. (1992). Practitioners' use of theory: Examples from a workgroup. *Health Education Quarterly, 19*(3), 331–340.

Centers for Disease Control and Prevention (CDC), U.S. Department of Health and Human Services (USDHHS). (2003). *CDCynergy 3.0: Your Guide to Effective Health Communication (CD-ROM Version 3.0).* Atlanta, GA: Author.

Centers for Disease Control and Prevention (2000). *Healthy plan-it: A tool for planning and managing public health programs. Sustainable Management Development Program.* Atlanta, GA: Author.

Centers for Disease Control and Prevention (CDC), U.S. Department of Health and Human Services (USDHHS). (no date). *Planned approach to community health: Guide for local coordinators,* Atlanta, GA: Author.

Chaplin, J. P., & Krawiec, T. S. (1979). *Systems and theories of psychology* (4th ed.). New York: Holt, Rinehart & Winston.

Crosby, R. A., Kegler, M. C., & DiClemente, R. J. (2002). Understanding and applying theory in health promotion practice and research. In R. J. DiClemente, R. A. Crosby, & M. C. Kegler (Eds.), *Emerging theories in health promotion practice and research: Strategies for improving public health.* (pp. 1–15). San Francisco: Jossey-Bass.

DiClemente, R. J., Crosby, R. A., & Kegler, M. C. (Eds.). (2002). *Emerging theories in health promotion practice and research: Strategies for improving public health.* San Francisco: Jossey-Bass.

Eng, E. (1997). *Room with a view for a change.* Keynote address to the Annual Meeting of the National Society of Public Health Education, Indianapolis, IN.

Fishbein, M., & Ajzen, I. (1975). *Belief, attitude, intention and behavior: An introduction to theory and research.* Reading, MA: Addison-Wesley.

Glanz, K., & Rimer, B. K. (1995). *Theory at a glance: A guide for health promotion practice* (NIH publication no. 95–3896). Bethesda, MD: National Institutes of Health, National Cancer Institute.

Glanz, K., & Rimer, B. K., & Lewis, F. M. (Eds.). (2002). *Health behavior and health education: Theory, research and practice.* San Francisco, Jossey-Bass.

Glanz, K., Lewis, F. M., & Rimer, B. K. (2002). Theory, research, and practice in health behavior and health education. In K. Glanz, B. K. Rimer, & F. M. Lewis (Eds.). *Health behavior and health education: Theory, research, and practice* (3rd ed, pp. 22–39). San Francisco: Jossey-Bass.

Green, L. W. (1974). Toward cost-benefit evaluations of health education: Some concepts, methods, and examples. *Health Education Monographs, 2* (Suppl. 1), 34–64.

Green, L. W. (1975). Evaluation of patient education programs. Criteria and measurement techniques. In *Rx: Education for the patient: Proceedings of the Continuing Education Institution, Southern Illinois University* (pp. 89–98). Carbondale, IL: Southern Illinois University Press.

Green, L. W. (1976). Methods available to evaluate the health education components of preventive health programs. In *Preventive Medicine,* USA (pp. 162–171). New York: Prodist.

Green, L. W. (1979). National policy on the promotion of health. *International Journal of Health Education, 22,* 161–168.

Green, L. W. (1980). Healthy people: The surgeon general's report and the prospects. In W. J. McNervey (Ed.), *Working for a healthier America* (pp. 95–110). Cambridge, MA: Ballinger.

Green, L. W. (1981a). Emerging federal perspectives on health promotion. In J. P. Allegrante (Ed.), *Health promotion monographs.* New York: Teachers College, Columbia University.

Green, L. W. (1981b). The objectives for the nation in disease prevention and health promotion: A challenge to health education training. In *Proceedings of the National Conference for Institutions Preparing Health Educators,* (DHHS Publication No. 81–50171) (pp. 61–73). Washington, DC: U.S. Office of Health Information and Health Promotion.

Green, L. W. (1982). Reconciling policy in health education and primary care. *International Journal of Health Education, 24* (Suppl. 3), 1–11.

Green, L. W. (1983a). New policies in education for health. *World Health,* (April/May), 13–17.

Green, L. W. (1983b). *New policies for health education in primary health care* (Background document for the technical discussions of the 36th World Health Assembly, May 1983.) Geneva: World Health Organization.

Green, L. W. (1984a). La educacion para la salud en el medio urbano. In *Conferencia InterAmericana de Educacion Para La Salud* (pp. 80–82). Mexico City: Sector Salud, SEP, and International Union for Health Education and World Health Organization.

Green, L. W. (1984b). Health education models. In J. D. Matarazzo, S. M. Weiss, & J. A. Herd (Eds.), *Behavioral health: A handbook of health enhancement and disease prevention* (pp. 181–198). New York: Wiley.

Green, L. W. (1984c). Modifying and developing health behavior. *Annual Review of Public Health, 5,* 215–236.

Green, L. W. (1984d). A triage and stepped approach to self-care education. *Medical Times, 111,* 75–80.

Green, L. W. (1986a, October). *Applications and trials of the PRECEDE framework for planning and evaluation of health programs.* Paper presented at the meeting of the American Public Health Association, Las Vegas, NV.

Green, L. W. (1986b). Evaluation model: A framework for the design of rigorous evaluation of efforts in health promotion. *American Journal of Health Promotion, 1*(1), 77–79.

Green, L. W. (1986c). *New policies for health education in primary health care.* Geneva: World Health Organization.

Green, L. W. (1986d). Research agenda: Building a consensus on research questions. *American Journal of Health Promotion, 1*(2), 70–72.

Green, L. W. (1986e). The theory of participation: A qualitative analysis of its expression in national and international health policies. In W. B. Ward (Ed.), *Advances in health education and promotion* (pp. 211–236). Greenwich, CT: JAI Press.

Green, L. W. (1987a). How physicians can improve patients' participation and maintenance in self-care. *Western Journal of Medicine, 147,* 346–349.

Green, L. W. (1987b). *Program planning and evaluation guide for lung associations.* New York: American Lung Association.

Green, L. W., & Allen, J. (1980). *Toward a healthy community: Organizing events for community health promotion* (PHS Publication No. 80–50113). Washington, DC: USDHHS, Office of Disease Prevention and Health Promotion.

Green, L. W., Glanz, K., Hochbaum, G. M., Kok, G., Kreuter, M. W., Lewis, F. M., Lorig, K., Morisky, D., Rimer, B. K., & Rosenstock, I. M. (1994). Can we build on, or must we replace, the theories and models in health education? *Health Education Research, 9*(3), 397–404.

Green, L. W., & Kreuter, M. W. (1991). *Health promotion planning: An educational and environmental approach* (2nd ed.). Mountain View: Mayfield.

Green, L. W., & Kreuter, M. W. (1999). *Health promotion planning: An educational and ecological approach* (3rd ed.). Mountain View: Mayfield.

Green, L. W., Kreuter, M. W., Deeds, S. G., & Partridge, K. B. (1980). *Health education planning: A diagnostic approach.* Palo Alto: Mayfield.

Green, L. W., Levine, D. M., & Deeds, S. G. (1975). Clinical trials of health education for hypertensive outpatients: Design and baseline data. *Preventive Medicine, 4,* 417–425.

Green, L. W., & McAlister, A. L. (1984). Macro-intervention to support health behavior: Some theoretical perspectives and practical reflections. *Health Education Quarterly, 11,* 323–39.

Green, L. W., Mullen, P. D., & Friedman, R. (1986). An epidemiological approach to targeting drug information. *Patient Education and Counseling, 8,* 255–268.

Green, L. W., Wang, V. L., Deeds, S. G., Fisher, A. A., Windsor, R., & Rogers, C. (1978). Guidelines for health education in maternal and child health programs. *International Journal of Health Education, 21* (suppl.), 1–33.

Green, L. W., Wilson, A. L., & Lovato, C. Y. (1986). What changes can health promotion achieve and how long do these changes last? The tradeoffs between expediency and durability. *Preventive Medicine, 15,* 508–521.

Green, L. W., Wilson, R. W., & Bauer, K. G. (1983). Data required to measure progress on the objectives for the nation in disease prevention and health promotion. *American Journal of Public Health, 73,* 18–24.

Janz, N. K., Champion, V. L., & Strecher, V. J. (2002). The health belief model. In K. Glanz, B. K. Rimer, & F. M. Lewis (Eds.), *Health behavior and health education: Theory, research, and practice* (3rd. ed, pp. 45–66). San Francisco: Jossey-Bass.

Kerlinger, F. N. (1986). *Foundations of behavioral research* (3rd ed.). Austin, TX: Holt, Rinehart & Winston.

Labonte, R., & Robertson, A. (1996). Delivering the goods, showing our stuff: The case for a constructivist paradigm for health promotion research and practice. *Health Education Quarterly, 23*(4), 431–447.

McDermott, R. J. (2000). Social marketing: A tool for health education. *American Journal of Health Behavior, 24*(1), 6–10.

McKenzie, J. F., Neiger, B. L., & Smeltzer, J. L. (2005). *Planning, implementing, and evaluating health promotion programs: A primer* (4th ed.). San Francisco: Benjamin Cummings.

McLeroy, K. R., Bibeau, D., Steckler, A., & Glanz, K. (1988). An ecological perspective for health promotion programs. *Health Education Quarterly, 15*(4), 351–378.

McLeroy, K. R., Steckler, A., Goodman, R., & Burdine, J. N. (1992). Health education research, theory and practice: Future directions. *Health Education Research: Theory and Practice, 7*(1), 1–8.

McLeroy, K. R., Steckler, A., Goodman, R., Burdine, J. N., & Gottlieb, N. (1993). Social science theories in health education: Time for a new model? *Health Education Research: Theory and Practice, 8*(3), 305–312.

National Association of County Health Officials (NACHO). (1991). *APEX/PH, Assessment protocol for excellence in public health.* Washington, DC: Author.

National Association of County and City Health Officials (NACCHO). (2001). *Mobilizing for action through planning and partnerships (MAPP).* Washington, DC: Author.

National Association of County and City Health Officials (NACCHO). (2000). *Mobilizing for action through planning and partnerships (MAPP)*. Retrieved February 19, 2004, from http://mapp.naccho.org/view_model.asp?image+MAPP+model.

National Cancer Institute (NCI). (2002). *Making health communication programs work* (NIH Publication No. 02-5145). Washington, DC: U.S. Department of Health and Human Services (USDHHS).

Neiger, B. L. (1998). *Social marketing: Making public health sense.* Paper presented at the annual meeting of the Utah Public Health Association. Provo, UT.

Neiger, B. L., & Thackeray, R. (2002). Application of the SMART model in two successful social marketing campaigns. *American Journal of Health Education, 33,* 291–293.

O'Donnell, M. P. (1996). Editor's notes. *American Journal of Health Promotion, 10*(4), 244.

Parcel, G. S. (1983). Theoretical models for application in school health research. *Health Education, 15*(4), 39–49.

Parvanta, C. F., & Freimuth, V. (2000). Health communication at the Centers for Disease Control and Prevention. *American Journal of Health Behavior, 24*(1), 18–25.

Patton, R. P., Corry, J. M., Gettman, L. R., & Graff, J. S. (1986). *Implementing health/fitness programs.* Champaign, IL: Human Kinetics.

Prochaska, J. O. (1979). *Systems of psychotherapy: A transtheoretical analysis.* Homewood, IL: Dorsey Press.

Prochaska, J. O., & DiClemente, C. C. (1983). Stages and processes of self-change of smoking: Toward an integrative model of change. *Journal of Consulting and Clinical Psychology, 51*(3), 390-395.

Prochaska, J. O., DiClemente, C. C., & Norcross, J. C. (1992). In search of how people change: Application to addictive behaviors. *American Psychologist, 47*(9), 1102–1114.

Prochaska, J. O., Johnson, S., & Lee, P. (1998). The transtheoretical model of behavior change. In S. A. Shumaker, E. B. Schron, J. K. Ockene, & W. L. McBee (Eds.), *The handbook of health behavior change* (2nd ed., pp. 59–84). New York: Springer Publishing Company.

Prochaska, J. O., Redding, C. A., Harlow, L. L., Rossi, J. S., & Velicer, W. F. (1994). The transtheoretical model of change and HIV prevention: A review. *Health Education Quarterly, 24*(4), 471–486.

Redding, C. A., Rossi, J. S., Rossi, S. R., Velicer, W. F., & Prochaska, J. O. (1999). Health behavior models. In G. C. Hyner, K. W. Peterson, J. W. Travis, J. E. Dewey, J. J. Foerster, & E. M. Framer (Eds.), *SPM handbook of health assessment tools* (pp. 83–93). Pittsburgh, PA: The Society of Prospective Medicine.

Rogers, E. M. (2003). *Diffusion of innovations* (5th ed.). New York: Free Press.

Rosenstock, I. M. (1966). Why people use health services. *Milbank Memorial Fund Quarterly, 44,* 94–124.

Ross, H. S., & Mico, P. R. (1980). *Theory and practice in health education.* San Francisco: Mayfield.

Rotter, J. B. (1954). *Social learning and clinical psychology.* New York: Prentice–Hall.

Simons-Morton, B. G., Greene, W. H., & Gottlieb, N. H. (1995). *Introduction to health education and health promotion* (2nd ed.). Prospect Hts., IL: Waveland Press, Inc.

Simons-Morton, D. G., Simons-Morton, B. G., Parcel, G. S., & Bunker, J. F. (1988). Influencing personal and environmental conditions for community health: A multi-level intervention model. *Family and Community Health, 1*(2), 25–35.

Smith, W. A. (1999). *What is social marketing?* Washington, DC: Academy for Educational Development.

Smith, W. A. (2000). Social marketing: An evolving definition. *American Journal of Health Behavior, 24*(1), 11–17.

Sullivan, D. (1973). Model for comprehensive, systematic program development in health education. *Health Education Report, 1*(1), (November/December), 4–5.

Timmreck, T. C. (2003). *Planning, program development, and evaluation* (2nd ed.). Boston: Jones & Bartlett.

Walsh, D. C., Rudd, R. E., Moeykens, B. A., & Moloney, T. W. (1993). Social marketing for public health. *Health Affairs, 12,* 104–119.

Weinstein, N. D. (1988). The precaution adoption process. *Health Psychology, 7,* 355–386.

Weinstein, N. D., Rothman, A. J., & Sutton, S. R. (1998). Stage theories of health behavior: Conceptual and methodological issues. *Health Psychology, 17,* 290–299.

Weinstein, N. D., & Sandman, P. M. (2002a). The precaution adoption process model. In K. Glanz, B. K. Rimer, & F. M. Lewis (Eds.), *Health behavior and health education: Theory, research, and practice* (3rd. ed, pp. 121–143). San Francisco: Jossey-Bass.

Weinstein, N. D., & Sandman, P. M. (2002b). The precaution adoption process model and its application. In R. J. DiClemente, R. A. Crosby, & M. C. Kegler (Eds.), *Emerging theories in health promotion practice and research: Strategies for improving public health.* (pp. 16-39). San Francisco: Jossey-Bass.

CHAPTER 5

Ethics and Health Education

Chapter Objectives

After reading this chapter and answering the questions at the end, you should be able to:

1. Identify and define the three major areas of philosophy.
2. Define *ethics*.
3. Explain the difference between ethics and morality.
4. Explain why it is important to act ethically.
5. Define *professional ethics*.
6. Explain and briefly describe the two major categories of ethical theories.
7. Identify principles that create a common ground for all ethical theories.
8. Outline a guide for making ethical decisions.
9. Identify ethical issues associated with the profession of health education.
10. Explain how a profession can ensure that its professionals will act ethically.
11. Define *code of ethics* and identify the source of the code available for health educators.

Key Terms

anonymity
beneficence
benevolence
confidentiality
code of ethics
consequentialism (teleology)
epistemology
ethical
ethics

formalism (deontology or nonconsequentialism)
goodness (rightness)
individual freedom (equality principle, principle of autonomy)
informed consent
justice (fairness)
metaphysics

moral
moral philosophy
nonmaleficence
privacy
professional ethics
teleology
truth telling (honesty)
value of life

In recent years, there has been an increasing interest in ethical questions in all walks of life. The interest has become so great that it is difficult to avoid the topic of ethics in everyday living. Newspapers and television networks are constantly covering stories that involve ethical issues, many of which are related to health. Examples include genetic engineering, abortion, the right to die, nuclear waste storage, the marketing of harmful products such as tobacco in developing countries, the reduction of welfare benefits, appropriate sexual behavior, and professional behavior, to name a few.

How is it that we determine what is ethical or unethical? By whose standards do we make such judgments? To answer these questions requires some background and perspective. In this chapter, we will provide the background and perspective to understand how ethics relates to the profession of health education. First, we will present key terms that relate to the study of ethics and examine the origin of ethics. Next we will look at reasons why people should work from an ethical base. We will then briefly look at the theories used to create ethical "yardsticks" and how these theories can be used to make ethical decisions. Within this context, a sampling of ethical issues facing health educators today will be presented. Finally, we will conclude with a discussion on how a profession, or an emerging profession, can ensure that its professionals will act ethically.

Key Terms and Origin

Ethics, the study of morality, is one of the three major areas of philosophy. The other two are **epistemology,** the study of knowledge, and **metaphysics,** the study of the nature of reality (Thiroux, 1995). Ethics, or **moral philosophy** as it is often stated, dates back two thousand plus years to Socrates (470–399 B.C.), "the ancient Greek philosopher, who spent his days in the Athenian marketplace challenging people to think about how they lived" (White, 1988, p. 7). Though philosophers do not sit in the marketplace (or malls) today to challenge people, the behavior, actions, and values of people are constantly being examined for their appropriateness.

You will note that the word *ethics* was described using the words *moral* and *morality.* "'Ethics' and 'morals' come to us from two words in ancient Greek and Latin, *ethos* and *mores;* both mean 'character.' When we ask if an action is ethical, we can think, 'Is it the sort of thing somebody with a 'good character' would do?'" (White, 1988, p. 8.). Thiroux (1995) has made a distinction between ethics and morals, saying that ethics "seems to pertain to the individual character of a person or persons, whereas morality seems to point to the relationships between human beings" (p. 3). Clearly, "both ethics and morality involve the human ability to make choices among values and to make decisions about right and wrong" (Feeney & Freeman, 1999, p. 5). Nevertheless, to avoid confusion throughout the rest of this chapter, we will use **ethical** and **moral** to mean the same thing. "The important thing to remember here is that moral, ethical, immoral, and unethical, essentially mean, good, right, bad, and wrong, often depending on whether one is referring to people themselves or to their actions" (Thiroux, 1995, p. 3).

White (1988) refers to the words *good, right, bad,* and *wrong* as the labels people use when making ethical judgments about human actions. Some authors have used these words to define ethics. Feeney and Freeman (1999) state, "Ethics is the study of right and wrong, duty and obligation" (p. 5). "It is a discipline practiced by everyone who ever wondered, 'why should I do this rather than that?'" (Mellert, 1995, p. 2). Penland and Beyrer (1981, p. 6) defined ethics as "the study of rightness and wrongness in human conduct." "Acting 'ethically' is connected *with* what a person is doing and *how* he or she is doing it" (White, 1988, p. 8).

Why Should People Act Ethically?

Because ethics is one of the three major areas of philosophy, a philosophical answer to the question of why people should act ethically is that to act ethically brings meaning or purpose to the life of an individual (McGrath, 1994). It provides a standard by which to live. Ethical living, in turn, provides for a better society for all. It is the right thing to do for society and self.

From a more practical viewpoint, observation has shown "that those who are ethical tend to lead healthier (both physically and psychologically), more emotionally satisfying lives" (McGrath, 1994, p. 131). "In fact, the ethical life promises rewards for everyone involved. Your friends and associates will obviously feel better about life and about you if you treat them decently. And they'll probably reciprocate, treating you the same way, which will make your life better" (White, 1988, pp. 84–85). In short, the ethical person is more mature, stronger, healthier, and more advanced and has a more fully developed personality than those who are not ethical (White, 1988).

Professional Ethics

Whereas personal values and morality may guide us in our everyday living, it is important to note that they may not be sufficient to guide our professional behavior. People come to their work with different personal experiences. Because of these different experiences, they do not hold the same values nor have they learned the same moral lessons. Even those who hold the same beliefs may not apply them in the same way in a professional setting (Feeney & Freeman, 1999). Thus, in a work setting, individuals are guided by professional ethics. **Professional ethics** focuses on the "actions that are right and wrong in the workplace and are of public matter. Professional moral principles are not statements of taste or preference; they tell practitioners what they ought to do and what they ought not do" (Feeney & Freeman, 1999, p. 6).

Ethical behavior is expected from professionals. "'Ethics' delineates what we consider acceptable and unacceptable conduct regarding professional practice in Health Science education. Ethical conduct is particularly important to professional health educators, since we belong to a profession with a mission to serve the individual" (Pigg, 1994, p. iii). Health education is a profession with much human interaction. Dorman (1994) adds, "As writers, reviewers, and scientists we must insist on the highest of ethical practices in publication and research. As practitioners, we must seek to actively practice ethical behavior in our service and teaching. Individually, we must aspire for a reputation which reflects a life of personal integrity. The wisdom of King Solomon probably puts it best: *'A good name is more desirable than great riches; to be esteemed is better than silver or gold'"* (p. 4).

Table 5.1   Summary of Ethical Theories

Category	Primary Reasoning	Examples of Such Theories
Formalism (also known as deontology or nonconsequentialism)	The end does not justify the means.	Natural law morality, deontological ethics, existentialism
Consequentialism (also known as teleology)	The end does justify the means.	Contractarian ethics, utilitarianism, pragmatism

Ethical Theories

Philosophers do not speak with a common voice about the standards of morality. Depending on the ethical theory espoused, one philosopher may see a certain behavior as moral or ethical, while another may see the same behavior as immoral or unethical. For example, one philosopher may see corporal punishment as a moral action to punish a person for murder, while the second philosopher sees the taking of another life, for whatever reason, as immoral. The purpose of this section is not to present a detailed description of ethical theories—that has been done elsewhere—but to categorize and summarize the better-known theories (see Table 5.1) and to suggest ways by which their content can be applied to health education practice.

The primary means by which ethical theories have been categorized has been to place them in the category of formalism (**deontology,** or **nonconsequentialism,** as some refer to it) or consequentialism (or **teleology** as some refer to it). **Formalism** includes "those theories which look at the nature of the individual act and determine morality from whether that act is right or wrong in itself" (Mellert, 1995, p. 130). For example, a formalist would argue that lying to a client or patient is wrong even if it is done to help that person. According to this theory, the mere act of lying is wrong, regardless of the benefits it may bring. "What is moral or immoral is decided on some standard or standards of morality other than consequences" (Thiroux, 1995, p. 84)—that is to say, the end (the consequences) *does not* justify the means (the act).

Consequentialism, on the other hand, evaluates the moral status of an act by looking at its consequences (White, 1988). If the act produces good or happiness, it is morally okay; if it does not, it is immoral. Using the same example of lying to a patient/client, if the consequences turned out okay, the consequentialist would see this act as morally okay. In short, this category of ethical theories states that the end *does* justify the means.

As can be seen from these descriptions of formalism and consequentialism, the primary point of contention is whether or not the means justify the end. "The ethical question in both systems is: 'What is the right thing to do?'" (Tschudin, 2003, p. 47). "Is there a way to reconcile these two approaches to ethics, or must we simply make a choice between them?" (Mellert, 1995, p. 133). Most people would say that neither category of ethical theory can answer all moral questions in their lives. There are times formalism provides guidance for the ethical way to act, while consequentialism is best in other situations. What this means is that each person must carefully study the ethical theory options, combine what is compatible and resolve what is inconsistent in those options, and attempt to work out a moral consensus for herself and society (Mellert, 1995). This is not an easy process. Many times, philosophical questions and problems are abstract or conceptual in nature. For example, is there ever a time when it is okay for a health educator to lie to his supervisor? Such questions are answered through philosophical thought, using reason, logic, and argument. Thus, the most important tool people can use to find these answers is the mind.

When analyzing an ethical problem, people need to depend more on thinking than feeling—using their minds and not their hearts (White, 1988). For example, if a person says, "I feel that abortion, no matter when it occurs, is morally wrong," that person is really saying there is something about abortion that makes her uneasy, unhappy, or distressed. This person is expressing a feeling, not a moral position. This person's feelings would be better stated if she were to say, "Abortion makes me feel upset." However, if a person states that abortion is immoral, then she should be prepared to provide specific reasons for holding this belief (White, 1988). For example, she may hold the belief that life begins at conception, and having an abortion is ending the life of another human being. It is for these reasons that answering ethical questions is a thinking, not a feeling, process. Or, as Penland and Beyrer (1981) have stated, "If ethics is to have personal meaning it demands thoughtful examination. The answers to ethical questions are found by looking within, examining our personal belief systems and values, and using our intelligence to integrate what we have learned and what we have experienced with what we believe and value" (p. 6).

Basic Principles for Common Moral Ground

As was shown in the previous section, formalists and consequentialists are not in agreement when it comes to the rationale to be used in making moral decisions. No single ethical theory can answer every ethical question to the satisfaction of all, yet, to live in a moral society, all must be able to work from a common moral ground. "We must search for a larger meeting ground in which the best of all these theories and systems can operate meaningfully with a minimum of conflict and opposition" (Thiroux, 1995, p. 172).

To help us with this common ground, Thiroux (1995) has identified five basic principles that can apply to human morality, regardless of the embraced theory. The principles do not provide the answers to how one should behave, but rather "help to direct the thinking towards achieving a consensus on what ought to be done in difficult circumstances" (Tschudin, 2003, p. 51). The first principle is the **value of life** principle. This is the most basic of principles. Without living human beings, there can be no ethics. Thiroux (1995) has specifically stated this principle as "human beings should revere life and accept death" (p. 180). This means that no life should be ended without very strong justification. This, for example, is why topics such as abortion, suicide, euthanasia, and capital punishment raise a number of ethical questions.

The second principle is the principle of **goodness (rightness).** "Good" and "right" are at the core of every ethical theory. Theorists may disagree on what is good and bad and right and wrong, but they all strive for goodness and rightness.

"'Good' should not only be in abstract but it should be seen in relation to (other) human beings. As an example, a person who is suicidal may no longer value his or her life as 'good,' but that person's mother may have a very different concept of the value of her child's life" (Tschudin, 2003, p. 56).

It should be noted that several others (e.g., Fox & Swazey, 1997; Jecker, 1997) have presented the principle of goodness as two related principles: (1) the principle of **nonmaleficence** and (2) the principle of **beneficence,** or **benevolence.** "Briefly, nonmaleficence refers to the non-infliction of harm to others. The principle involves a moral obligation to 'above else, do no harm.' It encompasses bringing intentional harm to others as well as the risk of bringing harm that is non-intentional. It also encompasses harm which may result from both action and inaction—acts of omission and commission" (Balog et al., 1985, p. 91). Further, nonmaleficence can "be broken into three components: not inflicting harm, preventing harm, and removing harm when it is present" (Greenberg, 2001, p. 3). "Beneficence means simply doing good. It holds that we have the responsibility for taking positive steps to help others, including acts which involve: doing good, removing evil and/or harm, and preventing harm or evil. Beneficence is generally thought to be more altruistic and more far reaching than nonmaleficence because it requires that we take positive steps to help others" (Balog et al., 1985, pp. 91–92). In the bioethical realm, nonmaleficence and beneficence make up the "benefit-harm ratio" in which, ideally, benefits outweigh costs and in which the "minimization of harm" rather than the "maximation of good" is more strongly emphasized (Fox & Swazey, 1997).

Thiroux's third principle is the principle of **justice (fairness).** This principle states "that human beings should treat other human beings fairly and justly in distributing goodness and badness among them" (Thiroux, 1995, p. 184). Does this mean that all people will always get their fair share of goodness and badness? No, but it does mean everyone will have an equal chance at obtaining the good (Thiroux, 1995). "The bottom line is that one has indeed acted justly toward a person when that person has been given what she or he is due or owed" (Balog et al., 1985, p. 90). "The ethical questions are: Who should receive the benefits from good human actions and how should they be distributed?" (Tschudin, 2003, p. 57). For example, should only those who are able to pay for it receive health education?

The fourth principle of this common moral ground is the principle of **truth telling (honesty).** At the heart of any moral relationship is communication. A necessary component of any meaningful communication is telling the truth, being honest. This may be the most difficult principle to live by. This is not to say that people will never lie or that lying might be justified, but there is a need for a strong attempt to be truthful. In the end, morality depends on what people say and do (Thiroux, 1995). Health educators working in a clinical setting may be faced with this principle when caught in a situation in which an ill child (and a minor by law) asks about his or her health problem, but the child's parent or guardian has strictly forbidden such communication.

The fifth principle is that of **individual freedom (equality principle** or **principle of autonomy).** "The word *autonomy* comes from the Greek words *autos* ('self') and *nomos* ('rule,' 'governance,' or 'law') and originally referred to as self-governance in Greek city-states" (Greenberg, 2001, p. 3). "This principle means

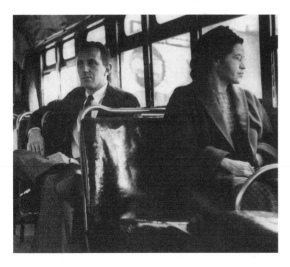 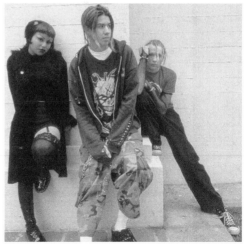

Individual freedom is an important principle of human morality. (l. Corbis; r. Michael Newman/PhotoEdit)

that people, being individuals with individual differences, must have the freedom to choose their own ways and means of being moral within the framework of the first four basic principles" (Thiroux, 1995, p. 187). This is to say that individual freedom is limited by the other four principles. This is a principle that health educators deal with on a regular basis, specifically as it relates to helping others engage in enhancing health behavior. Health educators need to respect the rights of others to deliberate, choose, and act (Balog et al., 1985).

With the grounding of the ethical theories and the establishment of these basic principles, let us examine the process of making ethical decisions.

Making Ethical Decisions

"Ethical decision making in health education, as in other areas, involves determining right and wrong within situations where clear demarcations do not exist or are not clearly apparent to the decision maker. . . . To be considered a professional health educator, one must possess requisite skill and knowledge in making individual decisions. And, in making decisions it is imperative that one has analyzed his or her decisions in terms of standards of right and wrong, good and bad" (Balog et al., 1985, p. 88). In order to decide and, in turn, act in an ethical manner, people must rely on their values, principles, and ethical thinking. To assist in this process, a number of authors (e.g., Balog et al., 1985; Feeney & Freeman, 1999; Fisher, 2003; Johnstone, 1999; Koocher & Keith-Spiegel, 1998; Mellert, 1995; Thompson, Melia, & Boyd, 2000; Tschudin, 2003) have presented guides for applying the concepts presented earlier in this chapter to everyday ethical decision making. Though the number of steps and labels used to identify the steps are different from guide to guide, they "have in common a process of moving from the present problematic to a fu-

---

Box 5.1   Steps in Ethical Decision Making

Step 1: Define the nature of the problem and seek answers to relevant informational questions.

Step 2: Contemplate the ultimate goals
and ideals for which you as a
moral person are striving.

Step 3: Consider the probable consequences of each alternative
under reflection.

Step 4: Consider the nature of the
alternatives.

Step 5: Reflect on yourself.

Step 6: Reflect on your society and your
environment.

Step 7: Apply the categorical imperative.

Step 8: Choose your alternative (Balog
et al., 1985) and act courageously and decisively.

Source: Adapted from Mellert, R. B. 1995.
Seven ethical principles. Dubuque, IA: Kendall/
Hunt.

---

ture more satisfactory situation" (Tschudin, 2003, p. 111). Because of the limitation
of space, we are presenting a single approach (Mellert, 1995) (see Box 5.1) to ethical decision making that is representative of these other guides.

The ethical decision-making process should begin long before any ethical
problems surface. The process begins when a person develops and sustains a professional commitment to doing what is right (Fisher, 2003). Such a commitment will
go a long way toward creating a work environment that can prevent many ethical
problems. This is not to say that all ethical problems will be avoided. Ethical problems can arise in situations in which two or more ethical principles appear to be in
conflict, in unforeseen reactions from those with whom health educators may work,
or in unexpected events (Fisher, 2003). However, having a commitment to doing
what is right becomes a form of "primary prevention" for many ethical problems.

Closely aligned with a commitment to doing what is right, is familiarity with
what the health education profession expects of practicing professionals. Stated differently, what are the expected norms for those who practice health education?
Such expectations can be found in the profession's code of ethics (see Appendix A).
With a commitment to doing what is right and knowing what is expected of a practicing professional, health educators are better prepared to make decisions when
confronted with an ethical problem.

The first step to take when confronted with an ethical decision is to "define the
nature of the problem and seek answers to relevant informational questions"
(Mellert, 1995, p. 156). Such questions include the following: What is possible and
what is not? Does a decision have to be made? If so, by when and in what context?
Are these decisions within the realm of your authority, or are they determined by
someone else with other responsibilities/authority/resources? Is there a legal question that must be answered? Balog et al. (1985) have referred to this step as analyzing the alternatives.

Second, "contemplate the ultimate goals and ideals for which you as a moral
person are striving. What are the most noble human aspirations that pertain to this
concrete situation?" (Mellert, 1995, p. 156). How should you as an ethical person
want to act in this situation? Consider the ethical theory you embrace and the prin-

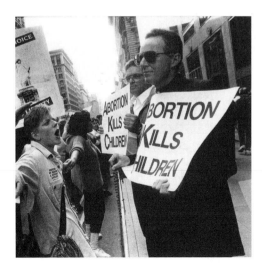

Social context plays an important role in ethical decision making. (Hazel Hankin/ Stock, Boston)

ciples for common ethical ground. How do these goals and ideals apply to this decision? Ultimate goals and ideals do not always apply to every decision and sometimes may not be appropriate, but, to the extent that they do apply, let them help with the decision.

Third, "consider the probable consequences of each alternative under reflection" (Mellert, 1995, p. 157). Look at both the short- and long-term consequences of each alternative. How will these consequences affect you, others, and the environment? In other words, weigh the strengths and weaknesses of the alternatives based on the consequences (Balog et al., 1985). Maybe the consequences are very different, or maybe they are not and, thus, may not be important in the final decision.

Fourth, "consider the nature of the alternatives" (Mellert, 1995, p. 157). Consider the formalist approach to the decision-making process in selecting an alternative. Does the alternative lead to an act or a behavior that is wrong, according to the natural law hypothesis? Would you be violating anyone's basic rights? Does it go against basic human ideals and intrinsic moral values? If you answer yes to these questions, you do not need to eliminate the alternative from further consideration but should give greater consideration to alternatives that do not violate this portion of your reflection.

Fifth, "reflect on yourself" (Mellert, 1995, p. 157). What impact will a proposed course of action have on you as a moral person? Will it enhance or detract from your moral stature? If it detracts, then maybe other alternatives should be considered. If you cannot accept a course of action "as part of your inner self and as data for your own moral growth, then there must be something morally questionable about it" (Mellert, 1995, pp. 157–158).

Sixth, "reflect on your society and your environment" (Mellert, 1995, p. 158). Will your action mesh with that of society and the environment? Moral acts are unselfish acts in that they do not prefer one's own interests at the expense of the interests of others (Mellert, 1995). Will society in general see your action as morally correct?

Seventh, "apply the categorical imperative" (Mellert, 1995, p. 158). Would you want your course of action to be a role model for others? If others were faced with the same decision, is this how you would want them to act?

Eighth, choose your alternative (Balog et al., 1985) and "act courageously and decisively" (Mellert, 1995, p. 158). You have put a great deal of effort and thought into this conclusion. You have acted responsibly; you should have no regrets and feel no guilt over your decision.

In considering these components in Mellert's guide, it is important to note that Mellert realizes that moral decision making does not occur in a vacuum. If it were, every decision would be resolved with the "right" alternative for all. Each decision is surrounded by the context in which it must be made. Mellert feels that, when working through the guide, a person must consider and be aware of the context. When making ethical decisions, people must have a sense of:

1. Place. Be aware of the appropriateness of an action in a particular environment. One action may be appropriate in one setting but not in another.

2. Time. Be aware of the history leading up to the decision and other similar decisions. Learn from past decisions.

3. Identity. Who am I? How does this moral decision relate to me?

4. Social relationships. Be aware that making moral decisions will impact social relationships. There is a good chance that not everyone will agree with your decision and action.

5. The ideal. When making a moral decision, aim for the most noble ideals of humanity.

6. The concrete. Never lose sight of the fact that choices arise from concrete events.

7. Seriousness. When making a moral decision, do so with an attitude that is appropriate to the situation.

Now let us see if we can apply Mellert's guide to the profession of health education. Consider the following ethical dilemma. You are the health educator responsible for the employee health promotion program of your organization. Based on the results of the health risk appraisals you administered, you are aware that one employee, "high up in the organization" (e.g., school principal, department manager), is a consistent abuser of alcohol. This person's supervisor is also aware of the situation but has decided to ignore it. The employee in question is well liked within the organization and is a good employee. To the best of your knowledge, alcohol has not impacted this person's work performance, but you feel it has the potential to do so. What should you do with this information? Consider the following questions:

Step 1. Nature of the problem

1. Do you have to do anything with this information?

2. What are your alternatives?

3. How soon do you need to make a decision? Are others in danger?

4. Are there others who can help you with this decision?

Step 2. The ultimate goals and ideals

1. How does this situation fit with the ethical theory you embrace?

2. What is the good, or right, thing to do?

3. Is individual freedom/autonomy a concern?

Step 3. Consequences of the alternatives

1. What are the short- and long-term benefits (or costs) of all involved for each alternative?
2. Will there be a big difference in the final outcome based on the alternative selected?
3. How will the consequences impact you, others, the environment, and the organization?

Step 4. Nature of the alternatives

1. Do any of the alternatives violate certain human ideals or intrinsic moral rules or values?
2. Would you be acting immorally?

Step 5. Reflection on yourself

1. Would you be enhancing your moral standing?
2. Can you accept (live with) your own action?

Step 6. Reflection on society and the environment

1. What impact will your decision have on society? The environment? In other words, how will others be impacted? Other workers? Members of this person's family?
2. Is your decision consistent with the way society in general would deal with this?
3. Is there a norm? Is it ethical?

Step 7. Categorical imperative

1. Have you acted as a role model?
2. Is this how you hope others would act in the same situation?

Step 8. Choose an alternative and act courageously and decisively

1. How will you handle the situation with the alcohol-abusing employee?
2. Do you even have a responsibility to act?
3. If so, with whom do you speak first? The employee? The supervisor?
4. Do you go above the supervisor and share the information with those at the next level?
5. Should you do nothing?
6. What is the morally right thing to do?
7. What if the employee is punished or even fired for the behavior?
8. What if the employee hurts someone else at home or on the job because of the alcohol use?
9. What if the newspaper acquires this information and shares it with the whole community?

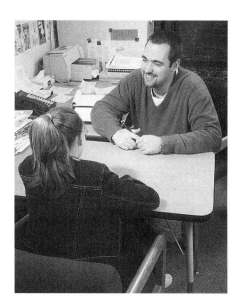

The professional-client relationship is an obligation that is often encountered by health educators. (Spencer Grant/PhotoEdit)

As you can see, moral decisions are not easy to make. They are not to be taken lightly and responsible action is important. Remember, this decision will not occur in a vacuum; the "ideal" decision may not be the best decision.

Ethical Issues and Health Education

As noted at the beginning of this chapter, ethical concerns interface with all aspects of our lives. That includes our professional lives too. "Professional ethics seeks to determine what the role of professions is and what the conduct of professionals should be" (Bayles, 1989, p. 13). "Health educators face a complex array of ethical dilemmas in professional practice" (Iammarino et al., 1989, p. 104). Although some of the ethical issues faced by health educators are very specific to the profession, such as the ethical issues surrounding getting clients to begin a health-enhancing behavior, the majority of concerns affecting most professions are similar (Hiller, 1987).

Bayles (1989) has organized the substantive obligations of professions and professionals, regardless of the profession, from which most professional ethical dilemmas arise. The following is a list of these obligations, with several questions that relate the obligations to the practice of health education.

1. **Obligations and availability of services.** The primary issue related to this obligation is the equality of opportunity for making professional services available to all citizens. Examples of ethical issues associated with this obligation include the right to legal counsel, access to health care, and refusal to accept clients for lack of ability to pay. (Who should receive health education? What about clients who are hard to reach? In what settings should it be offered? Should clients have to pay for health education, or should health education be denied if a person cannot pay? Should health educators ever terminate an intervention before it is complete? Is

---

Box 5.2   *Informed Consent: An Ethical Obligation*

The term **"informed consent"** is often associated with medical procedures or research projects, but it is also important in health education/promotion. The concept behind informed consent is that people—whether patients, research subjects, or participants in a health education/promotion program—should be given sufficient information from which to make informed choices about whether or not they want a certain medical procedure, or to participate in a research project or health education/ promotion program (NCI, 2004). From an ethical standpoint, "the idea of consent is based on the principle of respect for the person, and thus on the concept of human rights of life and liberty" (Tschudin, 2003, p. 172).

Valid informed consent requires: a) disclosure of relevant information to prospective participants about the program; b) their comprehension of the information, and c) their voluntary agreement, free from coercion and undue influence, to participate (OHSR, n. d.).

Though receiving a medical procedure or participating in a clinical trial often carries more risks than participating in a health education/promotion program, individuals should not be allowed to participate in any health education/ promotion program without giving their informed consent (McKenzie, Neiger, & Smeltzer, 2005). In practice, the informed consent process should include: 1) the health educator discussing the details of the program (i.e., purpose of the program, description of the intervention, risks and benefits associated with participation, alternative programs that will accomplish the same thing, and the freedom to discontinue participation at any time) with the prospective participant; 2) the participant having an opportunity to ask questions about the program; and 3) the participant signing a written informed consent document.

---

there ever a time when a health educator should use an intervention in which the possible outcomes are questionable?)

2. **Obligations between professionals and clients.** Once the services of a professional have been secured, a number of ethical issues can arise from the professional-client relationship. "The fiduciary model presents the best ethical ideal for the professional-client relationship" (Bayles, 1989, p. 100). In such a model, the professional is honest, candid, competent, loyal, fair, and discrete. At the same time, the client keeps commitments to the professional, is truthful to the professional, and does not request unethical acts from the professional. (Is there ever a time when health educators should not be candid or honest with their clients? How should health educators respond when their clients ask them about their personal behavior? Is there ever a time when a health educator should not obtain informed consent before proceeding with an intervention?) (See Box 5.2.)

3. **Obligations to third parties.** This obligation revolves around what others need to know about the professional-client relationship. Often professionals are confronted with the issue of whether or not to share client information with family members of the client, people in a supervisory capacity (e.g., teachers, employers), legal authorities (e.g., police, lawyers), or peers (e.g., professional colleagues). (What

---

Box 5.3   Privacy and HIPAA

One of the most basic concepts associated with providing a service (e.g., health education) to other people is that of privacy. **Privacy** has been defined as "the claim of individuals, groups, or institutions to determine for themselves when, how, and to what extent information about them is communicated to others" (Westin, 1968, p. 7). Thus, when people have agreed to participate in a health education/promotion program, it becomes the duty of the health educator to protect the information provided by participants.

The importance of privacy for health educators, and all others associated with health care, was further emphasized with the enactment of the Health Insurance Portability and Accountability Act of 1996 (officially known as Public Law 104-191 and referred to as HIPAA). HIPAA includes: 1) privacy standards for the use and disclosure of individually identifiable private health information; 2) transaction standards for the electronic exchange of health information; and 3) security standards to protect the creation and maintenance of private health information. The HIPAA regulations apply to protected health information (PHI), whether transmitted orally, in writing, or electronically, that is generated by an employer, a health plan, a health clearinghouse, or a health care provider, or in connection with financial or administrative activities related to health care (Fisher, 2003). Failure to implement the standards can lead to civil and criminal penalties (USDHHS, 2003).

The two techniques that are used to protect the privacy of program participants are anonymity and confidentiality. **Anonymity** exists when no one, including those conducting the program, can relate a participant's identity to any information pertaining to the program. In applying this concept, health educators would need to ensure that collected information had no identifying marks attached to it such as the participant's name, social security number, or any other less common information. In practice, because of the nature (the need to know about the participants) of most health education/promotion programs, anonymity is not often used. Its most common application in health education/promotion is in conducting research projects.

On the other hand, the concept of confidentiality is common in health education/promotion programs. **Confidentiality** exists when only those responsible for conducting a program can link information about a participant with the individual and do not reveal such information to others. Thus, health educators need to take every precaution to protect participants' information. Often this means keeping the information "under lock and key" while the program is being conducted, then destroying (e.g., shredding) the information when it is no longer needed.

---

duty does a health educator have to share information with a student's parents when the student has shared the information with the health educator in confidence? Is there ever a time when a health educator can share confidential information? How about with the insurance company of a client? With the client's employer?) (See Box 5.3.)

4. **Obligations between professionals and employers.** Employed professionals have obligations to employers that are similar to the obligation they have to their clients (see #2 above). "However, the obligation to obey employers is stronger than an obligation to clients. It includes acting as, and only as, authorized" (Bayles, 1989, p. 158). On the other hand, "employers' obligations to professional employees are universal, role related, and contractual" (Bayles, 1989, p. 159). Ethical issues related to this obligation often involve due process, confidentiality, and professional support. (Should health educators always implement "company" policy when they know it is wrong or could bring harm to a client? What if a health educator has a conflict of interest between his personal life and what his employer says he must do? Is there ever a time when health educators should publicly speak against their employers?) (See Box 5.4.)

5. **Obligations to the profession.** "These obligations rest on the responsibilities of a profession as a whole to further social values" (Bayles, 1989, p. 179). Issues associated with this obligation include conducting research, reforming the profession, and maintaining respect for the profession. (Is there ever a reason health educators should not behave in a professional manner? What duty does a health educator have to report the inappropriate behavior of a colleague? What obligations do health educators have to keep up-to-date on the content of their fields?)

Having identified problems that may cut across all professions, let us examine those that are more specific to health education. First, Penland and Beyrer (1981) state that ethical issues are defined by two criteria. "First they must be 'issues'; that is, there must be controversy related to the problem or topic. There must be 'two sides,' supported by people with two different viewpoints" (p. 6). Issues, by definition, are controversial. For example, the need for youth to know sexual information is not an issue; however, who should provide such information is an issue.

"The second criterion for an ethical issue in health education is that it must involve a question of right and wrong" (Penland & Beyrer, 1981, p. 6). "Can health education programs in the worksite change health behavior?" may be a controversial issue, but it does not deal with rightness and wrongness. Thus, it is not an ethical issue, but "does an employer have the right to make all employees attend the health education program?" is an ethical issue.

Now that we know what comprises an ethical issue, let us look at some of the ethical issues health educators are likely to face. The literature is abundant with examples of ethical issues in health education. Issues cited include abstinence-only and abstinence-plus sexuality education (Wiley, 2002), curriculum development (Barnes, Fors, & Decker, 1980; Penland & Beyrer, 1981; Richardson & Jose, 1983), the business of health promotion (McLeroy, Gottlieb, & Burdine, 1987), the economics of health promotion (Warner, 1987), ethics instruction (Modell & Citrin, 2002), government-sponsored health campaigns (Faden, 1987), health behavior change (Hochbaum, 1980; O'Connell & Price, 1983; Read & Russell, 1985; Wikler, 1978), health education research (Buchanan et al., 2002; Minkler et al., 2002), health promotion evaluation (Thurston, Vollman, & Burgess, 2003), health risk appraisals (SPM, 1999), the mission of health education (Penland & Beyrer, 1981), research/scientific inquiry/publishing (Barnes, Fors, & Decker, 1980; Breckon,

---

Box 5.4 Practitioner's Perspective: Ethics

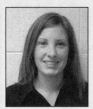

NAME: Brittany Mathers, B.S., B.P.H.E.

CURRENT POSITION/TITLE: Hepatitis C Surveillance Employee, Indiana State Department of Health

EMPLOYER: Ball State University through a grant from the Indiana State Department of Health

DEGREE/INSTITUTION/YEAR: B.S. and B.P.H.E., Queen's University, Kingston, Ontario, 2003

MAJOR: Health and Physical Education, and Biology

MINOR: Health

Describe an ethical issue that you have had to deal with as a health educator: For my first job in the health education field I was a Fitness and Lifestyle Counselor for business executives enrolled in an executive development program. In this position, I "coached" program participants on how to improve their current health status through lifestyle modification and provided the opportunity to participate in daily physical activities. Each evening, there would be a required social activity for the Fitness and Lifestyle Counselors, so we could continue to spread the health and wellness message. These evening activities however, were often held at local bars and clubs. The ethical issue I was faced with in this situation was supporting and providing opportunity for unhealthy behavior while trying to educate people on the importance of leading a healthy lifestyle. As a health educator, this portion of my job conflicted with both my personal beliefs and my professional ethical standards.

How did you handle the issue? Because I was required to attend the evening activities to fulfill my job, at first I didn't know how to deal with the situation. After several weeks, I spoke with my coworkers as well as my supervisor and expressed my concern. My supervisor was very supportive and recognized the ethical issue the Fitness and Lifestyle Counselors were faced with on a regular basis. As a result, our job description changed and attending the evening activities became optional.

Looking back on the issue, what might you have done differently? There are several things that I could have done differently in this situation. Looking back, I would ask more questions during the job

(Box 5.4 *continues*)

Harvey, & Lancaster, 1998; Iammarino et al., 1989; Margolis, 2000; Pigg, 1994; Price & Dake, 2002; Price, Dake, & Islam, 2001; Ross, Sundberg, & Flint, 1999; Seal, Bloom, & Somlai, 2000; Vitello, 1986), the selection of health educators (Barnes, Fors, & Decker, 1980; Penland & Beyrer, 1981), service by health educators (Price, Dake, & Telljohann, 2001), issues and special settings (Pigg, 1994; Roman & Blum, 1987), social marketing (Rothschild, 2000), the teaching of health (Telljohann, Price, & Dake, 2001), topical areas (Breckon, et al., 1998; Fennell & Beyrer, 1989), and the teaching of ethics (Odom, 1988; Patterson & Vitello, 1993). McLeroy, Bibeau, and McConnell (1993) have identified other areas of ethical concern, which

(Box 5.4 *continued*)

interview so that I had a better understanding of all the responsibilities the job entailed. Also, I would have immediately raised my concerns with my employer and not waited several weeks before I dealt with the situation. At that point in my career I was unfamiliar with the Code of Ethics for the Health Education Profession. Had I known the different responsibilities a health educator has to employers, this ethical issue could have been dealt with much sooner.

How frequently do you encounter ethical issues in your work? Ethical issues arise a lot in the health education field because of the nature of our work. Most issues, however, are dealt with without being recognized as ethical issues. For example, knowing the limits of your qualifications, respecting the privacy and dignity of others by keeping confidential information to yourself, accepting and acknowledging diverse opinions of others, and providing equal service to all people are ethical behaviors expected from a health educator on a daily basis. As a health educator, it is important to be aware and be familiar with different ethical issues in the field. Using good judgment and following a code of conduct helps to ensure an ethical workplace.

Have you had any training on how to deal with ethical issues? If yes, please describe it. **If no, do you think it should be included in the preparation of health educators?** During my undergraduate degree I took a biomedical ethics course. While this was my first introduction to ethics, it did not cover professional ethical issues a health educator faces, but rather ethical issues associated with health care. This course was an elective and thus, not all health education students were required to take it. I believe that training on how to deal with ethical issues should be included in the preparation of health educators, as this emerging profession requires high ethical standards.

What recommendations would you give to health education students to help them prepare for ethical issues like the one you described? My advice to health education students is to always use good judgment. If something does not seem right, it probably isn't. Don't be afraid to raise your concerns with your employer and co-workers as it is likely that others share similar feelings. I highly recommend students read and understand the Code of Ethics for the Health Education Profession. This document helps identify and guide ethical decisions a health educator may face. Time you invest now will certainly pay off in the future, because health educators will inevitably be faced with ethical situations.

reflect the inclusion of health education as a component of health promotion. The major categories of issues raised by McLeroy and colleagues (1993) include:

1. "Assigning individual responsibility to the victim for becoming ill due to personal failures" (p. 314)—for example, becoming ill because one does not exercise, or continues to use tobacco products

2. "Attempting to change individuals and their subsequent behaviors rather than the social environment that supports and maintains unhealthy lifestyles" (p. 314)

3. Using "system interventions to promote health behaviors" (p. 315)—for example, public policy strategies or coercive strategies to modify unhealthy actions

4. Overemphasizing behavior change as a program outcome instead of focusing more on changes in the social and physical environment

5. Overemphasizing the importance of health, forgetting that health is a means to an end, not an end in itself

6. Educating the public on the concept of risk and how to properly use risk factor information

7. Underemphasizing professional behavior, regardless of the health education setting—for example, keeping up-to-date, serving as a role model, and providing ethics education for the next generation of health educators

Ensuring Ethical Behavior

The majority of this chapter has been used to identify and deal with ethical issues and discuss why it is important to act ethically. What we have yet to discuss is how the profession can ensure that professionals will behave ethically. It cannot. Professionals who act unethically usually do so (1) for personal financial gain and reputation and (2) for the benefit of clients or employers without considering the effects on others (Bayles, 1989). However, a profession, and an emerging profession, can put procedures into place to work toward ethical behavior by all.

Some procedures put in place by professions are limited, in some form, to those who are in professional preparation programs and those who have already been admitted to the profession. Traditional ways of doing this have been through (1) selective admissions into academic programs, (2) retention standards to remain in academic programs, (3) graduation from academic programs, (4) completion of internships, (5) the process of becoming credentialed (i.e., certified or licensed to practice), and (6) continual updating to retain the credential. While proceeding through these steps, individuals may have to provide evidence of good moral character.

Once in the profession, professionals are expected to behave according to a system of norms. As noted earlier in this chapter, this system of norms (or professional moral consensus, as some refer to it) is often placed in writing and referred to as a code of ethics. More specifically, a **code of ethics** is a "document that maps the dimensions of the profession's collective social responsibility and acknowledges the obligations individual practitioners share in meeting the profession's responsibilities" (Feeney & Freeman, 1999, p. 6). Such a document is usually not only useful for the professional but also for those who use the services of the professional. An ethical code's principal function is to ensure minimal standards of practice for those for whom it was written (Thomasma, 1979). In other words, an ethical code sets standards "for honor, virtue, and dignity" (Iammarino et al., 1989, p. 101) and "helps professionals become aware of what is generally considered right or wrong professionally" (Richardson & Jose, 1983, p. 5). It also provides the consumers of health education services with an understanding of what they should expect from the provider.

Further, a profession should also have a means by which to deal with (discipline) professionals who violate the code of ethics. "A wide range of enforcement mechanisms are possible" (Taub, Kreuter, Parcel, & Vitello, 1987, p. 82). Such mechanisms may range from self-monitoring to a more formal process in which ethics cases are reviewed by a committee of peers. When self-monitoring is used, charges of the ethical violation "might be conveyed directly to the professional charged with the violation. That person would then be responsible for resolving the situation. This procedure works well when there is peer pressure for professionals to behave consistent with a clearly identifiable set of standards and rules of professional conduct" (Gold & Greenberg, 1992, p. 143). When ethical violations are reviewed by an ethics committee of the profession or as part of a professional organization, the "committees usually have the authority to recommend sanctions against members who are judged to behave unethically" (Gold & Greenberg, 1992, p. 143). First and/or minor violations of ethical behavior often carry disciplinary measures of "warnings." Repeated and/or major violations can lead to more serious penalties like limitations on the ability to practice and "even outright expulsion from the profession (that is, decertification or rescinding the member's license to practice)" (Gold & Greenberg, 1992, p. 145).

How does health education address these procedures for ensuring ethical behavior? Currently, the admission procedure into the profession of health education is not clear. Some colleges and universities preparing health educators have selective admission standards, but most have open admissions, meaning that students can enter the health education program if admitted to the institution. Once in the program, all academic institutions have retention standards and graduation requirements, however minimal they may be—minimum grades in certain courses or a grade point average of 2.0 on a 4-point scale. With regard to the amount of education required in the profession, a bachelor's degree is required to sit for the credentialing examination (CHES) (see Chapter 6); however, there is no consensus in the profession that a bachelor's degree should be the standard. Many feel a master's degree is more appropriate. Regardless of whether a bachelor's or master's degree is required to take the credentialing examination, the earned credential (CHES) is not universally accepted, either in or out of the profession, as necessary to practice health education.

The profession of health education has had a code of ethics for a number of years. The first was created in 1976 by the Society for Public Health Education (SOPHE). That code was later revised in 1983 and abridged in 1993. Though that code was developed more than twenty years ago, it was not universally adopted by the profession. In 1984, SOPHE and the Association for the Advancement of Health Education (AAHE; now known as the American Association for Health Education) appointed a joint committee to develop a profession-wide code of ethics. That committee was not able to create a profession-wide code of ethics. Further, in April 1994, AAHE developed another code, the "Code of Ethics for Health Educators." However, in 1995, the National Commission for Health Education Credentialing, Inc. (NCHEC) (see Chapter 6 for more on NCHEC) and Coalition of National Health Education Organizations (CNHEO) (see Chapter 8 for more on CNHEO) co-sponsored a conference, "The Health Education Profession in the Twenty-First Century: Setting the Stage," at which it was recommended that efforts be expanded to develop a profession-wide code of ethics. Soon after that conference the CNHEO began work on such a code. After several years of work, in 1999 the "Code of Ethics for the Health Education Profession" was created and approved by all members of CNHEO, thus replacing the earlier codes developed by SOPHE and AAHE (see Appendix A for a copy of the new code and more information on its development). However, like the codes before it, the new code does not include a formal procedure for enforcement. So currently, the profession has informal enforcement via "the subtle influences colleagues exert on one another" (Iammarino et al., 1989, p. 104).

As can be seen from this analysis, the health education profession is moving in the right direction but still has much opportunity to refine its ethical foundations.

SUMMARY

Ethical questions impact all aspects of life. Individuals on both a personal and professional level are constantly being confronted with ethical dilemmas. To deal with these situations, people must have a basic understanding of how to make an ethical decision. To prepare readers for this task, this chapter presented key terms, such as *philosophy, ethics,* and *morals;* the philosophical, practical, and professional viewpoints of why people and professionals should work from an ethical base; the two major categories of theories (formalism and consequentialism) used to create ethical "yardsticks" for making ethical decisions; a set of principles and a guide for ethical decision making; a sampling of the ethical issues facing health educators today; and a discussion about how a profession, or an emerging profession, can ensure that its professionals will act ethically.

REVIEW QUESTIONS

1. What are the three major areas of philosophy? What does each of them mean?
2. In your own words, how do you define *ethics*?
3. What do the definitions of *ethics* and *morals* share? How are they different?
4. Why is it important to act ethically?
5. What is meant by the term *professional ethics*?
6. How would you summarize the difference between the two major categories of ethical theories?
7. What are Thiroux's five principles that create a common ground for all ethical theories?
8. What should be included in a guide for making ethical decisions?
9. Name five ethical issues currently facing the profession of health education.
10. What can a profession do to ensure that its professionals will act ethically?
11. Define code of ethics.

CRITICAL THINKING QUESTIONS

1. If you were asked by one of your professors to help design a professional ethics course for health education majors/minors at your college/university, what would you suggest be included in the course? Why?
2. Several professions (e.g., medicine and law) have procedures for dealing with members' unethical behavior. In fact, if the offense is extreme enough a lawyer can be

disbarred and a physician could lose his or her license to practice medicine. Do you think the profession of health education should create a similar process to review unethical behavior and if necessary take away the certification of certified health education specialists (CHES)? Defend your response.

3. Do you think that all health education majors/minors should be required to take an ethics course while in college? Why or why not? If you responded yes to the question, do you think that a general ethics course open to all university students would be sufficient, or do you think the course should be specific to the profession? Why?

ACTIVITIES

Directions for activities 1–4. You will find four scenarios that include an ethical dilemma. Using the guide put forth by Mellert in this chapter, write a response to one of the scenarios. Include in your response a paragraph for each of the components of Mellert's guide. Your eight paragraphs should state your course of action.

1. You have been hired to work for the city health department to complete a project that was begun by your predecessor and funded with money from the National Institutes of Health (NIH). The grant requires the health department to develop X number of programs on the topic of hepatitis and then to present these programs to X number of people representing very specific priority groups in the community. After being hired, you discover that the administrator of the grant, your supervisor, has not adhered to the grant guidelines. Only half the number of programs have been developed as the grant required. Further, the number of presentations is less than required, and presentations have been given to people not in the identified priority groups. In addition, your supervisor has taken some of the travel funds allocated to pay for your travel to and from presentations and has diverted them into his personal travel fund to attend a national conference in Las Vegas. It is now time for you to develop your year-end report, which will be sent directly to NIH. Your supervisor has provided you with a copy of the original grant proposal and says to make sure your figures agree with those in the proposal. In other words, he expects you to "fudge" the data. What will you do?

2. As the health and fitness director of a large corporate wellness program, you have been asked to provide data to your supervisor that supports the effectiveness of your program. The trend in the company has been to cut programs that do not "carry their weight." The "bottom line" is important. In your review of the data related to your program, it is obvious that the data are not very strong. However, in fairness to you, the program has been in operation for only two years, and it is too early to see the type of results management is looking for. You are the only one who has access to the data, and no one will know if the data you submit are accurate. How will you handle this situation?

3. You are a high school health teacher. The board of education has just adopted a policy that prohibits the teaching or discussing of information related to contraceptives or abortion in the district. The only approach that can be mentioned in the classroom is abstinence. As a professional health educator, you have read that the abstinence approach is ineffective with a significant number of students. After class one day, one of your students approaches you and informs you that she is pregnant. She requests your help and asks for the name and location of an abortion clinic. She also asks that you not tell anyone else about this. What will you do?

4. You are the health educator for a large city hospital. Your supervisor has asked you to develop a program on "safer sex" practices for the gay and lesbian population. The

program is to be provided to each HIV-positive person who enters the hospital, and it is to be made available to lesbian and gay groups in the community. Because of your strong religious convictions, your personal values and beliefs are opposed to the gay/lesbian lifestyle and the "safer sex" approach. In addition, you feel very uncomfortable dealing with homosexuals in general and especially with anyone who is HIV-positive. How will you handle this situation?

5. Read thoroughly the "Code of Ethics for the Health Education Profession" presented in Appendix A, then provide written answers to the following questions.

   • What is your overall opinion of the code? Does it include everything you thought it would? Were there any surprises?

   • Is there anything in the code you feel should not be there? If so, what?

   • If you could add something else to the code, what would it be?

   • Do you think the profession should incorporate a means of enforcement in the code? Why or why not?

6. Select one of the ethical theories presented in Table 5.1 to study further. Find and read from other sources explaining the theory. Then write a three-page paper on the theory's application to the practice of health education.

7. Make an appointment to meet with one of your professors or with a practicing health educator. Inform him/her that you would like to spend about fifteen to twenty minutes discussing professional ethics. At the meeting ask him/her if he/she has ever observed a professional situation that involved an ethical dilemma. If so, ask him/her to describe the situation without revealing the parties who were involved. Then ask how the dilemma was resolved. After your meeting, summarize in writing the discussion and compare the steps taken in the situation to the components of Mellert's guide. Do you think the dilemma was handled properly? Why or why not?

WEBLINKS

1. **http://hsc.usf.edu/CFH/cnheo**

   Coalition of National Health Education Organizations (CNHEO)

   This is the home page for the CNHEO. The Coalition has as its primary mission the mobilization of the resources of the health education profession in order to expand and improve health education, regardless of the setting. At this site you can print out a copy of the Code of Ethics for the Health Education Profession.

2. **http://www.ethics.org/**

   Ethics Resource Center (ERC)

   The ERC is a nonprofit, nonpartisan educational organization whose mission is to strengthen ethical leadership worldwide by providing leading-edge expertise and services through research, education, and partnerships.

3. **http://www.usoge.gov/**

   U.S. Office of Government Ethics (OGE)

   The OGE, a small agency within the executive branch, exercises leadership in the executive branch to prevent conflicts of interest on the part of government employees, and to resolve conflicts of interest that do occur. This site provides a view of what an employer—the federal government in this case—expects in terms of ethical behavior.

4. **http://www.professionalethics.ca/**

   Professional Ethics

   This is a Canadian Web site that provides a wide variety of resources on various topics related to professional ethics. One special feature of this Web site is the presentation of a number of up-to-date articles on professional ethics. It also has links to several other ethics-related Web sites.

5. **http://www.hhs.gov/ocr/hipaa/index.html**

   United States Department of Health and Human Services (USDHHS)

   This is a page at the USDHHS Web site where you can get more information about the National Standards to Protect the Privacy of Personal Health Information.

6. **http://www.cancer.gov/clinicaltrials/understanding/simplification-of-informed-consent-docs**

   National Cancer Institute (NCI)

   This is a page at the NCI Web site where you can get more information about informed consent.

CASE STUDY

Sue accepted a position as a patient educator with the Franklin County Hospital after graduating with her bachelor's degree last spring. She is one of five health educators employed by the patient education department. About three months after Sue was hired, she observed Tom, the most experienced patient educator in the department, engage in what she believed was unethical behavior. Sue observed Tom accepting a really nice windbreaker (worth about $80) from a pharmaceutical company representative. In return, the pharmaceutical rep asked Tom to recommend the pharmaceutical company's glucometer during the diabetes education sessions he ran. Tom said that "that would be no problem." Do you agree with Sue—do you think this is unethical behavior? On what ethical principles do you base your response? Is there something in the "Code of Ethics for the Health Education Profession" (Appendix A) that supports your position? Say you agree with Sue; what would be your course of action? Do you think Tom's supervisor should be involved? Why or why not? Do you think Tom should be sanctioned by the profession? If so, how could it be enforced?

REFERENCES

Balog, J. E., Shirreffs, J. H., Gutierrez, R. D., & Balog, L. F. (1985). Ethics and the field of health education. *The Eta Sigma Gamma Monograph Series, 4*(1), 65–110.

Barnes, S., Fors, S., & Decker, W. (1980). Ethical issues in health education. *Health Education, 11*(2), 7–9.

Bayles, M. D. (1989). *Professional ethics* (2nd ed.). Belmont, CA: Wadsworth.

Breckon, D. J., Harvey, J. R., & Lancaster, R. B. (1998). *Community health education: Settings, roles, and skills for the 21st century* (4th ed.). Gaithersburg, MD: Aspen Publishers.

Buchanan, D., Khoshnood, K., Stopka, T., Shaw, S., Santelices, C., & Singer, M. (2002). Ethical dilemmas created by the criminalization of status behaviors: Case examples from ethnographic field research with injection drug users. *Health Education & Behavior, 29*(1), 30–42.

Dorman, S. M. (1994). The imperative for ethical conduct in scientific inquiry. In R. M. Pigg, (Ed.), Ethical issues of scientific inquiry in health science education. *The Eta Sigma Gamma Monograph Series, 12*(2), 1–5.

Faden, R. R. (1987). Ethical issues in government sponsored public health campaigns. *Health Education Quarterly, 14*(1), 27–37.

Feeney, S., & Freeman, N. K., (1999). *Ethics and the early childhood educator.* Washington, DC: National Association for the Education of Young Children.

Fennell, R. & Beyrer, M. K. (1989). AIDS: Some ethical considerations for the health educators. *Journal of American College Health, 38,* 145–147.

Fisher, C. B. (2003). *Decoding the ethics code: A practical guide for psychologists.* Thousand Oaks, CA: Sage Publications.

Fox, R. C., & Swazey, J. P. (1997). Medical morality is not bioethics: Medical ethics in China and the United States. In N. S. Jecker, A. R. Jonsen, & R. A. Pearlman (Eds.), *Bioethics: An introduction to history, methods and practice* (pp. 237–251). Sudbury, MA: Jones and Bartlett.

Gold, R. S., & Greenberg, J. S. (1992). *The health education ethics book.* Dubuque, IA: Wm. C. Brown Publishers.

Greenberg, J. S. (2001). *The code of ethics for the health education profession: A case study book.* Boston: Jones and Bartlett Publishers.

Hiller, M. D. (1987). Ethics and health education: Issues in theory and practice. In P. M. Lazes, L. Kaplan, & G. A. Gordon (Eds.), *The handbook of health education* (pp. 87–108). Rockville, MD: Aspen.

Hochbaum, G. M. (1980). Ethical dilemmas in health education. *Health Education, 11*(2), 4–6.

Iammarino, N. K., O'Rourke, T. W., Pigg, R. M., & Weinberg, A. D. (1989). Ethical issues in research and publication. *Journal of School Health, 59*(3), 101–104.

Jecker, N. S. (1997). Introduction to the methods of bioethics. In N. S. Jecker, A. R. Jonsen, & R. A. Pearlman (Eds.), *Bioethics: An introduction to history, methods and practice* (pp. 113–125). Sudbury, MA: Jones and Bartlett.

Johnstone, M. J. (1999). *Bioethics: A nursing perspective* (3rd ed.). Sydney, Australia: Elsevier Limited.

Koocher, G. P., & Keith-Spiegel, P. (1998). *Ethics in psychology: Professional standards and cases* (2nd ed.). New York: Oxford University Press.

Margolis, L. (2000). Commentary: Ethical principles for analyzing dilemmas in sex research. *Health Education & Behavior, 27*(1), 24–27.

McGrath, E. Z. (1994). *The art of ethics: A psychology of ethical beliefs.* Chicago: Loyola University Press.

McKenzie, J. F., Neiger, B. L., & Smeltzer, J. L. (2005). *Planning, implementing, and evaluating health promotion programs: A Primer* (4th ed.). San Francisco: Benjamin Cummings.

McLeroy, K. R., Bibeau, D. L., & McConnell, T. C. (1993). Ethical issues in health education and health promotion: Challenges for the profession. *Journal of Health Education, 24*(5), 313–318.

McLeroy, K. R., Gottlieb, N. H., & Burdine, J. N. (1987). The business of health promotion: Ethical issues and professional responsibilities. *Health Education Quarterly, 14*(1), 91–109.

Mellert, R. B. (1995). *Seven ethical theories.* Dubuque, IA: Kendall/Hunt.

Minkler, M., Fadem, P., Perry, M., Blum, K., Moore, L., & Rogers, J. (2002). Ethical dilemmas in participatory action research: A case study from the disability community. *Health Education & Behavior, 29*(1), 14–29.

Modell, S. M., & Citrin, T. (2002). Ethics instruction in an issues-oriented course on public health genetics. *Health Education & Behavior, 29*(1), 43-60.

National Cancer Institute. (2004). Simplification of informed consent documents: Recommendation. Retrieved May 21, 2004, from http://www.cancer.gov.

O'Connell, J. K., & Price, J. H. (1983). Ethical theories for promoting health through behavioral change. *Journal of School Health, 53*(8), 476–479.

Odom, J. G. (1988). The status of ethics instruction in the health education curriculum. *Health Education, 19*(4) 9–12.

Office of Human Subject Research (OHSR). (n.d.). *Guidelines for writing informed consent documents.* Retrieved May 19, 2003, from http://206.102.88.10/ohsrsite/info/sheet6.html.

Patterson, S. M., & Vitello, E. M. (1993). Ethics in health education. The need to include a model course in professional preparation programs. *Journal of Health Education, 24*(4), 239–244.

Penland, L. R., & Beyrer, M. K. (1981). Ethics and health education: Issues and implications. *Health Education, 12*(4), 6–7.

Pigg, R. M. (Ed.). (1994). Ethical issues of scientific inquiry in health science education. *The Eta Sigma Gamma Monograph Series, 12*(2).

Price, J. H., & Dake, J. A. (2002). Ethical guidelines for manuscript reviewers and journal editors. *American Journal of Health Education, 33*(4). 194–196.

Price, J. H., Dake, J. A., & Islam, R. (2001). Ethical issues in research and publication: Perceptions of health education faculty. *Health Education & Behavior, 28,* 51.

Price, J. H., Dake, J. A., & Telljohann, S. K. (2001). Ethical issues regarding service: Perceptions of health education faculty. *American Journal of Health Education, 32*(4), 208–215.

Read, D., & Russell, R. (1985). Is behavioral change an acceptable objective for health educators? *The Eta Sigma Gamma Monograph Series, 4*(1), 9–61.

Richardson, G., & Jose, N. (1983). Ethical issues in school health: A survey. *Health Education, 14*(2), 5–9.

Roman, P., & Blum, T. (1987). Ethics in worksite health programming: Who is served? *Health Education Quarterly, 14,* 57–70.

Ross, J. G., Sundberg, E. C., & Flint, K. H. (1999). Informed consent in school health research: Why, how, and making it easy. *Journal of School Health, 69*(5), 171–176.

Rothschild, M. L. (2000). Ethical considerations in support of marketing of public health issues. *American Journal of Health Behavior, 24*(1), 26–35.

Seal, D. W., Bloom, F. R., & Somlai, A. M. (2000). Ethical principles for analyzing dilemmas in sex research. *Health Education & Behavior, 27*(1), 10–23.

The Society of Prospective Medicine Board of Directors (SPM) (1999). Ethics guidelines for the development and use of health assessments. In G. C. Hyner, K. W. Peterson, J. W. Travis, J. E. Dewey, J. J. Foerster, & E. M. Framer (Eds.). *SPM handbook of health assessment tools* (pp. xxii–xxvi). Pittsburgh, PA: The Society of Prospective Medicine.

Taub, A., Kreuter, M., Parcel, G., & Vitello, E. (1987). Report of the SOPHE/AAHE joint committee on ethics. *Health Education Quarterly, 14*(1), 79–90.

Telljohann, S. K., Price, J. H., & Dake, J. A. (2001). Selected ethical issues in the teaching: Perceptions of health education faculty. *American Journal of Health Education, 32*(2), 66-74.

Thiroux, J. P. (1995). *Ethics: Theory and practice* (5th ed.). Englewood Cliffs, NJ: Prentice-Hall.

Thomasma, D. (1979). Human values and ethics: Professional responsibility. *The Journal of the American Dietetic Association, 75*(5), 533–536.

Thompson, I., Melia, K., & Boyd, K. (2000). *Nursing ethics* (4th ed.). Edinburgh, Scotland: Churchill Livingstone.

Thurston, W. E., Vollman, A. R., & Burgess, M. M. (2003). Ethical review of health promotion program evaluation proposals. *Health Promotion Practice, 4*(1), 45–50.

Tschudin, V. (2003) *Ethics in nursing: The caring relationship* (3rd. ed.). Edinburgh, Scotland: Butterworth Heinemann.

United States Department of Health and Human Services (USDHHS) (2003). *Medical privacy—National standards to protect the privacy of personal health information.* Retrieved May 22, 2003, from http://hhs.gov/hipaa/.

Vitello, E. M. (1986). Ethical issues: Questions in search of answers. *Health Education, 17*(5), 39–42.

Warner, K. E. (1987). Selling health promotion to corporate America: Uses and abuses of the economic argument. *Health Education Quarterly, 14*(1), 39–55.

Westin, A. F. (1968). *Privacy and freedom.* New York: Atheneum.

White, T. I. (1988). *Right and wrong: A brief guide to understanding ethics.* Englewood Cliffs, NJ: Prentice-Hall.

Wikler, D. I. (1978). Coercive measures in health promotion: Can they be justified? *Health Education Monographs, 6*(2), 223–241.

Wiley, D. C. (2002). The ethics of abstinence-only and abstinence-plus sexuality education. *Journal of School Health, 72*(4), 164-167.

CHAPTER 6

The Health Educator: Roles, Responsibilities, Certifications, Advanced Study

Chapter Objectives

After reading this chapter and answering the questions at the end, you should be able to:

1. Define *credentialing.*
2. Discuss the history of role delineation and certification.
3. Explain the differences among *certification, registration, licensure,* and *accreditation.*
4. List and describe the seven major responsibilities of a health educator.
5. Discuss the need for advanced study in health education.
6. Outline factors to consider in applying for master's degree programs.

Key Terms

accreditation

certification

Certified Health Education Specialist (CHES)

competencies

Competencies Update Project (CUP)

credentialing

graduate research assistantship

graduate teaching assistantship

licensure

M.A., M.Ed., M.P.H., M.S.

M.S.P.H.

multitasking

National Commission for Health Education Credentialing, Inc.

National Task Force on the Preparation and

Practice of Health Educators

needs assessment

objective

primary data

responsibilities

role delineation

secondary data

sub-competencies

Although education about health has been around since the beginning of human intelligence, health education as a profession is, relatively speaking, an infant. When any infant begins to mature, it takes on its own identity. This chapter is about the emerging identity of health education. It chronicles major historical events that have helped shape the identity of health education since the 1970s.

The current identity of health education is also presented in terms of roles, responsibilities, certification, and accreditation. Because the identity of health and health education is a work in progress and constantly changing, this chapter also discusses the importance of advanced study and continuing education in the health education profession.

Credentialing

Credentialing is a process whereby an individual or a professional preparation program meets the specified standards established by the credentialing body and is thus recognized for having done so. Credentialing can take the form of accreditation, licensure, or certification. It is important to be familiar with these terms to understand credentialing as it applies to health education.

Accreditation "is the process by which a recognized professional body evaluates an entire college or university professional preparation program" (Cleary, 1995, p. 39). Thus, the health education program at any particular institution may be accredited by one of several outside agencies to be discussed later in this chapter. For example, the health education program at Alpha University could be accredited by Beta Accrediting Group. Such a process takes place after the program at Alpha University creates a self-study document that shows how it meets the Beta Accrediting Group's standards and after an on-campus visit by representatives from Beta. Throughout the accrediting process, factors such as student-teacher ratio, curriculum, and faculty qualifications would be closely examined.

Licensure is "the process by which an agency or government [usually a state] grants permission to individuals to practice a given profession by certifying that those licensed have attained specific standards of competence" (Cleary, 1995, p. 39). Licensure applies to most medical professionals, such as doctors, nurses, dentists, and physical therapists. The only health educators who are licensed in the United States at the present time are school health educators.

Certification "is a process by which a professional organization grants recognition to an individual who, upon completion of a competency-based curriculum, can demonstrate a predetermined standard of performance" (Cleary, 1995, p. 39). Note that certification is granted to an individual, not a program, and it is given by the profession, not by a governmental body. Certification is available for all health educators, regardless of specialty area. One who is certified is recognized as a **Certified Health Education Specialist** and may use the initials **CHES** behind one's name and academic degree.

History of Role Delineation and Certification

Certification in health education got its formal start in about 1978. At that time, individual certification for health educators was not available, except for school health educators, who had to be licensed. Accreditation was available only for school health and public health professional preparation programs. Many public health programs outside schools of public health, and all community health programs, were not accredited, nor was accreditation available for these programs. This gave rise to a situation in which there were great discrepancies in professional

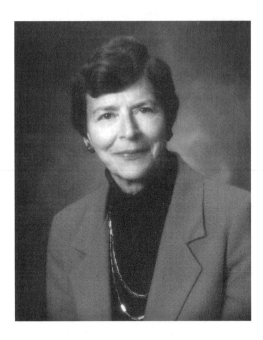

Helen P. Cleary—person most responsible for establishing certification for health education specialists. (Dr. Helen Cleary)

preparation. One program might look very different from another program. To say that an individual was a health educator had little meaning. In describing the situation, Helen Cleary, who was president of the Society for Public Health Education (SOPHE) in 1974, wrote the following:

> What I found in my travels [as SOPHE president] was a profession in disarray. Many, many health educators could neither define themselves nor their role. It was clear that the preparation of most was so varied that there was no common core. There was no professional identity, no sense of a profession. Numbers of competent, bright, young professionals were leaving health education for greener pastures. (Cleary, 1995, p. 2)

As a result of this situation, Cleary began to pursue the idea of credentialing health educators and/or health education programs. She soon discovered that, to undertake such a project, outside expertise and funding would be needed. Thomas Hatch, director of the Division of Associated Health Professions in the Bureau of Health Manpower of the Department of Health, Education and Welfare, expressed an interest in the project. Prior to funding the project, however, he needed assurances that members of the profession would work together to create a credentialing system. Hatch wanted to be certain that those who practiced health education in different settings would have enough in common to develop one set of standards.

In response to Hatch's concern, a conference was scheduled. The planning committee for the conference consisted of the presidents/chairpersons and/or their representatives of the eight organizations comprising the Coalition of Health Education Organizations, all of which had an interest in this project. The planning committee formulated two questions to be answered at the conference: (1) what are the commonalities and differences in the function of health educators practicing in

Table 6.1   Organizations Represented on the National Task Force
on the Preparation and Practice of Health Educators, 1978

American College Health Association
American Public Health Association, Public Health Education Section
American Public Health Association, School Health Education and Services Section
American School Health Association
Association for the Advancement of Health Education
Conference of State and Territorial Directors of Public Health Education
Society for Public Health Education, Inc.
Society of State Directors of Health, Physical Education and Recreation

different settings? and (2) what are the commonalities and differences in the preparation of health educators? (Cleary, 1995, p. 3). The conference, which has become known as the Bethesda Conference on Commonalities and Differences, was held in February 1978 in Bethesda, Maryland. After much discussion, those attending this conference concluded that health education was one profession and that a credentialing system was necessary. "It was the consensus of the participants that standards were essential if they were to provide quality service to the public and if they were to survive as a viable profession" (Cleary, 1986, p. 130). Further, those who had been on the planning committee for the conference were asked to continue as a task force to develop the credentialing system; thus, the **National Task Force on the Preparation and Practice of Health Educators** was born (see Table 6.1).

In January 1979, funding became available to embark on the project, and **role delineation** for health educators got under way. Alan Henderson was hired as the project director, and under his leadership a working committee of the task force began the difficult task of defining the role of the health education specialist. In describing this process, Cleary (1995) notes, "For the first time in the profession's history, specialists in school health education and in community health education faced each other across the table and learned that each was dealing with similar concepts, but using different terminology and, as well, applying them in different settings" (p. 5).

Once the initial phase of role delineation was completed, the next step was to verify and refine the role of a health educator. Funding for this became available in March 1980. A survey to verify the role was conducted of health education specialists working in all areas of health education. The results of this survey were very positive. There were no significant differences among practitioners in different settings.

In addition to the survey, a conference for college and university health education faculty members was held in Birmingham, Alabama, in February 1981. The conference provided the opportunity for academics to review the initial role delineation work and discuss its potential impact on the field. The planning committee for this conference was chaired by Warren E. Schaller from Ball State University. Two hundred thirty-eight academics from 125 institutions attended. Whereas many present were happy with the work and direction of the task force, others were not. The polar extremes of these differences centered around the health educator as an expert in content versus the health educator as an expert in process. This difference of opinion probably reflected the different types of professional preparation programs the faculty represented. Though these differences were very real, they were not divisive enough to alter the work of the task force.

The third step in the process was the development of a curriculum framework based on the verified role of a health educator. Initially, the task force decided to develop a curriculum guide. A curriculum guide is a fairly specific set of guidelines from which a curriculum is developed. Little room is left for interpretation, as the curriculum must meet the standards established in the guide. Betty Mathews from the University of Washington and Herb L. Jones from Ball State University were recruited to do the actual writing.

Once a draft copy of the guide was developed, it had to be pretested. Eleven regional workshops were held around the country to obtain feedback on the guide. Again, differences surfaced regarding whether health educators were specialists in content or process. Further, some felt entry-level preparation should be at the bachelor's degree level, while others believed it should be at the master's degree level. Feedback was also obtained from the professional associations and practitioners in the field.

To deal with some of the criticisms and to make the curriculum guide less prescriptive, it was ultimately transformed into a curriculum framework. A framework merely provides a frame of reference around which a curriculum can be developed. As Cleary (1995) notes, "It does not tell a faculty what to teach or how to teach it. It simply tells them what the students should know when they have completed the program of studies" (p. 9). Marion Pollock was the individual responsible for transforming the curriculum guide into a curriculum framework.

At this juncture, it was important to check with those in the profession to determine if they wanted to continue with the development of a credentialing system and, if so, what kind of a system they wanted. The Second Bethesda Conference was held in February 1986. Ninety-nine individuals attended the conference. Participants were divided into five groups and asked to respond to several predetermined questions. When reports from the groups were analyzed, four of the five were in favor of a certification system for individuals and some form of credentialing for professional preparation programs. They recommended that the task force continue to develop the credentialing system.

Over the next two years, the task force continued to work toward the development of a certification system for individual health educators. The Professional Examination Service (PES), which developed certification and licensure exams for many other professions, was contracted to assist with this process. Not only was its experience in test development vital to the process, but it was also willing to provide start-up funds to get the process off the ground.

By June 1988, the National Task Force on the Preparation and Practice of Health Education had been functioning for ten years. Much had been accomplished, yet there was still much to do. With the certification of individual health educators about to become a reality, it was time to establish a more permanent structure to coordinate and oversee the certification process. As a result, the **National Commission for Health Education Credentialing, Inc.,** was formed to replace the national task force. Its mission is "to improve the practice of health education and to serve the public and profession of health education by certifying health education specialists, promoting professional development, and strengthening professional preparation and practice" (National Commission for Health Education Credentialing, 2004a). This organization still oversees the health education credentialing process.

(Text continues on page 164)

Box 6.1 Practitioner's Perspective: CHES

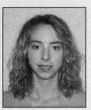

NAME: Julia A. Eminger, B.A., CHES
CURRENT POSITION/TITLE: Regional Program Director
EMPLOYER: Indiana Tobacco Prevention and Cessation Agency (ITPC)
DEGREE/INSTITUTION: B.A., Purdue University, 2002
MAJOR: Health Promotion, Health and Fitness
MINOR: Art and Design

Job Responsibilities: I oversee the ITPC community-based tobacco control grants in twenty counties in central Indiana. I provide technical assistance, conflict management, and resource development to the community-based tobacco control coalitions in each of these counties. I assist them with both programming and budgeting issues so that their efforts are consistent with their personal tobacco control work plan and the tobacco control goals of ITPC. I regularly participate in their local coalition meetings and provide personal strategy sessions. These meetings allow me to continuously assist them with the creation and implementation of effective local tobacco control efforts. I also oversee and provide assistance to two statewide grants with the Prenatal Substance Use Prevention Program and the Indiana Teen Institute. Plus, I am involved in state-level strategic planning and targeted initiatives in all areas of tobacco control, including prevention, cessation, media, enforcement, evaluation, and policies.

How I obtained my job: A professor from Purdue notified me of the opportunity to have an internship with a newly created state agency focusing on tobacco control. I became an intern at ITPC during the last semester of my senior year. During my internship, I was able to develop a strong working knowledge of tobacco control and the agency. One month after graduation, the Director of

Community Programs at ITPC, to whom I reported during my internship, informed me that the position of Regional Program Director was newly vacant. I applied for this position because I enjoyed my internship and the agency itself. With this position, I believed that I had the opportunity to work in a cutting-edge area of public health with experienced professionals.

What I like most about my job: I like working closely with the local county tobacco control coalitions. They vary in size, focus, and strength, giving me the opportunity to provide technical assistance and strategic planning on various levels. I am continuously developing trainings, materials, and other customized needs for the local partners. For instance, I have provided tailored training on tobacco control advocacy and coalition capacity to several coalitions in order to assist them in taking their community collaboration to a higher level of effectiveness. I also enjoy working on tobacco control initiatives at the state level. For example, I have had the opportunity to be on a small working group that has restructured our youth movement against big tobacco. The broad skills and experiences I have developed through this position have challenged me both personally and professionally.

What I like least about my job: Because the counties I work with are up to two

(Box 6.1 continues)

(Box 6.1 *continued*)

hours away, I travel often in order to develop close relationships with and to give personal attention to the local partners. My frequent travel schedule reduces the amount of time I have to stay up-to-date on the continuously changing tobacco control field and to work on state-level agency initiatives.

How CHES certification has helped me: I believe that the CHES certification has enhanced my credibility on the job and in the health education profession. I can prove to employers and other professionals that I have competency in health education intervention assessment, planning, implementation, and evaluation because I passed a standardized certification exam. My health education knowledge is evident with the CHES without having yet obtained a graduate degree. I feel more confident and effective as a health educator. I know that the knowledge I gained in college is lasting through the passing of the CHES exam and obtaining the required continuing education credits.

How my work relates to the responsibilities and competencies of a CHES: My work as a Regional Program Director is directly in line with the responsibilities and competencies of a CHES. Every local tobacco control coalition is working on a broad range of tobacco control initiatives. Therefore, I provide assessment, planning, implementation, and evaluation technical assistance at all times as each coalition has different focuses throughout a grant cycle. For instance, one coalition may need assistance planning a media campaign focused on educating the public about the dangers of secondhand smoke, while another coalition requests a valid and reliable instrument to determine the local support for a tobacco control policy. In order to provide the best technical assistance, I focus on coordinating the most effective and efficient types of services ITPC can provide to our state and local partners. I achieve this first through gathering the most relevant and effective resources for the issue needing to be addressed. Second, I communicate the tobacco control concepts through individual, small group, or large group meetings or interactive presentations that are tailored to the communication style of the participants.

Recommendations for those preparing to be health educators: I recommend that you focus on getting the best internship experience possible. I completed three internships during college to increase my skills and to determine the area of health education in which I wanted to work. I have interned at a health club, a university employee wellness program, and a state health agency. This broad range of experience made me marketable to obtain a job soon after graduation and helped me determine that I wanted to work for a nonprofit agency. Also, I highly recommend building strong relationships with your professors and internship supervisors. I was able to participate in two different research projects during college and obtained my first professional position because I had proven my high work ethic. Plus, I strongly suggest that you become a CHES as early as possible. By completing the exam right after graduation, I still had a strong working knowledge of health education that helped me pass the exam, along with quickly becoming more marketable as a professional. You will have great employment and graduate school opportunities in health education after college graduation by completing an internship, health education research, and the CHES certification.

With the PES in place to develop the certification exam and the National Commission for Health Education Credentialing in place to oversee the process, it was time to certify the first health educators.

Individual Certification

In October 1988, the charter certification period began. Charter certification allowed qualified individuals to be certified based on their academic training, work experience, and references without taking the certification exam. When a new certification program is initiated, charter certification is usually available for a limited period of time, after which anyone seeking certification must meet all criteria for certification and pass the examination. The initial requirements for charter certification in health education, through which 1,558 individuals obtained certification, were as follows:

Degree	Experience	References
Graduate degree with health education emphasis	At least four years' experience	Three references
Bachelor's degree with health education emphasis	At least seven years' experience	Three references
Bachelor's degree with other than health education emphasis	At least twenty-five years' experience	Three references

In 1990, the charter certification period ended, and the first examination was held. Six hundred forty-four candidates passed the first exam and became Certified Health Education Specialists.

The CHES voluntary professional certification program established for the first time a national standard for health education practice. The benefits of national certification include the following:

1. It attests that an individual possesses the knowledge and skills deemed necessary to practice in the field as delineated by the profession.

2. It assists employers in identifying qualified health education practitioners.

3. It assures consumers that services are provided by professionals who have met national standards.

4. It provides a system to assure that health education professionals participate in continuing education and professional development activities.

These are important benefits, and all health education students are strongly urged to obtain certification upon graduation (National Commission for Health Education Credentialing, 2004).

Currently, eligibility to sit for the CHES exam is based exclusively on academic qualifications. To sit for the exam, one must "possess a bachelor's, master's or doctoral degree from an accredited institution of higher education; *AND* (1) an official transcript that clearly shows a major in health education, e.g., Health Education, Community Health Education, Public Health Education, School Health Education, etc.; *OR* (2) an official transcript that reflects 25 semester hours (37 quarter hours) of course work with specific preparation addressing the seven responsibilities delineated in the FRAMEWORK" (National Commission for Health Education Credentialing, 2004b).

Graduate Health Education Standards

The roles and responsibilities document, *A Competency-Based Framework for Professional Development of Certified Health Education Specialists* (National Commission for Health Education Credentialing, 1996), defined the skills needed for the entry-level health education professional. Although many health educators with advanced degrees had obtained certification, it attested only to the fact that they had entry-level skills. The document provided guidance for professional preparation programs at the bachelor's degree level, but there was no such guidance available for professional preparation programs at the graduate level.

In June 1992, the Joint Committee for Graduate Standards was established by the Association for the Advancement of Health Education (now called the American Association for Health Education [AAHE]) Board of Directors. Committee membership was initially comprised of Society of Public Health Education (SOPHE) and AAHE members serving on their respective accreditation bodies. To obtain a broader perspective, committee membership was expanded to include members from the Council on Education for Public Health (CEPH) and the National Commission for Health Education Credentialing, Inc. (NCHEC). After much work, discussion, and review, the Joint Committee for Graduate Standards developed a draft document that contains additional responsibilities, competencies, and sub-competencies specific to graduate-level preparation.

In February 1996, the draft document was presented to a large group of college-level health educators at the National Congress for Institutions Preparing Graduate Health Educators, which was held in Dallas, Texas. The national congress was convened to "engage professional preparation programs in a review and dialogue about advanced competency-based preparation" (Joint Committee for Graduate Standards, 1996). One hundred thirty-four individuals representing more than one hundred colleges and universities attended the meeting. Throughout the three-day meeting, the graduate competencies were thoroughly discussed and debated. Recommendations for improving the graduate competencies were presented to the planning committee. Despite some dissension, the general mood was in favor of the competencies, and the planning committee was urged to move on with the approval process.

Following this meeting, revisions were made to the draft document, and the final version was presented to the AAHE and SOPHE boards of directors for approval. Approval was granted in March 1997.

Competencies Update Project

The initial Role Delineation Project began over twenty years ago. Since then, health education has evolved and matured, creating a need to reverify the competencies and sub-competencies of a health educator. Begun in 1998, the

Competencies Update Project (CUP) is nearing completion. It was conducted by the twenty-five-member CUP Advisory Committee (CUPAC) (National Commission for Health Education Credentialing, 2004c).

The overall purpose of the CUP project was to determine the degree to which the role of the entry-level health educator was still up to date, and to continue the development of advanced-level competencies. Specific objectives were to:

- "Determine the degree to which the responsibilities, competencies, and sub-competencies for entry-level health educators are still valid as determined by their ability to accurately reflect the current scope of health education practice and their generic applicability across practice settings."

- "Specify the role of the advanced-level health educator and further verify the responsibilities, competencies, and sub-competencies as determined by their ability to accurately reflect the current scope of health education practice and their generic applicability across practice settings."

- "Realign the responsibilities, competencies, and sub-competencies for entry- and advanced-level health educators to accurately reflect the current scope of health education practice and their generic applicability across practice settings (National Commission for Health Education Credentialing, 2004c, pp. 1–2).

The final CUP report is being developed as this book goes to press and a preliminary press release describing the project and its results was issued on November 5, 2004 (See Box 6.2). This report will be based on the largest national dataset ever created of practicing health educators. Over 4,000 health educators from every state in the United States and from all major employment settings completed the nineteen-page questionnaire. The response rate for the survey was 70% and the total database contains more than 1.6 million data points (Gilmore, Olsen, Taub, & Connell, 2003). The results of this project will ultimately impact and strengthen the curricula of health education professional preparation programs throughout the United States, certification at the individual level, accreditation/approval of undergraduate and graduate health education programs, and the professional development and continuing education of currently practicing health educators.

Program Accreditation

"Accreditation is a process by which a recognized professional body evaluates an entire program against predetermined criteria or standards" (Cleary, 1995). In most professions, colleges and universities that train students to enter a given profession are accredited by a recognized professional body that operates independently of the college or university. If a program does not meet the standards of the recognized professional body, it can lose its accreditation. A nonaccredited program might have difficulty recruiting new students and may be restricted in its participation in the profession. Therefore, accreditation helps ensure that all students entering the profession have similar training and preparation.

In health education, accreditation is available through three accrediting bodies. Health education programs that are affiliated with a college of education and train students for positions in school health may be accredited through the National Commission for the Accreditation of Teacher Education (NCATE). The Council on

Box 6.2 CUP Press Release

A Cooperative Project of the American Association for Health Education, American Public Health Association (Public Health Education & Health Promotion Section and School Health Education & Services Section), American School Health Association, Association of Schools of Public Health, Association of State & Territorial Directors of Health Promotion & Public Health Education, Coalition of National Health Education Organizations, Council on Education for Public Health, Eta Sigma Gamma, National Commission for Health Education Credentialing, Society for Public Health Education, Society of State Directors of Health, Physical Education, & Recreation.

Press Release

Date: November 5, 2004
Contact: Linda Lysoby, Executive Director, NCHEC

The National Commission for Health Education Credentialing, Inc., the American Association for Health Education, and the Society for Public Health Education, announce the completion of the National Health Educators Competency Update Project (CUP). This six-year, (1998–2004) multi-phased national study specifies the role and responsibilities of contemporary health education practitioners across the United States. The study results have implications for the professional preparation, practice, and certification of all health educators regardless of the setting in which they are employed.

Based on extensive data gathered from more than 4,000 practitioners and more than 1.6 million data points, CUP study provides a model of three levels of practice (entry, advanced 1, and advanced 2) with each subsequent level building upon the previous level(s). The 163 practitioner-validated Sub-competencies align with 35 Competencies and 7 Areas of Responsibility, which include:

- Assess individual and community needs for health education
- Plan health education strategies, interventions, and programs
- Implement health education strategies, interventions, and programs
- Conduct evaluation and research related to health education
- Administer health education strategies, interventions, and programs
- Serve as a health education resource person
- Communicate and advocate for health and health education.

The health education profession will benefit immediately and during the next decade from the research leadership provided by the project steering committee members: Dr. Gary Gilmore, University of Wisconsin at La Crosse, Chairperson, Dr. Alyson Taub, New York University, and Dr. Larry Olsen, New Mexico State University. Further inquiries for information and access to products referenced above should be directed to the National Commission for Health Education Credentialing, Inc. at P. O. Box 90158, Allentown, PA 18109-0158.

Education for Public Health (CEPH) accredits schools of public health, public health programs in non-schools of public health, and master's degree programs in community health education. Undergraduate programs in school or community health may elect to obtain approval through the Society for Public Health Education/American Association for Health Education (SOPHE/AAHE) process. However, as of June 2004, only sixteen institutions had chosen to obtain SABPAC (SOPHE/AAHE Baccalaureate Program Approval Committee) approval (SOPHE, 2004).

Having three accreditation approvals available is considered by many a weakness in the profession. As Cleary (1995) notes, "There were (and are) huge gaps and great discrepancies in the accreditation/approval process" (p.16). Professional preparation is not at all uniform in the profession (Cleary, 1986). Some programs focus more on content, such as drugs, sexuality, stress, and physical fitness, while other programs emphasize process courses, such as planning, implementing, and evaluating. Some programs stress individual behavior change, while others stress a socioecological or ecological approach to change. In 1987, the National Task Force on the Preparation and Practice of Health Educators attempted to develop a registry of health education programs. This effort, however, had to be abandoned. There was too much variety in faculty, administrative arrangements, courses, and philosophies of the various professional preparation programs to agree on criteria for inclusion in the registry (Cleary, 1995).

Currently there are 256 programs listed in the 2003 AAHE *Directory of Institutions That Prepare Health Educators*. Many of these programs are not accredited, and there is no professional body monitoring their efforts. The whole accreditation issue has recently been reviewed by the professional associations. On January 15–16, 2000, the Society for Public Health Education and the American Association for Health Education co-sponsored a meeting in Dulles, Virginia, to explore the issue of accreditation. Twenty-four professionals who were broadly representative of health education professional preparation programs or other stakeholders attended. Meeting participants reached consensus that a "coordinated accreditation system" was needed. The SOPHE/AAHE National Task Force on Accreditation in Health Education was established and charged to (1) "gather background information and refine plans for a comprehensive, coordinated quality assurance system that meets commonly accepted standards of accreditation, and (2) develop processes for ensuring profession-wide involvement in the discussion and design of such a system to foster its adoption and utilization" (Society for Public Health Education, 2000, p. 5).

The task force completed its work in the spring of 2004 and submitted its final report, including results and recommendations, to both the AAHE and SOPHE boards of directors (See Box 6.3 for the final results and recommendations). Both boards accepted the final report and have instituted a new committee to transition from the National Task Force recommendations to an implementation phase of the process. Dr. David Birch, Southern Illinois University, and Dr. Kathleen Roe, San Jose State University, are co-chairing this new transistion committee.

Responsibilities and Competencies of Health Educators

The "Responsibilities and Competencies for Entry-Level Health Educators" (see Appendix B) was developed from the *Framework for the Development of Competency-Based Curricula for Entry Level Health Educators* (National Task Force on the Preparation and

Practice of Health Educators, 1985). The Responsibilities and Competencies document lists the seven major **responsibilities** of health educators. In essence, these seven responsibilities specify the scope of practice for health educators. Under each of these responsibilities are three or four **competencies.** A competency "reflects the ability of the student to understand, know, etc." (National Commission for Health Education Credentialing, 1996, p. 12). Each competency is further delineated into two to four **sub-competencies.** A sub-competency "reflects the ability of the student to list, describe, etc." (National Commission for Health Education Credentialing, 1996, p. 12). Although not part of the original document, the National Commission for Health Education Credentialing has published a book that identifies several objectives for each sub-competency (National Commission for Health Education Credentialing, 1996). An **objective** "reflects the ability of the student to perform" (National Commission for Health Education Credentialing, 1996, p. 12). All prospective health educators, whether focusing their professional preparation on school, community, clinical, or worksite settings, should be able to demonstrate the various competencies, sub-competencies, and objectives on completion of their academic program of study.

The "Responsibilities and Competencies for Entry-Level Health Educators" document should be used by health education students on a regular basis during their professional preparation program. The National Commission for Health Education Credentialing (1996) suggests that the competencies be used "as a personal inventory to assess progress toward becoming a health educator; that is to determine which competencies and sub-competencies have been mastered. It is suggested that the student assess his or her progress at intervals during the student's course of study and do a final review at the completion of the health education program" (p. 7). Students who have been diligent in monitoring their progress and who can perform the competencies, sub-competencies, and objectives as indicated will have a much greater chance of passing the credentialing exam to become a Certified Health Education Specialist.

Because the seven major responsibilities identified in the "Responsibilities and Competencies for Entry-Level Health Educators" are the core of what a health educator does, it is important to have a basic understanding of what each responsibility entails. The following is a brief description of each responsibility.

Responsibility I: Assessing Individual and Community Needs for Health Education

Conducting a needs assessment is "perhaps the most critical part of program planning" (Anspaugh, Dignan, & Anspaugh, 2000, p. 74). A **needs assessment** is a "process by which those who are planning programs can determine what health problems might exist in any given group of people" (McKenzie, Neiger, & Smeltzer, 2005, p. 72). Other terms that can be used to describe this process of determining the needs of people to whom programs are directed include community analysis, community diagnosis, and community assessment (McKenzie et al., 2005). All health educators, regardless of the setting in which they are employed, must have the skills to assess the needs of those groups or individuals to whom their programs are directed. Therefore, a school health educator needs to base curriculum on the needs of the students, a health educator in the corporate setting needs to plan

---

Box 6.3 Results and Recommendations from the National Task Force on Accreditation in Health Education

1. That accreditation be the quality assurance mechanism for health education professional preparation institutions, and should replace existing approval processes in orderly transition.

2. That there be a unified accreditation system, comprising two parallel, coordinated accreditation mechanisms for community and school health education preparation institutions, which are responsive to the needs of the health education profession. These mechanisms must assure that common and specific competencies in health education are addressed at the undergraduate and graduate levels.

   a. That the National Council for the Accreditation of Teacher Education (NCATE) is the preferred accrediting entity to provide a single coordinated accreditation mechanism for school health education programs at the undergraduate and graduate levels. If a dual teacher certification program is in place, health education is to be reviewed as a separate program.

   b. That the Council on Education for Public Health (CEPH) is the preferred accrediting entity to provide a single coordinated accreditation mechanism for community/public health education programs at the undergraduate and graduate levels.

3. That the coordinated accreditation system should build upon the best practices of existing community and school health accreditation mechanisms.

4. That graduate professional preparation programs must assure that students perform all health education competencies, and that their performance reflect graduate-level proficiency.

5. That new designations should be created to distinguish the practice level of health educators at the undergraduate and graduate levels, parallel with other professional disciplines such as nursing and social work. We recommend that these designations be:

   a. Health Education Specialist (HES) for undergraduate-level practitioners from an accredited program.

   b. Master Health Education Specialist (MHES) for the graduate-level practitioners from an accredited program.

   (Box 6.3 continues)

---

programs based on the needs of the company's employees, and public health educators should base their health education efforts on the needs of the community they serve. Health education programs should not be based on the whim of the health educator or any small group of decision makers. Resources are too valuable to waste on programs that do not address the needs of the population being served. As McKenzie et al. (2005) notes, ". . . failure to perform a needs assessment may lead to a program focus that prevents or delays adequate attention directed to a more important health problem" (p. 73). Conversely, "We know our health education programs are on target when we base them on accurate needs assessment data and a careful interpretation of their meaning" (Doyle & Ward, 2001, p. 124).

(Box 6.3 *continued*)

6. That the National Commission for Health Education Credentialing (NCHEC) is an appropriate entity to oversee the process of individual certification at both the undergraduate and graduate levels. We further recommend that:

a. Persons who successfully complete the certification processes should be designated as a Certified Health Specialist (CHES) (undergraduate level) or Master's-level Certified Health Education Specialist (MCHES) (both master's and doctorate graduate level). Only students from accredited programs/ schools should be eligible for CHES and MCHES certification; however, those individuals who held the CHES certification prior to the implementation of this process would remain certified.

b. Appropriate deeming of those undergraduate-level practitioners holding CHES should be considered, with students currently from nonaccredited undergraduate programs/schools permitted to sit for CHES for a reasonable, multiyear period of time. After such time, only students from accredited undergraduate programs/ schools should be eligible to sit for CHES. A multiyear window of time should allow the new accreditation system to be fully functioning, while offering a transition period for programs/ schools to prepare and qualify for accreditation.

c. Appropriate deeming of those master's- or doctorate-level practitioners holding CHES be considered, with a window of time of up to 24 months to earn MCHES designation.

7. That the results of the work of the Task Force be articulated to the American Public Health Association, Association of Schools of Public Health, Association of Teachers of Preventive Medicine, Coalition of National Health Education Organizations, National Commission for Health Education Credentialing, and other relevant groups.

The implementation of the Task Force recommendations will require a profession-wide effort and the commitment of new resources over several years from a broad range of stakeholders beyond SOPHE and AAHE.

Source: Final Report of the National Task Force on Accreditation in Health Education. Presented to the AAHE Board of Directors, March 2004.

Ultimately, it is the well-conceived and -conducted needs assessment that determines if a health education program is justified and that defines its nature and scope (Gilmore & Campbell, 2005).

To conduct a needs assessment, health educators should know how to locate and obtain valid sources of information that pertain to their specific population or populations with similar characteristics. For example, this may entail a literature review or accessing information from local, county, or state health departments. In addition to examining such pre-existing information, which is called **secondary data,** it may be necessary for health educators to gather data of their own, known as **primary data.** They may have to conduct mail or telephone surveys, hold focus

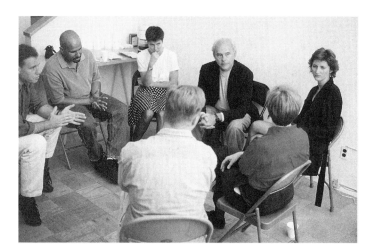

Health educators often need to hold focus groups to learn more about the needs of their priority population. (David Harry Stewart/Stone)

group meetings, or use a nominal group process. Once all of this information has been collected, the health educator must be able to analyze the data and determine priority areas for health education programming.

The following example of a situation experienced by a health education internship student demonstrates the importance of needs assessment. The student had been placed with the Shriners Hospital for Burned Children in Cincinnati, Ohio. The hospital had noted a problem with children being burned around campfires during the summer months, and asked the student to develop a fire safety program for young campers. Fortunately, the site supervisor required the student to conduct a needs assessment before planning the program. After conducting focus groups, interviewing camp counselors, and reviewing the literature, it was decided that campers were the wrong group to target with the program. What was needed was a program for the camp leaders and counselors. Had not the needs assessment been done, valuable time and resources would have been spent developing a program for the wrong target audience.

Responsibility II: Planning Effective Health Education Programs

Planning involves more than just determining a location and time for a health education program. Planning begins by assessing the health needs, problems, and concerns of the target population. Early in the planning process, it is important to recruit interested stakeholders, such as community leaders, representatives from community organizations, resource providers, and representatives of the target population, to support and help develop the program. Without the help of these stakeholders, it may be impossible to develop effective programs. To be effective in the planning process, the health educator should have strong written and oral communication skills, leadership ability, and the expertise to facilitate diverse groups of people reaching consensus on issues of interest.

As part of the planning process, health educators must be competent to develop goals and objectives specific to the proposed health education program. These goals and objectives are the foundation on which the program is established. Writing specific and measurable objectives is critical. No health education program should be initiated without objectives, or considered complete until an evaluation of the objectives is conducted. Mastering the ability to write good objectives is a skill one can only obtain through guided practice and experience. Once program goals and objectives are written, the next step is to develop appropriate interventions that will meet these goals and objectives.

Responsibility III: Implementing Health Education Programs

After the initial planning, including the needs assessment, goal and objective setting, and intervention development, it is time to implement the programs. For many health educators, implementation is the most enjoyable of the responsibilities, for it entails the actual presentation of the program.

To successfully implement a program, the health educator must have a thorough understanding of the people in the priority population. What is their current level of understanding regarding the issue at hand? What will it take to get the people to participate? Do they need financial assistance or childcare? What time of the day should the program be offered? What location or locations would be most convenient? While some of these questions can be answered from the initial needs assessment, it may also be necessary to obtain additional information about the target population before proceeding with implementation.

In conducting various health promotion and education programs, it is important that the health educator be comfortable using a wide range of educational methods or techniques. In school health, for example, it is not enough to simply lecture to students about "proper" health behaviors. A good health educator includes many teaching strategies such as brainstorming, debate, daily logs, position papers, guest speakers, problem solving, decision making, demonstrations, role playing, drama, music, and current events. In community health, most programs require going beyond developing and distributing a simple pamphlet on a given health topic. Again, a wide variety of strategies should be used, including television, radio, newspapers, billboards, celebrity spokespersons, behavioral contracting, community events, contests, incentives, support groups, and many more. As a general rule, health educators should always use multiple intervention activities when planning and implementing programs.

Once a program is in place and operating, the role of the health educator is not over. The health educator should continue to monitor the program to make certain everything is going as planned. If problems are noted, it may be necessary, even while the program is in progress, to revise the objectives or the intervention activities.

Responsibility IV: Evaluating the Effectiveness of Health Education Programs

In health education, it is critical that accurate evaluation be conducted to measure the success of programs. Without good evaluation, one does not know if the programs being implemented are meeting the specified goals and objectives. Programs that are not properly evaluated may be wasting valuable time, money, and other resources. Further, a program that is not evaluated, and thus cannot "prove its worth," may risk being cut back or even eliminated when resources are short and downsizing occurs.

To conduct an effective evaluation, the health educator must first establish realistic, measurable program objectives. As has already been mentioned, this is an important part of the planning process. Once objectives are in place, the health educator must develop a plan that will accurately assess if the program objectives have been met. Depending on the setting, this may involve developing and administering tests, conducting surveys, observing behavior, or other methods of data collection. Evaluation plans can be very simple or extremely sophisticated, depending on the program being evaluated, the expectations of the program planners, and the requirements of the funding agents.

After data have been collected, they must then be analyzed and interpreted. Reports need to be developed and distributed to the appropriate parties. Ultimately, the results of the evaluation should be used to modify and improve current or future program efforts.

Responsibility V: Coordinating Provision of Health Education Services

Considering the previous responsibilities, it should be obvious that a great deal of coordination is needed to bring a health education program to fruition. Therefore, coordination is another skill that is critical for health educators to possess. As a first step, health educators need to be aware of related programs to make sure there is not significant overlap in services. By knowing what others are doing, it is also possible to identify gaps in services where important needs may be unmet.

Health educators must facilitate cooperation among personnel, both within programs and between programs. Many public school systems, for example, have initiated coordinated school health programs. This involves coordinating the activities and services of school nurses, counselors, psychologists, food service personnel, physical educators, health educators, teachers, administrators, support staff, parents, and community health agencies. The ultimate goal is to develop both curricular and extracurricular programs to improve the health status of students, faculty, staff, and the community as a whole.

Similar examples can be seen in the community setting. For example, a health department decides to apply for grant funds to reduce the incidence of tobacco use in its community. The health educator may bring together individuals and/or groups with a vested interest in reducing tobacco use to form a coalition. Membership in the coalition might include representatives from the American Cancer Society, American Lung Association, American Heart Association, local medical society, local dental association, public health department, public school system, and YMCA/YWCA. Coordination and integration of the services offered by these various groups would be critical to the successful development of a grant proposal and ultimately to the success of the funded program. It may even be necessary for the health educator to conduct or coordinate in-service training programs to make sure all coalition members have similar levels of knowledge and sophistication related to tobacco prevention programs.

Responsibility VI: Acting as a Resource Person in Health Education

Health educators are often called on to serve as resource persons. It is not unusual for a student to seek out the health teacher for assistance when having a health-related problem. In the corporate setting, health educators get questions about topics ranging from nutritional supplements to cancer signs and symptoms, to the best type of shoe to wear for jogging. Because it is impossible for health educators to know all of the information that could be called for in a given position, they must have the skill to access resources they need. It may be necessary to visit the library; use computerized health retrieval systems; access health databases; find information on specific diseases, obtain local, regional, state, and national epidemiological data; and much more. As part of this process, it may be necessary for health educators to select or develop effective educational resources for dissemination.

Being able to retrieve information, however, is not enough. Health educators must establish effective consultive relationships with those seeking assistance, whether they be students, clients, employees, or other health educators. They must instill confidence in those seeking information and develop effective means of communicating information in a nonthreatening manner. In some situations, health educators may decide to market their skills, via consultation, to individuals or groups and may make serving as a resource person the primary focus of their career.

Responsibility VII: Communicating Health and Health Education Needs, Concerns, and Resources

Health educators must interact with various groups of people, including other health professionals, consumers, students, employers, employees, and fellow health educators. Obviously, health educators must be good communicators. They must be skilled in written communication, oral communication, and mass media use. Health educators need to feel comfortable working with individuals, small groups, and large groups, as the situation warrants. In essence, communication is the primary tool of the health educator.

It is often necessary for health educators to serve as filters between scientific information and their students or clients. The health educator must have the skill to translate difficult scientific concepts so that their constituents understand the information necessary to improve and protect their health. For example, health educators may be called on to help HMO patients incorporate the recommendations of their physicians. A physician may tell a patient to start an exercise program, reduce fat in the diet, or manage stress better. Although many patients have a general idea of what these recommendations mean, they do not have the knowledge or skills to implement the recommendations. Most physicians cannot take the time to explain in detail what these recommendations entail. It is often health educators who communicate the detailed information on exercising safely, teach the client to recognize high-fat foods by reading food labels, and instruct the patient in progressive neuromotor relaxation. This may involve conducting one-on-one instruction, developing a videotape for patients to watch, developing brochures for distribution to patients, teaching classes, or coordinating support groups—in other words, communicating with the clients.

Summary of Responsibilities and Competencies

The responsibilities, competencies, and sub-competencies required for entry-level health educators do not function independently but are highly interrelated. In conducting all of the responsibilities, one needs to be a good communicator. Conducting a good needs assessment requires the skills to identify and gather appropriate resources. Planning should be based on a valid and reliable needs assessment. When implementing programs, one needs to have good communication skills and serve as a resource person when asked to do so. Evaluation relies on goals and objectives established during the planning process. Coordinating people and programs is necessary in planning, implementing, and evaluating programs.

It is not sufficient to be proficient at one, two, or even six of the responsibility areas. All seven responsibilities are critical for effective health education to take place. It is beyond the scope of this book to provide the level of information necessary to teach the reader how to do these tasks. Rather, it is the intent of this text to familiarize readers with the responsibilities, competencies, and skills they will be taught in later classes and ultimately practice in their employment settings.

Multitasking

In addition to mastering the responsibilities and competencies of a health educator, it is often necessary for health educators to use several of these skills simultaneously on multiple ongoing projects. This requires health educators to be good at **multitasking**. In this context, multitasking refers to the skill of coordinating and completing multiple projects at the same time. Health educators must prioritize their activities to accomplish things that must be completed first, which usually precludes working on one project until it is finished.

While in college, health education students are often given a project at the beginning of a term. There is a specific amount of time to complete the project, and when the term ends the project is completed. In the work world, things do not function this way. Health educators work on multiple projects at the same time and each project is usually in a different stage of completion. Some students, when first exposed to multitasking, find it difficult. Organization is the key to successful multitasking. As an example of what can be done, one health education internship student used the visual concept of floating balloons to help her stay on task and organized while working on multiple projects. Using a bulletin board, unfinished projects and tasks were represented by floating balloons. Once completed, the balloons were placed at the bottom of the bulletin board in the hand of a stick figure that represented the health educator.

Technology

As in most professions, health educators must be familiar with and comfortable using technology. Health educators working in the smallest public health departments, to large voluntary agencies, to public schools, to sophisticated worksite fitness programs will need to know how to use the computer and other technology aids. Both the software and hardware are constantly changing, making it a challenge to learn and stay up to date. Entry-level health educators are expected to have these

---

Box 6.4 Entry-Level Technology Skills (Not Prioritized)

- Basic word processing/text editing skills including use of writing tools like spell checkers, electronic thesaurus, etc.
- Basic to advanced electronic spreadsheet use, beginning with elementary worksheets and progressing to more sophisticated "what-if" analyses
- Introductory statistical analysis software and data entry (assuming that statistics applications are also learned)
- Preparing effective PowerPoint presentations
- Critiquing components of computer-assisted health education software (health assessments to computer-assisted instruction)
- Electronic retrieval of quality health information—search engines, databases, and indexes of health literature

- Electronic health information media literacy, including evaluating the quality of health Web sites
- Utilizing a Web page editor to design and develop effective health-based Web pages. This would include skills needed to upload pages to a server and then marketing the site to specific Internet audiences.
- Professional electronic mail and discussion list etiquette
- Use of common technological innovations in health education such as digital video/photography, scanners, personal digital assistants, and computer-assisted interviews and surveys

Source: List provided by Dr. Ernesto Randolfi, Montana State University–Billings

Posted to HEDIR Electronic Listserve, 2002

---

skills by the time they enter their internships and certainly by the time they accept their first position. See Box 6.4 for a listing of entry-level computer skills.

Role Modeling

One final aspect of being a health educator involves the importance of being a role model. Being a role model is not listed anywhere in the roles and responsibilities of a health educator, but it has probably been discussed and debated more than any other aspect of being a health educator (Davis, 1999; Bruess, 2003). Some people feel that health educators should not be expected to be healthy role models. For example, one may feel that to do so would discriminate against health educators who are suffering from disease conditions that may cause obesity and preclude a regular exercise regimen. Some feel that being a healthy role model puts too much pressure on health educators and argue that there is no accepted definition for what "healthy" means. On the other hand, many in the profession believe that being a healthy role model is important to effectively carry out the responsibilities of the profession. Some even argue that, ethically, health educators must be role models.

The authors of this text tend to believe that role modeling is an important aspect of being a health educator, the purpose of presenting the issue is not to bring closure to the debate, but to stimulate health education students to enter the debate. Do you feel health educators should be role models? Do you think health educators who are not role models will be less effective in their work? What does it mean to be a role model? Are you a role model now or do you want to be a role model in the future?

Advanced Study in Health Education

After receiving a bachelor's degree in health education, the student should not stop the educational process. At the very least, health educators should continue to learn on their own. One way of doing so is to belong to and be active in one or more professional associations (see Chapter 8). Such memberships allows the opportunity to read professional publications and to attend state, regional, and national meetings of the associations. If one is a Certified Health Education Specialist, an average of fifteen continuing education contact hours are required each year (seventy-five over five years) to maintain certification. These may be obtained by reading professional journals and submitting responses to questions on selected articles, by attending various professional meetings and workshops, by taking additional coursework, or by participating in other professional development activities.

At some point, many bachelor's degree-level health educators should consider going on for a master's degree. In some areas of the country and in some health education settings, such as medical care and worksite health education, the master's degree is considered the entry-level degree. In other words, to be considered for employment in these settings, the health educator must hold an appropriate master's degree.

In school settings, the master's degree brings additional financial rewards and, in some states, progress toward more permanent teaching certificates. It is usually advised, however, not to complete a master's degree in teaching prior to obtaining one's first teaching position. The additional cost to a school district of hiring a new teacher with a master's degree versus a new teacher with a bachelor's degree may put the person with the master's degree at a disadvantage in the hiring process.

In community or public health settings, the master's degree may bring additional financial rewards, as well as promotions within the agency. It may also open the door to higher level positions with other community health agencies or public health departments.

Master's Degree Options

When considering a master's degree, one should first consider the type of degree one wishes to pursue. Typical choices include a Master's of Education **(M.Ed.),** Master's of Science **(M.S.),** Master's of Arts (**M.A.**), Master's of Public Health **(M.P.H.),** and Master's of Science in Public Health (**M.S.P.H.**) (Bensley & Pope, 1994). Some colleges and universities may offer only one degree option, while others may offer more than one, giving students the decision of degree choice.

The M.Ed. degree is typically found in institutions where the health education program is located in a College of Education or Teacher's College. Though many students in such programs may be focusing on school health, this does not mean that all persons with this degree designation have public schools as their career goal.

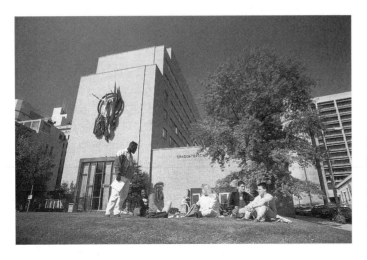

University of Pittsburgh School of Public Health—many health education positions require a master's degree. (University of Pittsburgh, PA)

Some colleges and universities offer the M.Ed. degree with such emphasis areas as community health and corporate health promotion.

The M.S. and M.A. degrees are usually found in universities where the health education program is located in colleges other than education. Because there is no accepted accreditation for these programs, they have much flexibility to develop programs that meet the needs of the local job market. They offer a variety of emphasis areas, including public health, community health education, and corporate health promotion. When considering differences between the M.S., M.A., and M.Ed. degrees, remember that the M.S. may be the more scientific or research-oriented degree, while the M.A. and M.Ed. may be more practitioner oriented.

As the name implies, the M.P.H. and M.S.P.H. are degree choices for those wishing to work in the field of public health. The M.S.P.H. degree is typically more research oriented than the M.P.H. degree; otherwise, the degrees are similar. The M.P.H. can be awarded in a variety of specialty areas such as an M.P.H. in nursing, M.P.H. in dietetics, or M.P.H. in epidemiology. It is the M.P.H. in health education that is of most interest to health educators. Most M.P.H. degree-granting colleges and universities are accredited by the Council on Education for Public Health (CEPH). Thus, the requirements to obtain an M.P.H. are more standardized than are the requirements to obtain the M.S., M.A., or M.Ed. degrees, which are typically not accredited by any professional body. To obtain M.P.H. accreditation, the curriculum must contain specific core courses. These include biostatistics, epidemiology, health planning, and environmental health. The M.P.H. has the reputation of being a more prestigious degree than the M.S., M.A., or M.Ed. There are, however, many more health educators with M.S., M.A., or M.Ed. degrees than with the M.P.H. degree. The 2003 AAHE directory lists 115 institutions that provide master's-level non-MPH degrees (AAHE, 2003). As of June 2004, there were 34 accredited schools of public health and 16 graduate programs in community health education. In addition, there were 39 graduate programs in community health/preventive medicine (Council on Education for Public Health, 2004).

Box 6.5 Practitioner's Perspective: Graduate-Level Study

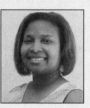

NAME: Jaime Holbrook

CURRENT POSITION/TITLE: Health Educator

EMPLOYER: Hamilton County General Health District, Cincinnati, OH

DEGREE/INSTITUTION: B.S., Central Michigan University, 1999; M.Ed., University of Cincinnati, 2001

MAJOR: Health Promotion and Education

EMPHASIS: Community Health

Job Responsibilities: In my work at the Hamilton County General Health District, I focus on injury prevention. I am currently the Coordinator for Hamilton County Safe Communities (HCSC), which is a traffic safety focused program. HCSC is funded through a grant from the Ohio Department of Public Safety. As Coordinator of HCSC I work with a 40-member coalition representing various agencies, including police, fire/EMS, hospitals, government, businesses, and community organizations. Through the coalition I coordinate many different community activities, mainly in the areas of seat belt usage, impaired driving, and speed reduction. I organize the HCSC *You Hold the Key* Teen Driving Program, which is run in several high schools throughout Hamilton County. I am also a Certified Child Passenger Safety Technician in which I conduct child safety seat inspections for the public. As part of the grant management, I am responsible or the budget and maintaining all records for purchasing and grant activities. As coordinator, I am required to develop

quarterly reports of grant activity, which must be submitted to the State.

What I like most about my job: In my current position I have a great deal of responsibility and autonomy that allows me to mold my own projects and to develop my own ideas. This freedom has helped me to learn a lot about program development and to really take pride in the projects that I work on. I also enjoy working with a vast array of professionals and being out in the field as opposed to mainly working from an office. I am able to network and meet many new partners, as well as actually make a difference in the community.

What I like least about my job: Being the coordinator of a grant, the most challenging task I face is managing the budget. This has been my first experience with budget management and I've learned that it is quite difficult to plan far enough in advance to ensure that funds are appropriately allocated and deal with

(Box 6.5 *continues*)

There are great variations between colleges and universities in the program requirements for the degree designations previously discussed. As bachelor's-level health education students begin to consider master's degree options, it would be wise to carefully examine program requirements and degree designation within the context of future career goals.

(Box 6.5 *continued*)

changes when adjustments are made to programs. Although this is one of the more stressful aspects of my position, it has been a great learning experience for me and definitely something that I feel all health educators should be exposed to.

How I obtained my job: I learned of the position opening through a jobs listserv that is run by one of my former UC professors as a service to past and present students. At the time I was searching for a new job, but I lived out of state. After learning about the job, I submitted my resume and had my first interview for the position over the phone. Once I had made it through the first round of interviews, I was asked to come to Cincinnati for a second interview with the Division Director, at which time I also was required to make a 50–60-minute presentation on the topic of my choice to the whole team. Shortly after my second interview was completed I was offered the position.

Why I decided to attend graduate school: My undergraduate degree was in health/fitness and after completing my studies I knew that I wanted to continue on in school. I felt that getting a graduate degree would give me a stronger background and better opportunities in the health field. I chose Community Health Education because it was an area that offered a lot of variety and I knew that I could work in many different arenas with this degree and not be forced to always do the same type of work.

My impressions of graduate school: Graduate school was a challenge and a great opportunity for me. Unlike undergraduate work, graduate school is focused on a particular topic so it allows you to learn in depth about your field instead of taking courses that may be unrelated. Although school was stressful because of the amount of coursework coupled with my responsibilities as a graduate assistant, I gained a great deal of practical knowledge about the field of health education. I was able to develop my professional skills, gain experience, and network with many professionals in the field, which helped me with obtaining a job.

Recommendations for Health Education students considering graduate study: I would recommend that when looking at graduate schools, research programs that will broaden the knowledge base you gained during your undergraduate work. Also, look for programs that have graduate assistantships, which provide free tuition and stipends, but also give you the chance to teach and/or do research in the field. Graduate school is a great way to expand your career opportunities and to sharpen your professional skills. Health education is a growing profession, so any added experience will only strengthen your career options in the future.

Selecting a Graduate School

Determining which college or university to attend is a decision that goes hand in hand with deciding which degree to pursue. In terms of practicality, factors such as cost, location, and size must be considered. For listings of graduate programs, see the American Association for Health Education's *Directory of Institutions Offering Undergraduate and Graduate Degree Programs in Health Education* (AAHE, 2003). This resource lists all institutions that self-report health education programs by state and type of degrees offered. The best listing of accredited programs in public health can be found online at the Council on Education for Public Health Web site, http://www.ceph.org.

Reputation is an important factor to consider when selecting a health education graduate program. There is a definite hierarchy among colleges and universities in the United States, and graduating from one of the more prestigious institutions may lend instant credibility to the graduate degree and enhance job opportunities.

Next, consider the reputation of the health education program at a given institution. To learn about various programs, bachelor's-level health educators can talk to other professionals in the field whom they admire and trust. A visit or call to their former college professors may also be a good source of information. After narrowing the list to several programs, it is wise to contact each program. Ask program administrators if they can provide written materials describing the program, application forms, admission requirements, a copy of the graduate catalog, and a list of recent graduates and where they have been employed. Much of this information may be obtained online. Contacting recent graduates is a good way to learn about a particular program.

Finally, do not overlook the college/university library as a resource. Most university libraries subscribe to a microfiche service that provides university catalogs. An overview of graduate health education programs can be obtained from this resource. In addition, many colleges and universities now have home pages on the World Wide Web that provide information about graduate programs and in some cases allow students to complete the application process electronically.

Admission Requirements

As an undergraduate health education student, it is not too early to be concerned about admission requirements to graduate school. Although admission requirements vary greatly from one university to another, one factor that has traditionally been important is the undergraduate grade point average (GPA). In general, a student should strive to achieve an overall undergraduate GPA of at least a 3.0 on a 4.0 scale to be sure of consideration by most graduate programs. Some institutions do not specify a minimum GPA (Bensley & Pope, 1994). Instead, they tend to use more individual and subjective criteria in their admission process. In either case, it is important for new health education students to attempt from the first term of their freshman year to achieve the best grades possible. Too often, low grades in the first two years of college prevent otherwise good students from being accepted into the master's degree program of their choice.

In addition to GPA requirements, most graduate programs require a completed application form, a letter of application, and several letters of reference. To be considered for admission, some programs also require students to submit scores from a standardized performance test such as the Graduate Record Exam or Miller Analogy Test. These scores may be a major component in the decision-making process, or they may simply be used in conjunction with other applicant information to provide a more well-rounded view of the prospective student.

Financing Graduate Study

Funding the graduate degree may not be as burdensome as funding undergraduate education. Many colleges and universities award assistantships or fellowships to graduate students on a competitive basis. Typically, these graduate awards pay all or part of the graduate tuition and provide students with a monthly stipend to cover living expenses during their graduate studies. In return, students agree to work for the health education program. If the award is a **graduate teaching assistantship** (or fellowship), the student teaches a specified number of undergraduate courses each term. These are usually introductory health education courses that meet general university requirements or are the first courses for health education majors. If the award is a **graduate research assistantship** (or fellowship), the student usually works closely with one or more faculty members on a particular research project. Students might be assigned to do library research, assist with data collection, enter data into the computer, or a host of other research-related activities.

Graduate assistantships and fellowships not only provide an excellent alternative for funding graduate education but also provide valuable health education work experience for the student.

SUMMARY

Since the late 1970s, many people have worked very hard and dedicated much time to defining and developing the roles and responsibilities of a health educator. The initial stages of this work have become known as the Role Delineation Project. As a result of this work, there is now an agreed-on set of responsibilities, competencies, and sub-competencies for health educators, regardless of whether they ultimately wish to work in schools, communities, clinics, or corporate settings. These responsibilities, competencies, and sub-competencies encourage college and university professional preparation programs to develop their curricula so that a standardized set of skills is taught to all health education students. Further, the responsibilities, competencies, and sub-competencies are the basis for establishing individual certification within the profession. In 1997, three additional responsibilities with accompanying competencies and sub-competencies were identified for graduate preparation in health education. In 1998, the Competencies Update Project (CUP) was initiated to review and update both the entry-level and advanced-level competencies.

Continued study in health education is necessary to stay current with health information and new techniques for conducting health education programs. All health educators should read professional journals, join one or more professional associations, and take an active role in their functioning. Certified Health Education Specialists (CHESs) must obtain continuing education credits to maintain their certification. For most bachelor's-level health educators, it would be advisable to consider a master's degree at some point in their career. Decisions concerning graduate study should not be taken lightly. Undergraduate health education students need to be aware of the admission requirements for graduate school and work to make sure they meet these requirements. Graduate assistantships or fellowships provide an excellent alternative to fund graduate education.

REVIEW QUESTIONS

1. Define *credentialing* and explain the differences among certification, registration, licensure, and accreditation.

2. Outline the major events of the Role Delineation Project.

3. Review the "Responsibilities and Competencies for Entry-Level Health Educators" (Appendix B). Do you think they are more focused on health content or the process skills needed to be a health educator? Defend your position and explain why you believe the health education profession has moved in this direction.

4. Identify two ways health educators can stay up-to-date in the field.

5. What is the difference among the following academic degrees: M.A., M.Ed., M.S., M.P.H., M.S.P.H.?

6. Briefly describe the process for applying to graduate school.

CRITICAL THINKING QUESTIONS

1. If Helen Cleary and her contemporaries had not begun the Role Delineation Project, and if there were no certification (CHES) available to health educators, how do you think the profession would be different today? Think in terms of professional preparation, recognition, employment opportunities, and so on.

2. Suppose an accreditation system were developed and implemented that required all health education professional preparation programs to meet the same guidelines and standards. How do you think such a system would impact the profession? What do you see as the potential positive outcomes and the potential negative outcomes of such accreditation?

3. You have been asked to serve as a student member to the Competencies Update Project Advisory Committee (CUPAC). At your first meeting you are asked to give your opinion on the entry-level and graduate standards as they currently exist. Do you feel they accurately represent professional practice? Why or why not? What changes do you think should be made in terms of eliminating competencies, adding competencies, and/or moving competencies from one level to the other?

ACTIVITIES

1. Read each competency and sub-competency of a health educator. Score each competency and sub-competency using the following scale:

   A. I currently have the skill to meet this competency/sub-competency.

   B. I am uncertain if I have the skill to meet this competency/sub-competency.

   C. I do not have the skill to meet this competency/sub-competency.

   After rating each competency and sub-competency, make a list of things you can do to enhance your skills. Keep this table, and periodically reevaluate your skills throughout your program of study.

2. Write to one or more universities you may wish to attend and request information on their graduate health education programs or go online to find this information. Try to learn about their admission requirements, degree options, and financial aid opportunities.

3. Make an appointment with a professor at your school to talk about graduate school. Ask about the schools the professor attended and the degree earned. Finally, ask for advice on what degree to earn and what school to attend.

WEBLINKS

1. **http://www.nchec.org/**

   National Commission for Health Education Credentialing (NCHEC)

   Use this Web site to learn more about becoming a Certified Health Education Specialist (CHES). The site provides helpful information about health education certification including application procedures.

2. **http://www.ceph.org/**

   Council on Education for Public Health

   The Council is responsible for accrediting programs in public health. A complete list of accredited schools and programs of public health can be found at this site.

3. **http://www.csuchico.edu/cjhp/2/1/index.htm**

   California Journal of Health Promotion.

   Read the article titled, "Improving the Quality of Professional Life: Benefits of Health Education and Promotion Association Membership" by Kathleen Young and Whitney Boling. This article clearly explains the benefits of professional association membership for keeping up-to-date with the profession. It also provides a list of health education professional associations to consider joining. While at this site, also read the article titled, "Graduate School in Health Education: A Challenge to Consider" by Michele Pettit. It provides insight and helpful points to ponder when considering graduate school.

CASE STUDY

Anita considers herself a school health educator. She graduated from college with a major in health education and an emphasis in school health. She is licensed by the state in which she lives to teach health education in the schools. She is also a Certified Health Education Specialist (CHES) and has been very vocal in advocating that all school health educators should be CHESs. Anita has been asked to provide a thirty-minute presentation at the state AAHPERD convention on the importance of CHES. This audience will be mostly school health educators. Your task is to help Anita develop the main points of her presentation. Why should school health educators become CHESs? Also, be the devil's advocate. What arguments is she likely to hear from those who are not certified and do not feel certification is important? How can she respond to these arguments? (Note: This same case study can be replicated with Anita being a community health educator, worksite health educator, or clinic/hospital health educator).

REFERENCE LIST

American Association for Health Education (2003). Directory of institutions offering undergraduate and graduate degree programs in health education. *American Journal of Health Education*. 34 (4), 219–235.

Anspaugh, D. J., Dignan, M. B., & Anspaugh, S. L. (2000). *Developing health promotion programs*. Boston: McGraw Hill.

Bensley, L. B., Jr. & Pope, A. J. (1994). A study of graduate bulletins to determine general information and graduation requirements for master's degree programs in health education. *Journal of Health Education, 25* (3), 165–171.

Cleary, H. P. (1986). Issues in the credentialing of health education specialists: A review of the state of the art. In William B. Ward (Ed.), *Advances in health education and promotion,* Greenwich, Conn: Jai Press, Inc., 129–154.

Cleary, H. P. (1995). *The credentialing of health educators: An historical account 1970–1990.* New York: The National Commission for Health Education Credentialing, Inc.

Council on Education for Public Health. (2004). U.S. Schools of Public Health and Graduate Public Health Programs Accredited by the Council on Education for Public Health. Available at: http://www.CEPH.org/

Davis, T. M. (1999). Health educators as positive health role models. *Journal of Health Education.* 30 (1).

Doyle, E., & Ward, S. *The process of community health education and promotion.* Mountain View, CA: Mayfield Publishing.

Gilmore, G. D., & Campbell, M. D. (2005). *Needs and capacity assessment strategies for health education and health promotion.* Boston: Jones and Bartlett.

Gilmore, G. D., Olsen, L. K., Taub, A., & Connell, D. (2003). National Health Education Competencies Update Project: Preliminary Results. Presented at the AAHPERD National Convention, April 2, 2003, Philadelphia.

Joint Committee for Graduate Standards (1996). National Congress for Institutions Preparing Graduate Health Educators. Program Booklet, 1.

McKenzie, J. F., Neiger, B. L., & Smeltzer, J. L. (2005). *Planning, implementing & evaluating health promotion programs* (4th ed.). San Francisco: Pearson, Benjamin Cummings.

National Commission for Health Education Credentialing. (1996). *A competency-based framework for professional development of certified health education specialists.* New York: National Commission for Health Education Credentialing.

National Commission for Health Education Credentialing. (1998). *Spring, 1998 Certified Health Education Specialist Examination Brochure.* [Brochure].

National Commission for Health Education Credentialing. (2004a). Mission Statement. Available at: http://www.nchec.org/aboutnchec/about.htm.

National Commission for Health Education Credentialing. (2004b). Eligibility for the CHES Exam. Available at: http://www.NCHEC.org/becomeches/eligibility.htm.

National Commission for Health Education Credentialing. (2004c). Competencies Update Project. Available at: http://www.NCHEC.org/aboutnchec/cup/press.htm.

National Commission for Health Education Credentialing. (2004). Why certify? Credentialing and benefits of certification. Downloaded 6/4/04 at http://www.nchec.org/whycert/certify.htm.

National Task Force on the Preparation and Practice of Health Educators (1985). *Framework for the development of competency-based curricula for entry level health educators.* New York, NY: National Commission for Health Education Credentialing, Inc.

Society for Public Health Education. (June 2004). SABPAC. Available at: http://www.SOPHE.org.

Society for Public Health Education. (2000). Future directions for quality assurance of professional preparation in health education. *News & Views, 27* (3).

CHAPTER 7

The Settings for Health Education

Chapter Objectives

After reading this chapter and answering the questions at the end, you should be able to:

1. Identify the four major settings in which health educators are employed.
2. Describe the major responsibilities for health educators in the four major settings.
3. Discuss the advantages and disadvantages of the four major settings.
4. Explain the qualifications and major responsibilities of health educators working in colleges and universities.
5. Identify a variety of "nontraditional" settings in which health educators may be employed.
6. State several action steps that can be taken to help procure one's first job in health education.

Key Terms

community health education
coordinated school health program
hard money
health care settings

networking
portfolio
public health agencies
school health education

service learning
soft money
voluntary health agencies
worksite health promotion

Today, most Americans live a healthier and longer life than ever before. Despite this fact, however, it is clear that many, if not most, Americans are not living at their optimal level of health. Hereditary, environmental, and behavioral factors predispose too many U.S. citizens to disease, suffering, disability, and premature death. Health education professionals are specially trained to help individuals and communities reduce their health risks. According to the U.S. Department of Labor

Bureau of Labor Statistics (2004), in 2002 there were over 43,000 health educators employed in the United States earning a mean annual wage of $39,190. The challenge for health educators is to help people reduce their risk and increase the probability of a long, happy, and productive life.

To meet this challenge, health educators conduct programs in a variety of settings (National Commission for Health Education Credentialing [NCHEC], 2004). The use of multiple settings is important, as it allows health educators to reach the greatest number of people in the most convenient, efficient, and effective ways possible. Although the goals of health education and the skills needed to carry out the responsibilities are nearly the same in all settings (English & Videto, 1997), the actual duties of a job may differ greatly from setting to setting.

Professional preparation programs in health education typically prepare students for employment in one or more of four major settings. These settings are schools, hospitals/clinics, community/public health agencies, and business/industry. On obtaining advanced degrees, students from any of these settings may seek employment as college or university health educators. In addition, health educators can work in a variety of nontraditional employment areas.

In this chapter, each of the four major settings for health education will be discussed. After a short introduction to the setting, a description of one day in the career of a health educator from that particular setting is presented. This is designed to give the reader a general idea of what a workday is like. Because of the great diversity in duties from health educator to health educator even within the same setting, it is impossible to say that this is a typical day. For most health educators, there is no such thing as a typical day. Following this is a section that describes additional responsibilities that might be assigned to health educators in the setting. Again, this is not intended to be an exhaustive list but is intended to further the reader's understanding of job responsibilities in that setting. Finally, each section will end with a listing of some advantages and disadvantages for that setting.

School Health Education

School health involves "all the strategies, activities, and services offered by, in, or in association with schools that are designed to promote students' physical, emotional, and social development" (American School Health Association, 2004). **School health education,** as the name implies, primarily involves instructing school-age children about health and health-related behaviors. The initial impetus for school health stemmed from the terrible epidemics of the 1800s and the efforts of the Women's Christian Temperance Movement to promote abstinence from alcohol in the early 1900s. Many states mandated school health education to inform students about these health hazards. Unfortunately, these mandates have seldom been strictly enforced. Further, teachers have often been underqualified, with only an academic minor or a few elective courses to prepare them for the health classroom. As a result, the quality of school health programs has often been compromised (Breckon, Harvey, & Lancaster, 1998; Naidoo & Wills, 2000).

Despite these limitations, the potential for school districts and the health instruction program in particular to impact students is tremendous. It is easier and more effective to establish healthy behaviors in childhood than it is to change

Table 7.1   Rules of Good Health—1922

1. Take a full bath more than once a week.
2. Brush teeth at least once a day.
3. Sleep long hours with window open.
4. Drink as much milk as possible, but no coffee or tea.
5. Eat some vegetables or fruit every day.
6. Drink at least four glasses of water a day.
7. Play part of every day outdoors.
8. Have a bowel movement every morning.

Source: Data from Bernice C. Regney, "Rules of the Health Game" in *Milk and Our School Children,* U.S. Dept. of the Interior, Bureau of Education, Health Education, No. 11. (1922).

Table 7.2   National Health Education Standards

1. Students will comprehend concepts related to health promotion and disease prevention.
2. Students will demonstrate the ability to access valid health information and health-promoting products and services.
3. Students will demonstrate the ability to practice health-enhancing behaviors and reduce health risks.
4. Students will analyze the influence of culture, media, technology, and other factors on health.
5. Students will demonstrate the ability to use interpersonal communication skills to enhance health.
6. Students will demonstrate the ability to use goal-setting and decision-making skills to enhance health.
7. Students will demonstrate the ability to advocate for personal, family, and community health.

Source: A work of the Joint Committee on National Health Education Standards. Reprinted by permission of the American Cancer Society, Inc. (1995).

unhealthy behaviors in adulthood. Each school day provides the opportunity to reach 53 million students. The 119,000 schools in the United States provide a laboratory where students can eat healthy foods, participate in physical activity, and learn how to take care of their health and well-being (Centers for Disease Control, 2004b). School health programs have demonstrated effectiveness when they are well planned, sequential, provided significant time in the curriculum, and taught by a trained health educator (Fisher et al., 2003).

The sophistication of school health education programs has increased dramatically over the years. Today's school health educator needs to be well trained and prepared to deliver a comprehensive and demanding curriculum. Comparing the 1922 "Rules of Good Health" with the 1995 National Health Education Standards (Joint Committee on Health Education Standards, 1995) clearly illustrates this point (see Tables 7.1 and 7.2).

When the school health education component is made a part of a broader, district-wide approach known as a **coordinated school health program,** the potential to impact students in a positive way is even greater. Allensworth and Kolbe

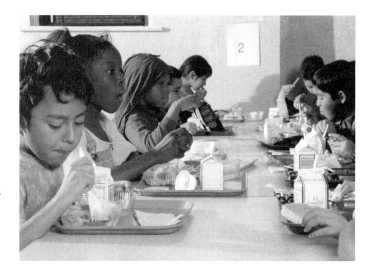

Food service is one component of a coordinated school health program. (David Buffington, Getty Images)

(1987) were first to envision a comprehensive and coordinated school health program. They defined it as:

> an integrated set of planned, sequential, school-affiliated strategies, activities, and services designed to promote the optimal physical, emotional, social, and educational development of students. The program involves and is supportive of families and is determined by the local community based on community needs, resources, standards and requirements. It is coordinated by a multidisciplinary team and accountable to the community for program quality and effectiveness. (p. 60)

In other words, a coordinated school health program coordinates and integrates various aspects of a school district to best impact the health of the students, faculty, staff, administration, and community as a whole. This includes food services, nursing services, school counseling and psychology, health instruction, physical education, administration, school environment, community involvement, and faculty/staff wellness (CDC, 2004).

A health educator choosing to work in the school setting will find a challenging and rewarding career. Given the number of school districts in the United States, it is obvious that a large number of people teach health education in the schools. Unfortunately, many of these people are not health education specialists. Some school districts have used biology, physical education, home economics or family life, and consumer science teachers to teach health. Even when certified health education teachers are employed, they may have only a minor in health education and are not fully prepared. A further problem confounding the employment situation in the schools is that the requirement for health education is usually less than for other academic subjects. Students typically need only one or two semesters of health education to graduate from high school, while they probably are required to complete four years of English. Thus, with such a minimal requirement, the number of health teachers needed and the resulting demand for health teachers are low. The bottom line is that, in many parts of the country, it is difficult to obtain a job in school health.

Those students who are really committed to being outstanding health teachers, however, should not be deterred from this career path. With time, dedication, and perseverance, those who really want to teach health in the schools can usually find employment. Substitute teaching, coaching, and volunteering are good ways to make oneself known in a school district and increase the likelihood of eventual employment. Students are encouraged to talk to their own professors to determine the job market for school health education in their area.

A Day in the Career of a School Health Educator

At 5:45 A.M. the alarm goes off and Ms. Bell's day is started. Ms. Bell teaches seventh- and eighth-grade health at a junior high school in a suburban school district. After going through the normal morning routine, she arrives at the school building around 7:00 A.M. There is a half hour before homeroom, so she picks up her mail and duplicates a test that she prepared the night before for her eighth-grade health class. In homeroom she takes attendance, gets a lunch count, listens to announcements over the loudspeaker, and collects money from a fruit sale fund-raiser. The fruit sale is being conducted by the PTA to raise money for new computers in the school. Essentially, homeroom involves administrative responsibilities and a considerable amount of paperwork.

At 7:45 the first period starts. This school has eight fifty-minute periods, with only four minutes between periods. The first three periods, Ms. Bell teaches seventh-grade health. Today's lesson is on refusal skills related to alcohol and drug use. Ms. Bell has written three scenarios students could find themselves in. The scenarios are open ended, so after each one Ms. Bell leads a discussion on how to use refusal skills to get out of a bad situation. She then asks students to role-play the situations to gain further practice in using refusal skills. Unfortunately, only two of her three classes will get this lesson today. The second-period class is one day behind due to an assembly that was held a week ago. Ms. Bell has to find a way to catch this group up with the rest of the classes.

Ms. Bell's fourth period is divided in half. The first half, she has study hall duty. It is her responsibility to take attendance and monitor the study hall. In today's study hall, two boys become unruly and nearly get in a fight. She sends them to the office for discipline, but the situation is quite upsetting.

The second half of fourth period is Ms. Bell's lunch time. She usually has twenty-five minutes to eat lunch and relax before fifth period begins. Today, however, she must use part of that time to drop by the office for a follow-up discussion with the assistant principal concerning the incident in study hall.

Fifth period, Ms. Bell teaches eighth-grade health. Today is a test day. While the students are taking their test, Ms. Bell works on a future lesson plan for the class.

Sixth period is Ms. Bell's planning period. Today she tries to make a phone call to the parents of one of her students who is having problems in health class, but no one is home. She then grades the test papers from her previous class and records the grades. She averages the grades and starts to develop interim reports for the fifth-period class, but she runs out of time. Seventh and eighth periods are also eighth-grade health classes. While students take their tests, Ms. Bell works on grading papers from the previous classes and writing her interim reports.

(Text continues on page 194)

Box 7.1 Practitioner's Perspective: School Health Education

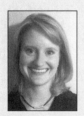

NAME: Kate Mathay

CURRENT POSITION: Health Teacher

EMPLOYER: Centerville City Schools

DEGREE/INSTITUTION: B.S. in Education, B.S. in Health Promotion and Enhancement, Miami University, 2001

MAJORS: Health Education; Health Promotion and Enhancement

EMPHASIS: Nutrition

Responsibilities: My primary responsibility is educating students in areas of health, while following my school system's curriculum and the Ohio State Standards for Health Education. Topics of study include disease prevention, sex education, alcohol, and other drugs. Other daily requirements consist of maintaining accurate records, and creating an open line of communication with parents and staff regarding students' progress and behavior in my class. This includes phone calls, e-mails, Web page development, and parent conferences. I am also responsible for active participation on staff committees, intramural coaching, and working on community-wide events. My school district requires a minimum of 15 hours of in-service training throughout the school year, and expects that I will attend state and national conferences in my field. Finally, my most important responsibility is to be an effective teacher. This requires being a role model for my students, staying current with what they're involved in, keeping up to date with the latest health information and teaching strategies, and constantly evaluating and improving myself and my lessons.

Obtaining my position: My principal once confided in me that I had the job before I even interviewed for it. At the end of my senior year in college, I learned of an opening at the middle school level and decided to apply for the job. The day before I started the interview process, I walked into my principal's office, introduced myself, and made it known that I wanted the job. I highly suggest you do the same, because it was this initiative that won her over.

Before this interview took place, I strived to make myself marketable for the employment world. My university offered a service to critique your interview skills. This gave me practice and experience with some of the more difficult questions. I spent a great deal of time talking with people in the field about job options and openings, checking every Web site I could, and attending job fairs at my university and the surrounding communities. I learned that you have to be willing to go anywhere, sell yourself to anyone, and be open and flexible with your future.

What I enjoy most: There is not a single day that is the same as the last when you are a teacher. I can never predict exactly how the day will flow, what will happen, how my lesson will work, or how my students will respond. A fire drill could go

(Box 7.1 *continues*)

(Box 7.1 *continued*)

off right in the middle of the lesson I spent hours preparing. You will not find that in an office job. Furthermore, my coworkers are phenomenal. I learn from them constantly, commiserate with them on a daily basis, and spend a great deal of time with them outside of school as well. They keep me coming to work in the middle of January when there is no break in sight.

That being said, my students play a large factor in my enjoyment as well. I relish the times when my kids' faces light up because of their success. They make me laugh with their innocence and self-expression. I am reminded everyday that what I do is meaningful and important. Some students spend more time with the adults of their school than with the adults in their home. If I don't make a difference with these students, no one will. This can be a daunting, but gratifying, task.

What I enjoy least: The most frustrating part of my job is dealing with the one student, or group of students, who don't care. They don't want to be there, they don't care what you or anyone else has to say, and there is no one at home to reprimand them for their attitudes and lack of performance. Most often, their home life is such that school is the last of their concerns, and the environment is not conducive to studying or completing projects. This lack of parental support, lack of internal motivation, and lack of resources can create an arduous teaching experience.

The second difficulty I have discovered through the years comes not from the day-to-day tasks, but from the "powers that be." Earning and maintaining a license to educate, and proving you are effective, requires jumping through more hoops than I ever thought possible. What makes these "hoops" even more exacerbating is when you consider the source. Many of the laws and regulations surrounding education come from politicians who never had any formal training in the field. While I can appreciate the desire to have the best teachers in our classrooms, the Knights of the Round Table did not put forth this much effort to prove their worth.

Recommendations: If you want to "like" your job and be good at it the first time around, find another career. In teaching, you have to be effective and make a difference with *every* child. It's not enough to like them or to give them a smile each day. You have to show quantitative results in every child's learning. To do this I recommend you pay attention to things like Gardner's *Learning Styles,* Bloom's *Taxonomy,* and the State Standards. I suggest you use curricula that are proven to be effective, but add your own creative spark to the lessons. Stay enthusiastic, current with the trends, and involved in your students' lives. And most importantly, continue to evaluate yourself. Yes, your administration will evaluate you, and there will be those hoops to jump through, but the best assessment comes from your students, your coworkers, and yourself. It is not necessary to reinvent yourself every September, but you must stay fresh, stay on top of what is new, and stay effective.

School ends for the students at 2:57 P.M. After monitoring the hall while students leave the building, Ms. Bell hurries to the cafeteria for the monthly teachers' meeting. General information and announcements are presented by the principal. The meeting ends at 4:00 P.M.

In addition to her teaching responsibilities, Ms. Bell coaches the junior high girls' volleyball team. Practice usually goes from 3:15 to 5:00. Today's practice will go from 4:00 to 5:00 due to the teachers' meeting. After practice, Ms. Bell waits until the last girl leaves the locker room, then returns to her classroom to prepare for the next day's classes. She leaves the school at around 5:30 P.M.

After dinner and her family responsibilities, Ms. Bell spends twenty minutes on the phone with the student's parents who were not at home earlier in the day. She then finishes grading the tests she gave in class and continues working on interim reports. It will take her at least one more evening to finish the interims. At 11:00 P.M. she turns off the light and goes to bed.

Additional Responsibilities

In addition to the lesson planning, grading, parent meetings, disciplining, coaching, and the various administrative duties, teachers may have still more responsibilities. They may be involved in curriculum development, the review of materials for classroom use, the chaperoning of dances or other after-school activities, fund-raising, and the advising of student groups such as yearbook, debate, or student council. School health educators should also be active members of their professional organizations. This allows them to network with other health educators and to stay up-to-date in the field. Finally, school health educators should be strong advocates for school health (Utah State University, 1996). They must make certain that fellow faculty, administrators, school boards, and the community as a whole are aware of the unique contributions of a school health program. (See Table 7.3.)

Community/Public Health Education

Community health education, as defined by the Joint Committee on Health Education and Promotion Terminology (2002), is

> a theory-driven process that promotes health and prevents disease within populations (p. 97).

Community health programs target individuals, local communities, states, and the nation. There is a reciprocal relationship between these various targets. Over the years, it has become clear that the health of a community is closely linked to the individual health of community members. Likewise, the collective behaviors, attitudes, and beliefs of everyone who lives in the community profoundly affect the community's health. Indeed, the underlying premise of *Healthy People 2010* is that the health of the individual is almost inseparable from the health of the larger community, and that the health of every community in every state and territory determines the overall health status of the nation. This explains why the vision for *Healthy People 2010* is "Healthy People in Healthy Communities" (U.S. Department of Health and Human Services, 2000a).

Table 7.3   Advantages and Disadvantages of Working
in School Health Education

Advantages

- Health educators have the ability to work with young people during their developmental years.
- Health educators have the potential to prevent harmful health behaviors from forming instead of working with older people after such behaviors have been formed.
- Health educators have the opportunity to impact all students, because health education is usually a required course.
- A graduate degree is not needed for entry-level employment.
- There is good job security.
- Summer months are free and there are nice vacation periods in December and in spring.
- Benefits are good.

Disadvantages

- Good health educators usually spend many long hours at their job, including weekends and evenings that may compensate for the long vacation periods.
- Health educators may have relatively low status in a school district when compared with teachers of more traditional subjects such as math, science, and English.
- Pay is low when compared with professionals in other fields, but comparable when compared with that of other health educators.
- Discipline problems are often seen as a major disadvantage.
- Summer "free time" may be consumed with summer employment and/or returning to college for additional required coursework.
- It is difficult dealing with conservative school boards, parents, and community groups when teaching controversial issues such as sex education and drug education.

The most likely sources of employment for community health educators are voluntary health agencies and public health agencies. **Voluntary health agencies** are created by concerned citizens to deal with health needs not met by governmental agencies (McKenzie, Pinger, & Kotecki, 2002). As the name implies, they rely heavily on volunteer help and donations. There are usually paid staff members who are responsible for administration, volunteer recruitment and coordination, program development, and fund-raising. Health educators are hired to plan, implement, and evaluate the education component of the agency's programs. They often, however, are involved in other aspects of the agency as well. Voluntary health agencies are usually funded by such means as private donations, grants, fund-raisers, and possibly United Way contributions. Examples of voluntary health agencies include the American Cancer Society, American Heart Association, and American Lung Association. Most of these large, well-known voluntary agencies have national, state, and local divisions.

Public health agencies, or official governmental health agencies, are usually financed through public tax monies. Government has long been responsible for doing for the people as a whole what individuals could not do for themselves. Thus, governments provide police protection, educational systems, clean air and water, and many other important services. Departments of public health, thus, are formed to coordinate and provide health services to a community. Health departments may

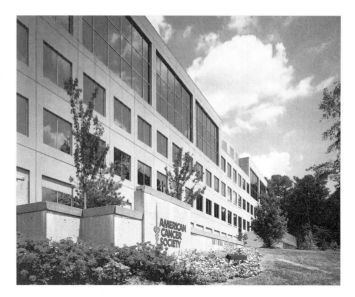

The American Cancer Society is a nationwide voluntary health organization dedicated to eliminating cancer as a major health problem by preventing cancer, saving lives from cancer, and diminishing suffering from cancer through research, education, advocacy, and service. Health educators often work for voluntary agencies like the American Cancer Society. (American Cancer Society/California Division)

be organized by the city, county, state, or federal government. They operate primarily with paid staff and typically provide health education services as part of their total program. Table 7.4 contains a list of agencies that have programs for which community/public health educators may be employed.

More diversity in terms of job responsibilities exists in the community/public health education setting than in the other major settings in which health educators are employed. This is due to the large number of community and public health agencies that exist and the vast differences in their missions, goals, and objectives. In some community/public agencies, health educators serve administrative functions such as coordinating volunteers, budgeting, fund-raising, program planning, and serving as liaisons to other agencies and groups. In other community/public agencies, the health educator may be more involved in direct program delivery to the clientele of that agency and/or the community at large. Most frequently, however, health educators are involved in a little bit of everything.

A Day in the Career of a Community Health Educator

Mr. Fischer is the health educator for a local division of the American Cancer Society (ACS). In that role, he has the responsibility of conducting health education programs in a four-county area of the state. Mr. Fischer usually arrives at the office between 8:30 and 9:00 in the morning. This morning, however, he had an 8:00 A.M. meeting with a local coalition that is trying to encourage school districts to implement comprehensive school health education into their curricula. This is an important issue, as the ACS has made comprehensive school health education one of its major priority areas at the national level. Mr. Fischer has been responsible for forming this coalition and was recently elected to serve as its chairperson. As such,

Table 7.4   Possible Sources of Employment in Community/Public Health Education

State, local, city health departments
U.S. Public Health Service
U.S. Food & Drug Administration
U.S. or state departments of agriculture
U.S. or state departments of transportation
County extension services
U.S. Department of Health and Human Services
U.S. Centers for Disease Control
National Institutes of Health
U.S. or state penal institutions
Voluntary health agencies
Private foundations

he sets the agenda, runs the meetings, takes minutes, and always plans for juice and bagels to be served.

It is 9:30 when Mr. Fischer finally arrives at his office. He spends the next half hour opening his mail, responding to e-mail, and returning telephone calls. From 10:00 to 11:00 is the biweekly staff meeting, which is run by Mr. Fischer's supervisor, who is director of the local ACS unit. In these meetings, staff members provide updates on projects for which they are responsible. Issues and problems facing the local unit are discussed, with the intent of involving the group in identifying potential solutions. Information from the state and national levels is also provided.

From 11:00 to 12:00, Mr. Fischer has time to sit at his desk and work on the Great American Smokeout. This is a yearly campaign to help smokers quit smoking for at least one day and hopefully for the rest of their lives. Mr. Fischer is responsible for this event. He has to recruit local sponsors to donate money or prizes for the event, plan a variety of activities to promote the event, contact local media to cover the various events, distribute materials to numerous participating groups, coordinate volunteers to assist with or run various events, develop letters of understanding with each group assisting with the event, and provide letters of thanks to all groups and individual volunteers who assist with the event after it is over. Twice during this hour, Mr. Fischer is interrupted by phone calls from individuals needing information on various cancers. Mr. Fischer writes down their request on a referral slip, along with their name and address. Twice a week he has a volunteer who comes in and mails all of the information that has been requested.

At 12:00 Mr. Fischer heads out for lunch. He usually eats lunch at his desk while working, but today he is speaking to the local Rotary Club about the Great American Smokeout. Although Mr. Fischer enjoys public speaking, he does not have enough time to handle all of the requests and frequently coordinates volunteers to speak on behalf of the ACS.

Mr. Fischer returns to his office shortly before 2:00. He takes another hour to answer phone calls and emails that have come in since the morning and writes some correspondence related to the Great American Smokeout and the Coordinated School Health Coalition. From 3:00 to 5:00, Mr. Fischer is on the phone, calling

Box 7.2 Practitioner's Perspective: Voluntary Health Agency

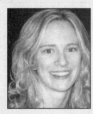

NAME: Sarah Kirsch

CURRENT POSITION: Health Promotions Director

EMPLOYER: American Cancer Society

DEGREE/INSTITUTION/MAJOR: BS, University of Cincinnati, 1997, in Health Education with Exercise Emphasis; MS, American University, 2000, in Health Promotion Management

Job responsibilities in my current position: In my current position I have many responsibilities, including the following:

- Supervise day-to-day office operations and coordinate the work of two Health Promotion Specialists to ensure success of projects in seven southwest Ohio counties.
- Provide leadership for volunteers by recruiting, training, planning and consulting in the implementation and evaluation of all American Cancer Society programs.
- Evaluate volunteer success and recommend modifications of volunteer activities as needed.
- Attend program trainings and updates, along with numerous conferences and workshops to continually increase my knowledge and skills within the health education field specifically related to the American Cancer Society.

- Help build and lead county-wide task forces or coalitions in order to accomplish a greater number of organizational initiatives.
- Continually update community cancer assessments in all seven counties.
- Work with businesses within the seven counties to educate employees on the importance of early detection and prevention.
- Develop strong relationships with hospitals in seven counties to increase patient referrals to health promotion programs and gain support for task forces.
- Write grants for school health projects, tobacco education, and cancer prevention programs.

How I obtained my current position: While in graduate school, I spent time

(Box 7.2 *continues*)

volunteers to participate in a fund-raiser called Jail and Bail. With this fund-raiser, volunteers are notified in advance that they will be picked up and escorted to "jail," where they will have to stay behind bars until they can raise bail. The jail is actually a temporary structure located at the local mall. Bail is raised by calling friends and acquaintances, requesting donations to the ACS. This is a good fund-raiser and a lot of fun, but it takes considerable staff time to prepare for the event.

Mr. Fischer leaves the office at 5:00 to have dinner with his family. Tonight, however, he has to be back at the office at 7:30 for a meeting of the Youth Education Committee. As the name implies, this committee of volunteers is responsible for all local ACS programs dealing with youth. As the health educator, Mr. Fischer has to be present for all of their monthly meetings. In addition to the Youth Education Committee, there are also board meetings, volunteer recognition nights,

(Box 7.2 *continued*)

volunteering for a community outreach program in the area of health education. I enjoyed working in a community-type setting, where I had the opportunity to interact with many different people in various situations. After completing graduate school I decided to move back to Cincinnati from Washington, DC. I saw a job posting in the *Cincinnati Enquirer* for the American Cancer Society. It seemed like a perfect fit because it would give me the opportunity to work in several communities with many people throughout southwest Ohio. It would also give me the chance to utilize the skills I had learned in health education and promotion to help prevent people from contracting cancer, or losing their life to the disease that took two of my grandparents' lives. After submitting my resume for review, I was given a phone interview, followed by two personal interviews. I began my job in September of 2000 overseeing all American Cancer Society programs and services in southwest Ohio.

What I like most about my current position: Working with a voluntary health organization is incredibly satisfying and rewarding. I am inspired each day by the strength and courage of the many individuals I meet or work with who are battling cancer themselves or have a close family member who is battling cancer.

What I like least about my current position: In my position I come into contact regularly with many people who have cancer or have had cancer. Although more and more people are surviving cancer today, there are still a significant number who lose their battle. The most difficult part of this job, and what I like least about it, is when I feel helpless because I cannot help someone. It is very difficult to see someone lose his or her life to the disease you are trying to work so hard to prevent.

Recommendation for those preparing to be health educators: I believe it is important to spend a great deal of time in the field experiencing many areas of health education. Learning in the classroom is very important, but hands-on experience will help you find the best fit for your personality and will afford the greatest opportunity to use your skills. This will also give you the chance to begin networking and developing relationships that can help you build your career as a health educator.

Adult Education Committee meetings, and numerous other speaking engagements and responsibilities that require Mr. Fischer to work in the evenings. He averages one or two nights a week on the job. In addition, he occasionally has to work on weekends during special ACS events.

Additional Responsibilities

As can be seen from the Mr. Fischer example, community/public health educators are involved in numerous and varied activities. Planning, implementing, and evaluating programs and events are major tasks, but, in conducting these tasks, health educators get involved in fund-raising, coalition building, committee work, budgeting, general administration, public speaking, volunteer recruitment, grant writing, and media advocacy. (See Table 7.5.)

Table 7.5 Advantages and Disadvantages of Working in Community/Public Health Education

Advantages

- Job responsibilities are highly varied and changing.
- There is a strong emphasis on prevention.
- There is usually a high community profile.
- Health educators work with multiple groups of people.
- There is a high degree of self-satisfaction.

Disadvantages

- Pay may be low, particularly in voluntary agencies.
- When hired directly by a community or public health agency, job security tends to be good. In such situations, the health educator is said to be employed on **hard money**. Sometimes, however, these agencies hire health educators on money secured through grants, which is known as **soft money**. In these situations, positions are terminated when grant funding is discontinued; so, job security can be a concern.
- Relying heavily on volunteers can be frustrating. While most volunteers are great, some do not demonstrate the same level of commitment as might a paid employee.
- There never seems to be enough money to run all the programs that need to be offered in the way they should be offered.

Table 7.6 Worksite Health Promotion Activities

Smoking cessation	Cancer risk awareness	Lending libraries
Stress management	Cardiovascular risk	Physical examinations
Weight loss	awareness	Smoke-free policies
Exercise/physical fitness	Skin cancer screenings	Counseling hot lines
Nutrition	Flu shots	Hypertension screenings
Safety	Health fairs	HIV/AIDS prevention
First aid & CPR	Bulletin boards	Paycheck stuffers
Mammography screenings	Newsletters	

Worksite Health Promotion and Education

The Joint Committee on Health Education and Promotion Terminology (2001) defines **worksite health promotion** as "a combination of educational, organizational and environmental activities designed to improve the health and safety of employees and their families" (p. 103). Since the mid-1970s, business and industry in the United States have been offerin worksite health promotion programs for their employees. These on-site programs offer an additional setting for health educators and allow them to reach segments of the population that had not been easily accessible in the past.

Health promotion programs at worksites differ greatly from site to site (U.S. Department of Health and Human Services, 2003) Some are very extensive, include elaborate facilities, and are conducted by full-time staff members hired by the company; others are minimal programs that may include only a brown bag lunch speaker's program or a discount at the YMCA or health club. For a list of worksite health promotion activities, see Table 7.6.

Box 7.3 Practitioner's Perspective: Community Health Educator

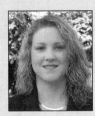

NAME: Melissa Schulte, BS, CHES

CURRENT POSITION/TITLE: Health Education Specialist

EMPLOYER: County of Fresno, Department of Community Health

DEGREE/INSTITUTION/YEAR: Bachelor of Science, California State University, Fresno, 1999

MAJOR: Health Science, Community Health Option

How I obtained my job: In preparation for a job as a health educator, I completed an internship program. Through this internship, I learned about many of the local health agencies and organizations where many health education professionals are employed. I maintained contact with my internship coordinator, who knew many other health education professionals in the community. After several submissions of applications and resumes to various agencies, the Fresno County Department of Community Health offered me a position as a Health Education Specialist.

How I utilize health education in my job: For the last four years, I have been a general practitioner in health education. My responsibilities include program planning and development, implementation and evaluation for different health programs. One of my primary tasks is determining the need for health programs through research and needs assessments and acquiring funding resources to support those programs.

What I like most about my job: The position I hold is unique in that I do not focus on one specific health issue, as do many of my colleagues. I am fortunate in that I am able to learn about many health issues and present background research and needs assessments to my colleagues in order for them to establish health programs.

What I like least about my job: The one drawback to my position is that, although I participate in nearly every component of a health education program, I do not see a single program from planning and development through implementation and final evaluation. In many cases, I see many programs in various stages of development and implementation at one time. This can create a situation where balancing all of the various programs' immediate needs is challenging. This continual challenge, however, intrigues me and pushes me to higher levels of competency in my work.

Recommendations for those preparing to be health educators: As students, we learn the components of health education programs. That information will provide the foundation of your work. The learning does not stop with the acquisition of your degree. Some words of advice for you: Know the community in which you intend to work. Complete an internship program. Find a mentor in the field. Your internship should provide you with many contacts in the field who are willing to serve as mentors. Find your passion and excel to serve the people in your community. Prepare for and take the Certified Health Education Specialist exam. This designation provides a distinction between you and your uncertified counterparts to potential employers, colleagues and clients that you have met national standards for your profession.

The role of health educators/health promotion specialists in the future: Health educators will continue to play a

(Box 7.3 *continues*)

(Box 7.3 *continued*)

valuable role in the community as well as the health care system. As health care costs increase, the desire to prevent or reduce the risk for health conditions that have high rates of morbidity and mortality will also increase. Health educators will assist the health care system by planning and implementing effective health education and health promotion programs to address lifestyle behaviors that modern medicine does not adequately address with patients. Health educators will also work to incorporate participation in these activities into individual health insurance-paid benefits. Together, the public health and health care systems will work together to improve the health status of all people.

The proportion of employers who provide worksite health promotion programs has increased over the years. It is reported that health improvement programs of some kind are now being offered by over 80% of worksites with 50 or more employees and almost all large employers with more than 750 employees (U.S. Department of Health and Human Services, 2003). Despite these impressive numbers for large employers, more needs to be done. Many of these large employers have only minimal health promotion offerings. The majority of U.S. employees work in small and medium-sized companies that are much less likely to offer any health promotion opportunities. Certain types of employers, such as retailers, seldom offer health promotion programs, and any employer with a high rate of workforce turnover has no motivation to offer health promotion programs (Linnan, 2004). Further, only 28% of employees aged 18 and over participate in employer-sponsored health promotion activities (U.S. Department of Health and Human Services, 2000b).

The United States was expected to spend $1.66 trillion on health care in 2003. Health care expenditures are projected to account for 17.7% of the gross domestic product (GDP) by 2012, which would be up from the 14.1% of the GDP in 2001 (U.S. Department of Health and Human Services, 2003). Much of these health care costs are picked up by business and industry in the form of health insurance premiums. Reduced health care costs and insurance premiums have been considered potential benefits of worksite health promotion programs. Other advantages, however, also exist. According to the Wellness Councils of America (1999), the advantages of worksite health promotion are "no longer a matter of speculation." Based on the worksite wellness literature, they cite six documented benefits associated with worksite wellness programs, including improved employee morale, reduced turnover, reduced absenteeism, increased recruitment potential, health care cost containment, and improved employee health status. An additional benefit noted by Breckon, Harvey, and Lancaster (1998) is that health promotion programs improve company image. When companies involve themselves in the health of their employees and the broader health issues of a community, the general public's perception of the company may be enhanced.

Though positions exist in the worksite health promotion setting that are strictly health promotion/education, more frequently expertise in exercise testing and prescription is required. This is because many worksite health promotion programs are based in a fitness center. It is often the fitness center that is the most visible aspect of a worksite health promotion program and attracts many employees to health promotion activities. Therefore, skills related to exercise are important, and these skills are not part of the competencies required by a health educator. As a result, health educators preparing for employment in worksite health promotion should strongly consider a minor or second major in exercise science. Beyond exercise expertise, a master's degree is also required for many entry-level health promotion/education positions in business and industry. In addition to the Certified Health Education Specialist (CHES) credential, certifications more specific to exercise are available from the American College of Sports Medicine and may be required at some worksite settings. Certifications for specific aspects of worksite health promotion, such as aerobic dance, first aid, and CPR, and for smoking cessation instructors are also available and encouraged. In general, the more degrees, certifications, and credentials one has, the better one will compete in the job market.

A Day in the Career of a Worksite Health Educator

The day begins early for Alisa. The fitness center opens promptly at 5:00 A.M. so that employees who start work at 6:00 A.M. can have time to work out prior to beginning their shift. Alisa has to be there at 4:45 A.M. to open the doors, turn on the lights, and greet the first members. The first two hours of her day are spent working the floor. This means she greets members as they enter the facility; walks around the machines, providing instruction where needed; chats with the members; answers health-related questions; and basically makes everyone feel important and welcome. By 7:00, all of the shift workers have left the fitness facility and, by 9:00, the managerial employees have cleared out.

From 9:00 to 11:00 is a slow time in the center. A few retired employees and their spouses use the machines, but this is basically the time for Alisa to get other tasks done. She begins by laundering the dirty towels and folding those that come out of the dryer. Next she provides the routine maintenance to the machines. This involves cleaning them with disinfectant and applying a lubricant to the moving parts. Once this is completed, Alisa has about an hour to work at her desk. Today she is writing an article on the different types of dietary fats to be included in the Wellness Center newsletter she publishes each month. The newsletter is distributed to all active employees and retirees of the company. Alisa is always amazed at how important writing skills are to her position in worksite health promotion.

Between 11:00 and 12:15, Alisa teaches two aerobics classes for the employees. The first is a beginners' class for new members. The second is supposed to be a more advanced class. Unfortunately, many of the shift employees have no choice in their lunch time, so Alisa ends up with some very advanced members in the beginners' class and some beginners in the advanced class. This is frustrating and could be avoided if there were another fitness center employee. There are, however, only two employees in the center, and Rob, the other health educator, must work the floor with the lunch crowd while Alisa teaches. Alisa is going to pursue the possibility of hiring a part-time aerobics instructor just for the lunch hours. This would allow her to offer a beginning and an advanced class at each time slot.

Box 7.4 Practitioner's Perspective: Worksite Health Promotion

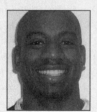

NAME: Tajuan Stoker
EMPLOYER: TriHealth (Contracted to Luxottica Retail)
TITLE: Health and Fitness Coordinator
DEGREE: BS, Health Education, University of Cincinnati, 2001
MAJOR: Health Promotion and Education with an Emphasis in Exercise and Health

Job Responsibilities: I am employed by the TriHealth Corporation, but am contracted through TriHealth to work at the Luxottica Retail corporate headquarters. At Luxottica, it is my responsibility to coordinate the day-to-day operation of the fitness center, including new member pre-screenings/fitness assessments, equipment orientations, and membership advising. I am to maintain membership enrollment, schedule Bodycrafters fitness classes and maintain fitness center equipment and amenities. I also promote employee wellness by conducting health assessments and screenings, and planning various programs for Bodycrafters members. In addition, I work with Luxottica Retail security to maintain member and facility safety.

What I like most about my position: There are many pluses to my position at Luxottica Retail. The first one is that I do not continuously do the same activities day in and day out. My projects change from week to week; for example, I am currently developing an employee running club to promote the health and fitness of Luxottica employees. Next month or maybe even next week I will have a different project. I enjoy changing projects as this keeps the job interesting for me as well as for the associates. Another plus is getting to know the people and watching them change their health behaviors. I love to see the excitement in people's eyes when they have lost a pound or can run on the treadmill for a longer period of time. This energizes me and helps keep me interested in my job. It makes me realize that this field of Health Promotion and Education really does help people make changes that improve their life.

What I like least about my position: The biggest negative about my position

(Box 7.4 *continues*)

From 12:15 to 1:00, Alisa runs an ongoing support group for employees trying to lose weight. All participants bring a brown bag lunch that is supposed to contain food appropriate for a weight-loss diet. They weigh in weekly, and Alisa provides each participant with a voluntary body composition (fat vs. lean) analysis every three months. At least twice a week, Alisa prepares a twenty-minute lecture on a weight-loss topic or invites a guest speaker from the community

At 1:00 the employees are back at their work stations, and there is again a quiet time in the health promotion center. Alisa spends the next hour eating lunch at her desk and working on a new incentive program for employees to join the health promotion center that will be offered next month. She has to develop all of the brochures, promotional material, and registration forms and arrange for the purchase of incentive items.

(Box 7.4 *continued*)

is that I do not have the opportunity to educate all the Luxottica Retail store employees on the importance of exercise and health first hand. There are over 22,000 Luxottica Retail store associates who do not have the opportunity to participate in a corporate fitness center and who do not receive the same level of health and fitness services as the associates do here at the Cincinnati office. Besides that, my position as a health and fitness coordinator through TriHealth is great, and I love it.

What helped me obtain this position: Internship, internship, internship, I cannot say it enough. This may be one of the most important aspects of your education program. Many schools do not require their students to do internships, or even provide their students with the resources to help them find an internship, but thankfully UC did. I completed my internship at Luxottica Retail my senior year. It was the most helpful experience that I could have had. During my internship I had the chance to work and participate first hand in the fitness and wellness activities of Luxottica Retail. This experience prepared me for future jobs in the health promotion field by teaching me what to expect from associates and em-

ployers. I also got the chance to use a lot of the information and skills that I learned through the classes that I took in college. For example, the program planning and program implementation classes were invaluable.

My advice to students reading this book is to find a good internship and apply yourself to doing the best job possible. If you can do a good job during the internship and can leave a lasting impression on the company, they may consider hiring you when you finish, or [the internship] can at least be used as a strong reference in the future. When the position of Health and Fitness Coordinator was created at Luxottica, my internship site supervisor, Amy Pawlak, remembered me and recommended me to TriHealth. Through my internship, I built strong business relationships and left a lasting impression on my employer. I would advise anyone doing an internship to take it very seriously, but also to enjoy yourself at the same time. Remember, the internship is a learning process and you may not get everything right, but try your best and leave a positive impression.

At 2:00 she has a meeting with upper management of the company. She has been advocating for the company to establish a no-smoking policy for the past five years. Two years ago, the company did restrict smoking to specified smoking areas, which was a major accomplishment. Today she will present a proposal to phase out all smoking over a one-year period. Alisa would be responsible for offering several smoking cessation classes over the twelve-month period prior to the no-smoking policy taking effect.

By 2:30 she is back in the health promotion center. The second shift employees are in the center now ahead of their shifts, so Alisa is again working the floor. Today she has to do initial fitness assessments on three new employees. This involves running the employees through a standardized series of tests. Based on the results of these tests, she prescribes an individualized exercise program for each

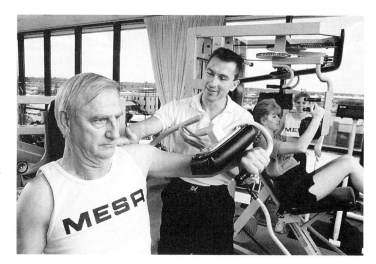

Health educators are employed by business and industry to provide programs to improve the health of employees. (Charles Thatcher/Stone)

employee. She then takes the employees through the fitness center and teaches them how to use the equipment and maintain a record of their progress.

By 3:30 Alisa is finished with the assessments. Because she had the early shift, opening the facility, she is finished for the day. Rob, who came in later, will stay and close the facility at 8:00.

Additional Responsibilities

The responsibilities involved in working in a corporate health promotion center are many and varied. In some facilities, maintaining records such as who is using the center, which programs are most popular, fitness assessment results, and health profiles is a major task. There are always many little things that need to be done, such as the creation and updating of bulletin boards, equipment maintenance, and towel distribution and laundering. Many times, annual health fairs, companywide health screenings, and flu shot programs are the responsibility of the health promotion staff.

Being a health educator in a worksite setting is not easy. It is imperative that worksite health education professionals stay up-to-date with health information and the operational processes of running a worksite program. As noted by the American College of Sports Medicine (2003), "the worksite health promotion professional needs to have a good handle on where to find the information, knowledge, resources and expertise that are needed to access the underlying foundations on which programs are built, the operational processes that allow programs to flourish, and the motivation to continually keep a heads-up attitude toward new and innovative strategies that allow well-established programs to maintain their cutting edge" (p. xi). See Table 7.7 for a listing of the advantages and disadvantages of employment in worksite health education.

Those who combine health education with a fitness background may find employment in settings beyond the business world. See Table 7.8 for a partial listing of employment opportunities for those with both health education and exercise training.

Table 7.7   Advantages and Disadvantages of Working in Worksite Health Education

Advantages

- It affords excellent opportunities for prevention. It provides access to individuals who may not participate in community programs.
- Health educators work with multiple and diverse groups of people, including everyone from upper management to shift workers.
- Most health educators in the corporate setting enjoy their positions and report a high degree of job satisfaction.
- Pay is usually higher than in other health education settings. Benefits are usually good, but they vary considerably from employer to employer.
- Health educators have access to fitness facilities for personal use.

Disadvantages

- Hours are long and irregular. To cover employees on all shifts in a company may necessitate health educators' working hours very early in the morning or late in the evening. It is not unusual to work more than eight hours a day.
- Upward mobility may be a problem. Typically, there are only one or two managerial positions in health promotion at any given worksite. This makes it difficult for health educators to move up. In addition, those holding managerial positions as directors of health and fitness have nowhere to move up in a company unless they are willing to get out of the health promotion field.
- Health promotion programs and fitness centers often seem to be low on a company's priority list. Such programs are often the first to receive budget cuts in difficult times and often seem to be short the staff necessary to run optimal programs.
- Some companies subcontract their health promotion and fitness programs to outside vendors. Some of these outside vendors hire part-time employees, pay lower wages, and provide few or no benefits.
- Health educators have strong pressure to be extremely fit and healthy role models for other employees.

Table 7.8   Employment Opportunities in Health Education with an Emphasis in Exercise and Fitness

Corporations, business, and industry	Entrepreneurial enterprises (aerobics studios, consulting, club owner, personal training)
Corporate/industrial parks	
YMCAs/YWCAs	Fitness product/service companies (sales and marketing)
Private health and fitness clubs	
Special-population clubs (women, elderly, etc.)	Condos and apartment complexes
Community parks & recreation programs	Hotels
Colleges/universities	Spas
Hospitals	Resorts and cruise lines
Sports medicine centers	

Health Education in Health Care Settings

Positions are available for health educators in a variety of **health care settings,** including public and for-profit hospitals, free-standing medical care clinics that provide both routine and emergency services, home health agencies that provide in-home care designed to replace or reduce the need for more expensive hospitalization, and physician organizations such as health maintenance organizations (HMOs) and preferred provider organizations (PPOs) (Breckon, Harvey, & Lancaster, 1998).

In hospitals and other health care settings, health educators have been hired to direct health and fitness programs for company employees, much the same as in other worksite settings (Breckon, Harvey, & Lancaster, 1998). Sometimes these programs are also open as an outreach service to community members. Other times, health educators are responsible for developing and conducting health and fitness programs specifically designed for community members.

Health educators have also been used in health care settings to provide patient education. For example, a patient is diagnosed with heart disease. That patient is then referred to the health educator for information about exercise, nutrition, weight control, stress management, smoking cessation, and so on. This could involve one-on-one education or counseling sessions with the patient, or it might involve group programs in which multiple patients receive the same program at the same time.

Unfortunately, patient education has not emerged as a major source of employment for health educators. Although it seems like an ideal activity for health educators, health insurance companies do not typically reimburse for the services of a health educator. Thus, many patient education positions have gone to nurses who can also serve other functions in the health care setting. Although health insurance companies are certainly concerned about reducing health care costs, their strategies to date have been more short term. The impact of health promotion and education programs may not be seen for years, and cause-and-effect relationships are difficult to establish. Therefore, without the availability of third-party payment, there is a major disincentive for hospitals, clinics, and private practice physicians to offer health promotion and education services to their patients. In response to this problem, the American Association for Health Education (AAHE) has made third-party reimbursement its number-one advocacy priority (AAHE, 1999).

Of all health care settings, HMOs have been most receptive to hiring health educators. The first HMOs were established in the 1970s as a result of federal money that was made available to help with start-up costs and to study the effectiveness of this health care delivery mechanism. In essence, patients belonging to an HMO pay one set fee for all their medical services in a given year. It therefore benefits the HMO to provide preventive health services and health education programs to keep their patients healthy. The fewer services a patient uses, the greater the cost benefit to the HMO. In the initial HMO legislation, one of the criteria for establishing an HMO was providing health education. Unfortunately, there were no stipulations on the professional preparation of the health education provider. Often, nurses or other individuals with no health education preparation or experience were given the responsibility of providing health education programs. As a result, some HMOs have developed outstanding health education programs with health educators, while others do very little.

There is, however, reason to be optimistic about future employment opportunities in health care settings for health educators. With changes in the medical care system rapidly occurring, the increased emphasis on cost-cutting measures, and movement toward more managed care, it is likely that prevention will take a higher profile in the future. As these changes occur, health educators will be the best

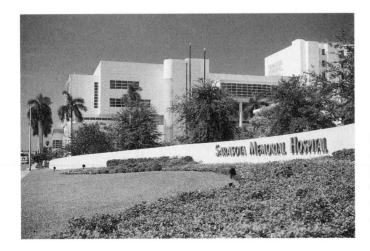

Hospitals employ health educators to provide programs for employees, patients, or the community at large. (Ed Bohon/The Stock Market)

prepared professionals to assume responsibility for helping individuals adopt healthy lifestyles.

A Day in the Career of a Health Care Setting Health Educator

Mary's day begins at 8:30 A.M., when she arrives at the hospital, picks up her mail, and proceeds to her office. She is the only health educator employed by this large metropolitan hospital, but she does have a secretary/assistant who works closely with her to carry out the duties of the position.

At 9:00 Mary has to attend the weekly staff meeting. This is a meeting with all department heads at the hospital. Much of the agenda does not concern Mary directly, but it is important for her to know what is going on in all departments. At today's meeting, it was decided to have an open house for the public to see the newly renovated obstetrics wing of the hospital. Mary is given the responsibility of planning and advertising this event.

At 10:00 Mary has an appointment with the administrative head of the Cardiac Rehabilitation Program at the hospital. The purpose of the meeting is to begin planning the development of two brochures that will eventually be distributed to all cardiac rehabilitation patients. One brochure will be on stress-management strategies, and the other on different types of dietary fat. They brainstorm ideas, and Mary agrees to develop a rough draft of the content of the brochures for the administrative head to review prior to their next meeting. They will also discuss graphics, layout, and production at the next meeting.

At 11:00 Mary leaves the hospital to drive to one of the local malls. The mall has decided to conduct a three-day health fair, and the hospital has agreed to be a cosponsor of the event. Today is a planning meeting for all of the agencies and businesses that will participate. In addition to serving on the planning committee, Mary is responsible for setting up the hospital's display and coordinating nurses and physicians to work in several screening stations. During the health fair, Mary will be at the hospital's booth all day, handing out materials, answering questions, and promoting the hospital's community outreach health promotion programs.

Box 7.5 Practitioner's Perspective: Health Care Educator

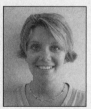

NAME: Jennifer R. Flanagan, AS, BS, RRT, CHES

CURRENT POSITION/TITLE: Health Educator

EMPLOYER: Ball Memorial Hospital Family Medicine Residency Center

DEGREE/INSTITUTION/YEAR: AS and BS, Ball State University, 1997 and 2000

MAJOR(S): Respiratory Therapy and Health Science

Job responsibilities: I have several responsibilities as the health educator at Family Medicine Residency Center (FMRC). FMRC serves as a training facility for physicians who are specializing in family medicine. There is a strong emphasis on their education. My work involves preparing the resident physicians to be effective patient educators. More specifically, I maintain a patient education room that houses various resources to assist the physicians while they see patients in their clinic. I also work with the residency's patient education committee to coordinate community outreach events and evaluate and select patient education material for the clinic. In addition, I provide individual health education to patients through physician referrals.

How I got my job: Before I graduated, one of my professors told our class about this job opening. I submitted my resume and was offered an interview. During the interview I was able to give examples of my work in the health education field by using several of my class projects. I also gave examples of how some of my experiences as a respiratory therapist had prepared me for this position.

What I like most about my job: I love the atmosphere in which I work. There is a strong emphasis on education. I love to

(Box 7.5 *continues*)

After lunch, Mary returns to the hospital around 1:00 and spends the next two hours working on the hospital's health and wellness newsletter. As a public service and to promote the hospital, Mary is responsible for developing a newsletter every other month that is mailed to all households in the hospital's immediate service area. Each edition of the newsletter features one department in the hospital and contains several additional articles about health and wellness. Mary writes much of each newsletter, using information she obtains from the Internet and from a variety of health journals and newsletters to which she subscribes. She designs and formats the newsletter with a desktop publishing program she has on her computer. She marvels at how important the computer is to her everyday functioning.

At 3:00 Mary leads a weight-loss support group for hospital employees. Most of the participants are nurses and housekeeping staff from either the first or second shift. At each session, participants weigh in, share their experiences over the previous week, and listen to a thirty-minute presentation designed to enhance their weight-loss program. Mary is responsible for each week's presentation. In addition, she provides participants with healthy recipes, exercise tips, motivational incentives, and recognition awards.

(Box 7.5 *continued*)

learn and share that knowledge with the physicians and patients. I find it very rewarding to provide patients with education and assistance to improve their health. I also enjoy the variety of my ob. Every day is different and that keeps it exciting.

What I like least about my job: There is very little that I don't like about my job, but there are several areas that can be challenging. I am the only health educator working with 29 physicians and 20+ office and nursing staff. It can be a challenge to implement new patient education programs that are not viewed as more work for the staff.

How my work relates to the responsibilities and competencies of a CHES: My work as a health educator requires me to use several of the responsibilities and competencies. I serve as a resource person for the physicians and nurses on patient education and health promotion issues. I work with various committees within FMRC to plan, implement, and

evaluate health education programs. When working directly with patients, I assess individual needs for health education to provide effective education. I am also involved with coordinating health education services between the community and the FMRC.

Recommendations for those preparing to be health educators: I would strongly recommend two things for anyone preparing to be a health educator. First, take advantage of special projects and assignments that you do for classes by trying to apply them to real situations. It is the best way to understand what you are learning and you can use this work to demonstrate your competence as a health educator. Second, talk to your professors about opportunities to network in the community. Volunteer for community health agencies that employ health educators. You not only get to see health educators in action, but you also gain valuable work experience.

After class, Mary answers phone calls and ties up loose ends until it is time for her to go home at 5:00. It is not unusual for Mary to take some work home in the evenings or on weekends. Tonight, however, Mary must return to the hospital at 7:30 P.M. to teach a stress-management class for the community. The stress class is part of the hospital's ongoing community outreach program. Each month a different health topic is taught, and Mary is responsible for either teaching the class or lining up the instructor for the class.

Additional Responsibilities

Health educators working in health care settings are involved in numerous and varied activities. The actual responsibilities can differ greatly from one health care setting to another. Planning, implementing, and evaluating programs and events are certainly major tasks. Health educators may also be involved in grant writing, one-on-one or group patient education services, publicity, public relations, employee wellness activities, and various collaborative efforts with other hospital staff, community agencies, or departments of public health.

Table 7.9 Advantages and Disadvantages of Working in a Health Care Setting

Advantages

- Job responsibilities are highly varied and changing.
- There is increased credibility due to the health care connection.
- There is usually a high community profile.
- Health educators work with multiple groups of people.
- Wages and benefits are good.
- There is a high degree of self-satisfaction.

Disadvantages

- Health education may have low status and low priority within health care settings.
- Jobs are difficult to obtain.
- Turf issues over educational responsibilities can develop.
- Hours may be long and irregular.
- Some medical doctors may be difficult to work with.

Administration is a major responsibility of many health educators working in hospitals. They are often hired as managers, directors, or coordinators of programs. Hospitals often adopt a "team" approach to health education, in which doctors, nurses, physical therapists, and other health specialists are all part of the team. Health educators plan and coordinate the programs and serve as resources for the other team members, who actually present the programs. In this type of position, the health educator provides little direct client service (Breckon, Harvey, & Lancaster, 1998). (See Table 7.9.)

Health Education in Colleges and Universities

Colleges and universities are another source of employment for health educators. Within the college setting, there are typically two types of positions health educators hold. The first is an academic, or faculty, position and the second is a health educator in a health service or wellness center.

As a faculty member, the health educator typically has three major responsibilities: teaching, community and professional service, and scholarly research. The amount of emphasis on each of these major responsibilities is dependent on the institution. In very large research institutions, faculty may spend most of their time writing grants and conducting research. In smaller four-year colleges, teaching may be the major responsibility. In addition to the major responsibilities, faculty may be asked to advise students, serve on committees, coordinate or lead student groups, attend professional conferences, and accept administrative duties.

The minimum qualification for working as a faculty member in the college/university setting is usually a doctoral degree in health education. Though some junior colleges and small four-year schools may hire faculty with only a master's degree, most faculty positions require the doctorate for tenure track positions. In addition, depending on the position for which one is applying, it may be necessary to have had prior experience or training in school health, community/public health, or worksite health promotion. Holding or being eligible for a Certified Health Education Specialist (CHES) credential is often listed as a preference or requirement for faculty positions.

As a health educator in a university health service or wellness center, the major responsibility is to plan, implement, and evaluate health promotion and education programs for program participants. In some universities, the program participants are students, while in others it is the faculty and staff. Many times programming responsibility is for both groups. In addition to program planning, the health educator may be responsible for maintaining a resource library; one-on-one advising with students; developing and coordinating a peer education program; speaking to residence hall, fraternity, and sorority groups; conducting incentive programs; and planning special events.

The minimum qualifications for working in a university health service or wellness center typically include a bachelor's or master's degree in health education. Students interested in working in this setting are advised to work as a volunteer or consider completing a practicum or internship in the campus wellness center while an undergraduate. Many universities have peer education programs in which undergraduate students are trained by the professional health educator to conduct programs for their peers. This type of experience is invaluable, whether or not a student is subsequently employed in a university health service or wellness center. It would also be a good idea to obtain the CHES credential for work in this area.

International Opportunities

Health education professionals may wish to consider working in foreign countries for all or a portion of their careers. There is great need for professionals with health education skills in many developing countries. These positions often require special dedication, as the living and working conditions may be more challenging than those experienced in the United States. For those so inclined, however, the rewards in terms of personal satisfaction and accomplishment can be tremendous. Further, the experience gained by planning, implementing, and evaluating health promotion and education programs in foreign countries can be invaluable to one's professional development.

Working in developing countries many times requires the health educator to examine different health problems and to try different approaches. For example, instead of helping people reduce high-fat and -cholesterol diets, as in the United States, the health educator may be helping people deal with problems of starvation, malnutrition, and parasitic and bacterial infections. Instead of dealing with heart disease and lung cancer, the health educator in a developing country may be facing schistosomiasis, diarrhea, and ascaris and tapeworm infections.

Consider the case of Sofia. Sofia was working as a community health educator for the health department in a rural community of about two thousand people in a developing country. The water source for this community consisted of several large ponds. These ponds were the only source of drinking water and were also used for bathing, clothes washing, and care of animals. Many people were getting sick with

---

Box 7.6 Practitioner's Perspective: University Wellness Center

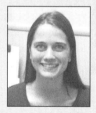

NAME: Christina Berg, MPH

CURRENT POSITION/TITLE: Director of Wellness Services

EMPLOYER: Boise State University

DEGREE/INSTITUTION/YEAR: Master's in Public Health, Community Health Education, University of Wisconsin–La Crosse, August 1998–May 2000; Bachelor of Arts in Organizational Communication, Psychology minor, University of Wisconsin–Eau Claire, August 1991–December 1995

How I obtained my job: My formal education provided me with a strong health promotion/public health background, as well as training, management, and leadership skills. Mind/body and complementary therapies training, with the addition of foreign travel, helped foster a holistic, well-rounded view of health. Internships, activity involvement, and prior work experiences offered programming and collaborative experiences in college, worksite, and community settings. Such experiences developed my evaluation and grant-writing skills, as well as my ability to teach and present. Solid administrative and interpersonal skills are crucial to success in my position. The capacity to facilitate group projects and strategically plan, along with create and disseminate educational materials using various communication mediums, also are desired traits. Direct experience working with student and employee wellness programming was key to my hire, since my position requires me to do both.

How I utilize my health education background in my job: Concentrated strategies to promote and facilitate healthy lifestyle choices can often determine the success of a student's college experience, which in turn can influence behaviors beyond college. My health education background allows me to initiate programming geared to positively impact academic success and improve retention rates by using the best practices and evaluating the strategies that have

(Box 7.6 *continues*)

---

severe diarrhea, and there had been several deaths among the elderly and very young. To alleviate this problem, it was decided to develop an educational campaign to get people to boil their water prior to consumption. Sofia was given the responsibility for developing this campaign. There was no local newspaper or radio stations, and no billboards, and many of the people could not read. After consulting with local leaders, it was decided that the best way to spread the information would be to use a "mobile communication system." This was accomplished by hooking up an old stereo system to a car battery and driving around the community, broadcasting information about the importance of boiling water. In addition, Sofia set up several demonstrations around the community about how to boil water effectively. These sessions were also advertised via the "mobile communication system."

As can be seen from Sofia's experience, health educators working in foreign countries must be able to develop creative, innovative programs to solve identified health problems. Most often, these programs must be low-cost, easily developed and

(Box 7.6 *continued*)

been implemented. Specific examples are as follows:

Wellness Services provides a holistic approach to health promotion and prevention for a diverse campus population at Boise State University. Our focus includes:

1. Contributing to the overall education of students and employees in the areas of lifestyle and behavior change, promoting physical, psychological, emotional, spiritual, and social health

2. Providing educational opportunities to build awareness and skills necessary to improve and maintain health, as well as address the environmental context in which health behavior decisions are made

3. Advocating for a healthy campus community and providing leadership on policy and program development

4. Engaging stakeholders in addressing campus-wide health issues by developing collaborative campus and community partnerships

What I like most about my job: As a director and educator, I feel my job is purposeful, allowing me to make a difference. Each day is always an adventure. Never a dull moment, with opportunities to continuously grow, learn, and give. I also enjoy mentoring student workers and interns, as well as working collaboratively with colleagues and community constituents.

What I like least about my job: The occasional politics and struggle for funding.

Recommendations for those preparing to have a job like yours: Recommendations would include the following:

1. Gain valuable experience through work/internship/assistantship opportunities.

2. Polish both oral and written communication skills.

3. Sharpen managerial and leadership skills.

4. Travel abroad to learn about health and different ways of living in other cultures.

5. Stay familiar with the literature to keep abreast of best practices.

6. Obtain a master's degree.

implemented, acceptable to the social norms of the community, and available to all aspects of the public. It is imperative that these programs be developed in conjunction with the local people being served. It is also helpful when programs are sponsored by organizations seen as credible by the priority population.

One of the best ways to begin a career in international health is to volunteer with the Peace Corps. Health education professionals are in demand by the Peace Corps, and students should begin the application process early in their senior year. Many colleges and universities are visited by Peace Corps recruiters every year, and talking to one of these Peace Corps volunteers is a good place to start. Faculty members on your campus may have been former Peace Corps volunteers, and talking to these individuals can provide valuable insight into the Peace Corps experience.

There are many advantages to volunteering with the Peace Corps. The Peace Corps provides volunteers with some of the best language and technical training in the world. Each Peace Corps volunteer is granted a monthly allowance for housing,

Table 7.10   International Health Organizations

National Council for International Health
American Association for World Health
World Health Organization (WHO)
Pan American Health Organization
U.S. Agency for International Development (A.I.D.)

food, clothing, and miscellaneous expenses. Free dental and medical care are provided, as well as free transportation to the placement setting and twenty-four vacation days per year. After completing the two-year experience, volunteers are given a post-service readjustment allowance of $6,075. They are also given preference for federal jobs and have enhanced scholarship and assistantship opportunities at more than fifty major colleges and universities. In addition, a successful Peace Corps experience may serve as a stepping stone to paid positions in other international health organizations (see Table 7.10).

Nontraditional Health Education Positions

In addition to the traditional settings for health education that have been described in this chapter, there are a variety of nontraditional jobs health educators may wish to consider. These positions may or may not carry the title of health educator. In some cases, they require the health educator to use the skills and competencies in different or unique ways. Further, it is often necessary for health educators to sell themselves to get these positions, as the persons doing the hiring may be unfamiliar with the skills and training of a health educator.

Given health educators' knowledge of health and fitness, sales positions related to health are a real possibility. Pharmacy sales, fitness equipment sales, and the sales of health-related textbooks are all areas in which health educators have found employment. Life and health insurance are two additional options to consider in the area of sales.

By emphasizing the communication competencies that are part of the professional training in health education, the health educator may seek employment in journalism, TV, or radio. Many television stations have a regular health or medical reporter who does feature stories on health-related issues. Newspapers may have a health column that could and should be written by a health educator. Again, it is necessary for health educators to sell themselves to obtain these positions. Taking elective classes in media, communications, and journalism and doing one's internship in these settings may also assist those interested in this career field.

Health educators should always be alert to unique job opportunities, many of which may not even carry the title of health educator. One health educator, for example, was hired by a state mental hospital as a "Teacher II." His job was to teach drug education to patients who had a history of drug problems and sex education to patients who had a history of sex problems. The remainder of his work schedule involved tutoring patients in math and science who were studying to obtain their high school general equivalency diploma.

Landing That First Job

At first, it may seem unusual to discuss landing one's first job while still an undergraduate in an introductory course, but this is the best time to consider the issue of future employment. There are several actions students can take during their undergraduate years to enhance their chances of obtaining employment. By following the suggestions made in this section, a student will be far ahead of those who wait until the end of their bachelor's degree program to address these issues.

No matter in what setting a health educator hopes to eventually work, landing the first job can be a frustrating experience. Students often find themselves in a dilemma. Employers want their new employees to have had "experience," but where are students supposed to get experience if they can't get hired? There are several possible answers to this question. One way to gain experience is to obtain part-time or summer employment in one's preferred health education setting. Typically, there are many more students looking for this type of employment than there are employment situations. Should such an opportunity be available, however, it is an excellent way to gain experience prior to graduation. Another way to obtain experience is to volunteer time in the chosen health education setting. Most professional health educators working in the field are more than willing to accept and use the volunteer time of health education students. In addition to experience, volunteering also begins the important process of **networking.** Networking involves establishing and maintaining a wide range of contacts in the field that may be of help when looking for a job and in carrying out one's job responsibilities once hired.

Some health education/promotion programs now offer **service learning** opportunities to their students (Cleary et al., 1998). Organized service learning opportunities provide course credit for students to work with a community agency to meet an identified community need. They provide hands-on, practical, real-world experience that students cannot obtain from the classroom. They are also beneficial in broadening one's professional network, which is so important in the health education field. Take advantage of as many service learning opportunities as possible. The experience and networking gained through service learning can give new health education professionals a tremendous advantage in the job market.

Carefully planning internships and practicums can help students obtain their first professional position. Required field experiences are often the best way to obtain practical experience in one's chosen setting. Students should consider what they would like to be doing five years after graduation and select an experience that closely matches that goal. Often students are hired by the agency after completing their practicum or internship experience.

In addition to obtaining experience, students should strive to obtain an excellent academic record. When there is heavy competition for an open position, one of the first strategies in making hiring decisions is to examine grade point average. This is not to say that the person with the highest grade point average is always the best person or will always get the job. But, when there are fifty applications for one job, grade point average is an easy way to begin limiting the field.

Develop a well-organized, professional-looking portfolio. A **portfolio** is a collection of evidence that enables students to demonstrate mastery of desired course or program outcomes. In health education, the responsibilities, competencies, and

Box 7.7 Practitioner's Perspective: Employer of Health Educators

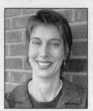

NAME: Mary Singler

CURRENT POSITION/TITLE: Health Promotion Manager

EMPLOYER: Northern Kentucky Health Department

DEGREES/INSTITUTIONS: BS, Health Education, and BA, Broadcasting, Eastern Kentucky University; M.Ed., Health Education, University of Cincinnati, 1996

MAJOR: Health Education

Recommendations for those preparing to be health educators: I am Manager of the Health Promotion Department for the large and growing Northern Kentucky Health Department. Both my bachelor's and master's degrees are in Health Education, and I am a Certified Health Education Specialist. I have worked as a health educator in a private not-for-profit agency, in a multinational for-profit organization, as a supervisor/health educator, and now a manager of a health promotion unit for a government agency. In five years my unit has grown from two health educators and a health educator/supervisor to thirteen health educators and two full-time managers. In this job and in my past positions, I've frequently been responsible for hiring health educators.

One of the first things I look for in a potential candidate's resume is a health education/promotion degree. The second thing I look for is certifications, evidence of community participation, or evidence of a strong interest or passion in something related to health and wellness. I read the cover letter and it makes a difference to me if someone has put time and thought into their letter. I immediately throw away any resume with spelling or grammar errors.

Grades don't matter to me as much as experience and good referrals. I look to see if students have gotten experience through past job and/or volunteer activities. When trying to fill a position, I usually talk to a few key people in my professional community to let them know I am looking for candidates. If they refer someone to me, I give that resume a little more attention. If I see a resume that indicates a workplace or school that I have worked with in the past, I may ask my contact at that insti-

(Box 7.7 *continues*)

sub-competencies should be emphasized. Many health education/promotion programs now require portfolios as part of their professional preparation programs. Even if the portfolio is not required, students should develop a portfolio on their own. Thompson and Bybee (2004) note that a portfolio is a "living document that is ever-changing with the increasing depth of knowledge and experience of the individual" (p. 52). They go on to identify five basic elements that should be included in any portfolio: 1) table of contents, 2) resume, 3) education and credentials, 4) samples of work, and 5) references. The samples of work could include such exhibits as student papers or course projects, audio- or videotapes of students giving a presentation, analyses of student work by professors and/or outside reviewers, student goal statements, reflections, and summaries (Cleary & Birch, 1996, 1997). Students may also want to consider developing the portfolio in an electronic format instead

(Box 7.7 *continued*)

tution if they know the potential candidate I am thinking about interviewing.

Being in the "network" and doing a good job in one's internship is really important. I use interns and practicum students from several universities in Ohio and Kentucky. A few years ago, when I worked for a different organization, one practicum student was late to almost every meeting I held and completely missed one very important meeting. This practicum student has now graduated and has applied for two health education positions my organization has posted. I have never even asked him for an interview. He doesn't know that I see every resume he sends my Human Resource Department. The point is, your network is smaller than you think. Do a good job—or a bad job—and people will remember the work you did.

Once you get the interview, do your research. Look the organization up on the Internet, get the job description, and get the profile of the organization. If the job posting lists a specific focus area like "tobacco prevention," look up what the CDC recommends in that area. It is very impressive when a candidate comes in well prepared for an interview. Prepare a portfolio and bring it to the interview. Practice showing your work before your interview, then use your portfolio to showcase your experience during the interview.

While you are academically preparing to be a health educator, don't just go to school; prepare to get a job! Take advantage of volunteer opportunities in your profession, obtain certifications, and join professional organizations. Start thinking about where you might want to do your internship well before you need to choose an internship experience and choose your internship experience wisely. Find an organization that has a good reputation and offers diverse, worthwhile internship experiences.

Last, but not least, don't hide your passion for the health education profession. Participate in a professional organization, volunteer experience, or credentialing process that truly interests you. You will learn *and* contribute, and this combination breeds success. Walk your talk: Eat right, exercise, and live a healthy lifestyle. Do your best work because it will matter in the future, and live a healthy lifestyle because it is part of your professional identity.

Welcome to the beginning of a professional career that can be fascinating, interesting, worthwhile, and personally rewarding.

of the more traditional notebook or binder. In addition to providing more flexibility in the way exhibits are presented and displayed, utilizing an electronic format also provides the opportunity to showcase one's creativity and to demonstrate technology skills to potential employers (McKenzie, Cleary, McKenzie, & Stephen, 2002). Imagine the impact when a new health educator provides a well-developed, attractive portfolio to a prospective employer.

Beyond the portfolio, consider what certifications are going to be important in landing your first job and carefully plan to make sure they are awarded either prior to graduation or as soon after graduation as possible. All professional health educators should pursue the CHES credential. In the future, this may be a prerequisite for many health promotion and education positions. Other certifications should be obtained depending on work setting and need.

Get to know your faculty. They are a great source of information about jobs and how to compete for them successfully. Often employers contact faculty directly, asking for the names of students who might be interested in a particular position. Unless a faculty member knows a student by name and knows that the student is in the job market, there is little the faculty member can do.

Most colleges and universities have placement centers that provide a variety of services to students. They may assist with developing the resume, maintain a list of job openings, provide workshops or handouts on interviewing skills, and establish reference files for students. It would be a good idea to contact the placement center well before graduation to determine when and how to access its services.

A final suggestion is to join one or more of the professional associations (see Chapter 8). Employers are typically impressed when they see that a young professional has been a member of a professional association and perhaps has attended one or more professional meetings. "Professional meetings and conferences are filled with opportunities.... Where else can you find hundreds, even thousands, of education professionals from all over the world coming together to share cutting-edge knowledge through presentations, sessions, workshops, socials, and other events, than [at] professional meetings and conferences?" (Dixon-Terry, 2004, p. 16). If your campus has a chapter of Eta Sigma Gamma, the professional health education honorary, try to get involved. Eta Sigma Gamma recognizes high academic achievement, provides opportunities to obtain valuable leadership experience, and allows students to plan, implement, and evaluate various service projects and social activities.

Students who follow the above suggestions will be better positioned to obtain initial employment in the health promotion and education profession. This is a good time to be a health educator and the future looks even brighter than the present. Floyd and Allen (2004) note, "As the field of health education continues to expand, the number and type of careers will continue to expand. Health education professionals must be willing to implement innovative and quality school and non-school programs for an increasingly diverse population in increasingly diverse settings. The future of health education is here" (p. 36).

SUMMARY

There are many settings in which a health educator can seek employment. In this chapter, we have discussed in detail health education positions in schools, community/public health agencies, worksites, health care facilities, colleges and universities, and international settings. In addition, we have examined the potential for employment in nontraditional settings and have considered what introductory-level undergraduate students can do to help themselves obtain their first job.

REVIEW QUESTIONS

1. Identify four major settings and two nontraditional settings in which health educators are employed.

2. Compare and contrast the roles and responsibilities of health educators working in schools, community/public health agencies, worksites, and health care facilities. How are all of these settings similar? How are they different?

3. What is the difference between a position funded with hard money and a position funded with soft money? Which position is preferable and why?

4. Explain why it might be said that health education has never reached its real potential in the health care setting. What factors have kept health education positions at a minimal level in this setting?

5. What is networking and why is it important in health education?

6. What can introductory-level health education students do now that might help them land their first job after graduation?

CRITICAL THINKING QUESTIONS

1. Select any health education setting and give specific examples of how a health educator working in that setting would need to utilize all seven responsibilities of a health educator (i.e., when thinking about assessment at the worksite setting, a health educator might have to assess the health needs of employees, assess the current health behaviors of employees, assess how responsive employees would be to a given health promotion program, assess upper management support for a given program, etc.).

2. If you were in a position to hire a new health educator, what qualities, traits, and experiences would you look for in making your hiring decision? Compare this with the qualities, traits, and experiences you currently possess. Make a list of things you could do to enhance your marketability prior to graduation.

ACTIVITIES

1. Select the one setting you think you would most like to work in. Develop a short essay describing why you prefer this setting to other health education settings.

2. Visit a health education professional who works in the setting in which you would most like to be employed. Develop a job description for this person's position that explains the qualifications and responsibilities needed for the job.

3. Examine the classified ads of a major city Sunday newspaper. Circle in red those jobs you find that specifically ask for a health educator. Next look through the same classified ads and circle in blue those that do not ask for a health educator but that require the same competencies and skills of a health educator.

4. Interview someone who is responsible for hiring health educators. Find out what that person looks for in a letter of application, a vita, and a personal interview.

5. Contact the placement office at your institution. Determine what services it offers and when these services should be accessed.

WEBLINKS

1. **http://www.bls.gov**

   U.S. Bureau of Labor Statistics

   Go to this Web site and do a search for "health educators." Review the various documents you find to determine workforce size, average salaries, states with most health educators employed, states with highest average salaries, metropolitan areas with highest average salaries, and other important information about health educators.

2. **http://www.peacecorps.gov/index.cfm**

   PeaceCorps

   This Web site provides information about the Peace Corps, what volunteers do, where the Peace Corps is active, benefits of Peace Corps service, how to become a Peace Corps volunteer, and much more.

3. **http://www.welcoa.org**

   Wellness Councils of America

   Click on "Free Resources" at the top right corner of the home page to connect to many valuable information sources about worksite health promotion.

4. **https://www.aahperd.org/iejhe/template.cfm?template=current/mckenzie3.html**

   This URL will link you to a 2002 article by McKenzie, Cleary, McKenzie, and Stephen titled "E-Portfolios: Their Creation and Use by Pre-service Health Educators." The article explains the advantages of electronic portfolios over traditional notebooks and binders. It also provides guidance on how to develop electronic portfolios.

5. **http://www.csuchico.edu/cjhp/2/1/index.htm**

   This is the URL for Volume 2, Issue 1 of the California Journal of Health Promotion. Once there go to the article by Eleanor Dixon Terry titled "Attending Professional Health Education Meetings: What's In It for the Student and New Professional." Click on the page numbers to download the article in an Adobe Acrobat format. This is an excellent article with good advice for students or new professionals attending their first professional health education meeting.

CASE STUDY

Carlos has been working as a school health educator for fifteen years since graduating from college. Recently, the local branch of the American Heart Association approached him about accepting a position as their health educator. Carlos is unsure what he should do. Compare the similarities and differences between the two positions. Make a list of advantages and disadvantages for each position. If you were in Carlos's position, what decision would you make and why?

REFERENCES

Allensworth, D., & Kolbe, L. (1987). The comprehensive school health program: Exploring an expanded concept. *Journal of School Health, 57,* 409–412.

American Association for Health Education. (August, 1999). Board of Directors Meeting—Minutes. Reston, VA.

American College of Sports Medicine. (2003). *ACSM's worksite health promotion manual.* Champaign, IL: Human Kinetics.

American School Health Association. (2004). What is school health? Retrieved May 14, 2004, at http://www.ashaweb.org/whatis.html

Breckon, J., Harvey, J. R., & Lancaster, R. B. (1998). *Community health education: Settings, roles, and skills for the 21st century.* Gaithersburg, MD: Aspen Publishers, Inc.

Centers for Disease Control and Prevention. (2004a). Coordinated school health program. Retrieved May 28, 2004, at http://www.cdc.gov/HealthyYouth/CSHP/index.htm

Centers for Disease Control and Prevention. (2004b). Schools: The right place for a healthy start. Retrieved May 14, 2004, at http://www.cdc.gov/HealthyYouth/about/healthyyouth.htm

Cleary, M. J., & Birch, D. A. (1996). Using portfolios for assessment in the college personal health course. *Journal of Health Education, 27* (2), 92–96.

Cleary, M. J., & Birch, D.A. (1997). How prospective school health educators can build a portfolio to communicate professional expertise. *Journal of School Health,* 67 (6), 228–231.

Cleary, M. J., Kaiser-Drobney, A. E., Ubbes, V. E., Stuhldreher, W. L., & Birch, D. A. (1998). Service learning in the "third sector:" Implications for professional preparation. *Journal of Health Education, 29* (5), 304–311.

Dixon-Terry, E. (2004). Attending professional health education meetings: What's in it for the student and new professional? *California Journal of Health Promotion, 2* (1). 16–21.

English, G. M., & Videto, D. M. (1997). The future of health education: The knowledge to practice paradox. *Journal of Health Education, 28* (1), 4–7.

Fisher, C., Hunt, P., Kann, L., Kolbe, L., Patterson, B., & Wechsler, H. (2003). Building a healthier future through school health programs. In *Promising practices in chronic disease prevention and control: A public health framework for action.* Atlanta, GA: Department of Health and Human Services.

Floyd, P. A., & Allen, B. J. (2004). *Careers in health, physical education and sport.* Belmont, CA: Wadsworth-Thompson Learning, Inc.

Joint Committee on Health Education Standards. (1995). *National Health Education Standards: Achieving Health Literacy.* Atlanta, GA.: American Cancer Society.

Joint Committee on Health Education and Promotion Terminology (2001). Report of the 2000 Joint Committee on Health Education and Promotion Terminology. *American Journal of Health Education, 32* (2), 89–104.

Kuttner, R. (1999). The American health care system—employer-sponsored health coverage. *The New England Journal of Medicine, 340* (3).

Linnan, L. (2004). The future of workplace health in America. Wellness Councils of America. Retrieved, June 2, 2004, at http://www.welcoa.org/freeresources/index.php?category=8

McKenzie, J. F., Cleary, M. J., McKenzie, B. L., & Stephen, C. E. (2002). E-portfolios: Their creation and use by pre-service health educators. *International Electronic Journal of Health Education, 55,* 79–83.

McKenzie, J. F., Pinger, R. R., & Kotecki, J. E. (2002). *An introduction to community health.* Boston: Jones & Bartlet.

Naidoo, J., & Wills, J. (2000). *Health promotion: Foundations for practice* (2nd ed.). Edinburgh, Scotland: Bailliere Tindall.

National Center for Health Statistics. (1997). *Employer-Sponsored Health Insurance: State and National Estimates.* Hyattsville, MD: U.S. Department of Health and Human Services.

National Commission for Health Education Credentialing (2004). What is a certified health education specialist? Retrieved May 15, 2004, at http://www.nchec.org/

Seffrin, J. A. (1994). Americans' interest in comprehensive school health education. *Journal of School Health,* 64 (10), 397–399.

Thompson, S. E., & Bybee, R. F. (2004). Professional portfolios for health educators and other allied health professionals. *California Journal of Health Promotion, 2* (1), 52–55.

U.S. Department of Health and Human Services. (2000a). *Healthy People 2010: Introduction.* Available at: http://www.health.gov/healthypeople/Document/HTML/Volume1/intro.htm

U.S. Department of Health and Human Services. (2000b). *Healthy People 2010* (Conference Edition, in Two Volumes). Washington, DC.

U.S. Department of Health and Human Services. (September 2003). *Prevention makes "cents."* Retrieved June 2, 2004, at http://aspe.hhs.gov/health/prevention/prevention.pdf

U.S. Department of Labor Bureau of Labor Statistics (2004). Occupational employment and wages, 2002. Retrieved May 14, 2004, at http://stats.bls.gov/oes/2002/oes211091.htm

Utah State University (March 16, 1996). Careers in Health Education. Available at: http://www.ed.usu.edu/coe/hper/advising/careers.html

Wellness Councils of America. (1999). Making a Case for Worksite Wellness: The Benefits of Worksite Wellness. Available at: www.welcoa.org/thecase/thecase_benefits_list.html

CHAPTER 8

Agencies/Associations/ Organizations Associated with Health Education

Chapter Objectives

After reading this chapter and answering the questions at the end, you should be able to:

1. Define each of the following terms and give several examples of each: *governmental health agency, quasi-governmental health agency, nongovernmental health agencies.*

2. Briefly describe the levels of governmental agencies and provide several examples of each.

3. List and explain the four primary activities of most voluntary health agencies.

4. Explain the purpose of a professional association/organization.

5. Identify the benefits derived from membership in a professional organization.

6. Identify the primary professional associations/organizations and coalitions associated with health education.

7. Describe the process by which a person can become a member of a professional association/organization.

Key Terms

American Academy of Health Behavior (AAHB)

American Alliance for Health, Physical Education, Recreation and Dance (AAHPERD)

American Association for Health Education (AAHE)

American College Health Association (ACHA)

American Public Health Association (APHA)

American Red Cross (ARC)

American School Health Association (ASHA)

Coalition of National Health Education Organizations, USA (CNHEO)

Directors of Health Promotion and Education (DHPE)

Eta Sigma Gamma (ESG)

governmental health agencies

International Union for Health Promotion and Education (IUHPE)

local public health agency

National Wellness Institute, Inc. (NWI)

nongovernmental health agencies

philanthropic foundations

Key Terms, *continued*

professional health
    associations/organizations

quasi-governmental health
    agencies

Society of State Directors of
    Health, Physical
    Education, and Recreation
    (SSDHPER)

Society for Public Health
    Education, Inc. (SOPHE)

voluntary health agencies

There are many health agencies, associations, and organizations with which health educators interact. Most of these agencies/associations/organizations were created to help promote, protect, and maintain the health of individuals, families, and communities. For many health educators, these agencies/associations/organizations will be places of employment. These groups regularly hire health educators to plan, implement, evaluate, and coordinate their educational efforts. Health educators not employed by these groups will find them to be valuable sources of up-to-date information and materials. This chapter classifies the agencies/associations/organizations into three major categories: governmental, quasi-governmental, and nongovernmental. Because information on most of these agencies/associations/organizations that support the efforts of health education/promotion is available elsewhere (Green & Ottoson, 1999; McKenzie, Pinger, & Kotecki, 2005; Miller & Price, 1998; & Reagan & Brookins-Fisher, 2002) and because this text was written primarily as an introduction to the profession, the primary emphasis of this chapter is on the professional health education associations/organizations.

Governmental Health Agencies

Governmental health agencies are health agencies that have authority for certain duties or tasks outlined by the governmental bodies that oversee them. For example, a **local public health agency** (often referred to as a local health department) has the authority to protect, promote, and enhance the health of people living in a specific geographical area. It is given this authority by the county, city, or township government that oversees it. Governmental agencies, which are primarily funded by tax dollars (they may also charge fees for services rendered) and managed by government employees, exist at four governmental levels: international, national, state, and local (city and county). Table 8.1 provides examples of governmental agencies and their governing bodies.

Quasi-Governmental Health Agencies

Quasi-governmental health agencies are so named because they possess characteristics of both governmental health agencies, and of nongovernmental agencies. They obtain their funding from a variety of sources, including community fund-raising efforts such as the United Way, special allocations from government bodies, fees for services rendered, and donations. They carry out tasks that are often thought of as services of governmental agencies, yet they operate independently of governmental supervision.

Table 8.1   Governmental Agencies and Their Governing Bodies

Level/Agency	Governing Body
INTERNATIONAL LEVEL	
World Health Organization (WHO)	United Nations (UN)
Pan American Health Organization (PAHO)	An independent agency
NATIONAL LEVEL	
Centers for Disease Control and Prevention (CDC)	U.S. government, Department of Health and Human Services (HHS)
Food and Drug Administration (FDA)	U.S. government, Department of Health and Human Services (HHS)
STATE LEVEL	
State health department	Individual state governments
State environmental protection agency	Individual state governments
LOCAL LEVEL	
Local public health agencies (LPHA)	City, county, or township governments
Local school districts	Local school boards

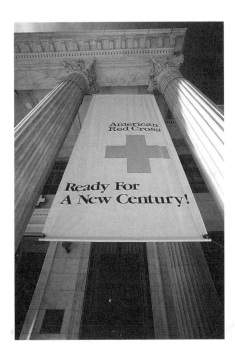

The American Red Cross is one of the best examples of a quasi-governmental agency. (Robert Rathe/Stock, Boston)

Probably the best known quasi-governmental health agency is the **American Red Cross (ARC)**. It was founded in 1881 by Clara Barton as an outgrowth of her work during the Civil War. Today, the ARC has several "official" responsibilities given to it by the federal government, such as providing relief to victims of natural

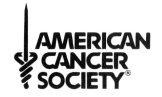 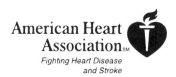 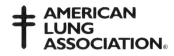

The three largest voluntary health agencies are the American Cancer Society, the American Heart Association, and the American Lung Association. (Symbols courtesy of the American Cancer Society and American Lung Association.)

disasters (Disaster Services) and serving as the liaison between members of the active armed forces and their families during family emergencies (Services to the Armed Forces and Veterans). The ARC also provides many nongovernmental services such as its blood drives and safety services classes such as water safety, first aid, and CPR.

Nongovernmental Health Agencies

Nongovernmental health agencies operate, for the most part, free from governmental interference as long as they comply with the Internal Revenue Service's guidelines for their tax status (McKenzie, Pinger, & Kotecki, 2005). They are primarily funded by private donations, or, as is the case with professional and service groups, membership fees. The nongovernmental agencies can be categorized into the following subgroups: voluntary, philanthropic, service, religious, and professional.

Voluntary Health Agencies

Voluntary health agencies are some of the most visible health agencies in a community. Voluntary health agencies are an American creation and grew out of unmet needs in communities. When governmental or quasi-governmental agencies were not in place to meet the needs of communities, interested citizens came together to form voluntary agencies. Such was the case with the American Cancer Society, the American Heart Association, the American Lung Association, the Alzheimer's Association, and the Sudden Death Syndrome Alliance. The number of voluntary agencies seems endless, with agencies for about every disease and part of the body impacted by a disease or an illness. Most voluntary agencies have four primary purposes: (1) raise money to fund research and their programs, (2) provide education to both professionals and the public, (3) provide service to individuals and families affected by the disease or health problem, and (4) to advocate for beneficial policies, laws, and regulations that impact the work of the agency and in turn the people it is trying to help. Some of these organizations obtain their money from community fund-raising efforts like the United Way, but most raise their money through writing successful grant proposals, carrying out specific special events (i.e., dance-athons, golf outings), conducting door-to-door solicitation or direct mail campaigns, and other receiving donations.

Philanthropic Foundations

Philanthropic foundations play an important role by funding programs and research on the prevention, control, and treatment of diseases and other health problems. *Philanthropy* means "the effort to increase the well-being of humankind, as by charitable donations" (Pritchard, 2001, pp. 632–633). Philanthropic foundations differ from voluntary health agencies in two primary ways. First, they were created with an endowment and, thus, do not have to raise money. Second, they are able to finance long-term projects that may be too expensive or risky to be funded by other agencies. Examples of some philanthropic foundations that have supported work by health educators are the Ford Foundation, the Robert Wood Johnson Foundation, and the Rockefeller Foundation.

Service, Fraternal, and Religious Groups

Each of the many different service, fraternal, and religious groups has also been important to health educators. Even though none of these groups has the primary purpose of enhancing the health of a community, they often get involved in health-related projects. It is not uncommon for health educators to interact with these groups as part of community coalitions or when they are seeking resources to fund or enhance their programs. Examples of service and fraternal groups (and their health-related projects) include the Kiwanis Club (Quest: Skills for Living), Fraternal Order of the Police (food and clothing donations for the needy), Lions (preservation of sight), Shriners (children's hospitals), and American Legion (community recreation programs).

Religious groups have also contributed to the work of health educators' projects, both on a global level (e.g., the Protestants' One Great Hour of Sharing, the Catholics' Relief Fund, and the United Jewish Appeal) and on a local level (e.g., food pantries, sleeping rooms, soup kitchens).

Professional Health Associations/Organizations

As noted at the beginning of this chapter, the primary focus of this chapter is the professional health associations/organizations. The mission of **professional health associations/organizations** is to promote the high standards of professional practice for their respective profession, thereby improving the health of society by improving the people in the profession (McKenzie, Pinger, & Kotecki, 2005). The mission is carried out by advocating for the profession; keeping the members up-to-date via the publication of professional journals, books, and newsletters; and providing the members with an avenue to come together at professional meetings. At these meetings, members have the opportunity to share and hear the new research findings, network with fellow professionals, and find out more about the latest equipment and published materials in the field. In addition, professional associations/organizations provide their members with "perks" such as reduced rates on various types of insurance, participation in tax-deferred annuity programs, discounts (annual national conventions, car rental, eye wear, long-distance telephone calls, publications, travel), job placement, and a variety of other associated items (see Box 8.1).

Professional associations/organizations are member driven and comprised, for the most part, of health professionals who have completed specialized education and

---

Box 8.1 Benefits of Joining a Professional Association/ Organization as a Student Member

- Opportunity to interact, collaborate, and network with other professionals in the profession
- Opportunity to meet and interact with health education students and faculty from other colleges and universities
- Develop professional colleagues
- Have a professional identity
- Professional guidance and mentoring
- Leadership development
- Learn more about how the profession and the association/organization operate
- Keep up to date on happenings in the profession and new health information
- Opportunity to participate in the association's/organization's electronic listserv
- Opportunity to grow professionally and personally while being supported and encouraged by others

- Be exposed to current research and pedagogy of the profession through meeting attendance and reading the publications of the association/organization
- Make professional contacts for future practicums, internships, or jobs
- Get connected to job banks
- Opportunity to make a presentation at a professional meeting
- Opportunity to serve the profession through an association/organization
- Discounted registration fees for professional meetings and publications
- If certified, opportunity to earn continuing education contact hours (CECHs) for recertification of the Certified Health Education Specialist credential and other licensures

Source: Adapted from Society for Public Health Education, Inc. (n.d.).; and Young, & Boling. (2004).

---

training and who are eligible for certification/licensure in their respective professions. These associations/organizations are funded primarily by membership dues, but it is becoming more common for these associations/organizations to seek grant funds (*soft money*) to help promote their missions. Most of these associations/organizations hire staff for day-to-day operations, but the officers of the associations/organizations are usually elected professionals.

In the remaining portions of this chapter, we will present information on the national professional associations/organizations that help promote the health education profession. The reader should also be aware that many of these national associations/organizations have affiliates and other related groups at the regional and/or state level. For example, the American Public Health Association is a national organization, but there are also state associations such as the Ohio Public Health Association, or the Indiana Public Health Association. In addition, there are also some state-only organizations that are not affiliated with any national organization. (Ask your instructor if there are any such organizations in your state.) Often it is these regional or state affiliates/organizations that health education students become members of first because of their proximity to campus, opportunities to get involved in a professional organization, less expensive membership dues, and local networking benefits. Table 8.2 and Appendix C contain information about the following organizations.

The American Alliance for Health, Physical Education, Recreation and Dance. The American Alliance for Health, Physical Education, Recreation and Dance (AAHPERD) is an alliance of six national associations [American Association for Active Lifestyles and Fitness (AAALF), American Association for Health Education (AAHE), American Association for Leisure and Recreation (AALR), National Association for Girls' and Women's Sports (NAGWS), National Association for Sport and Physical Education (NASPE), National Dance Association (NDA)] and six district associations (Central, Eastern, Midwest, Northwest, Southern, and Southwest). (Note that the district associations are comprised of AAHPERD members located in the states represented by these parts of the country. Also, states have an affiliate organization of AAHPERD—for example, the Ohio Association of Health, Physical Education, Recreation and Dance. A professional can be a member of both the state and national organizations, or just one or the other.) AAHPERD is several generations of professional organizations removed from its beginning in 1885, when "Dr. William G. Anderson invited a small group of professionals to meet with him to discuss mutual interests and concerns related to physical training. The purposes of the embryo association, resulting from this meeting, were simply stated: to disseminate knowledge, to improve methods, and to bring those interested in the subject into close relationship with each other" (Anderson, 1985, p. 94). The association continued to grow and turned into the American Physical Education Association (APEA) in 1937. In that year, the APEA "accepted an invitation from the National Education Association (NEA) to merge with its School Health and Physical Education Department to become an NEA Department with three divisions: health, physical education, and recreation" (Anderson, 1985, p. 1). The merger resulted in the formation of the American Association for Health and Physical Education. The word *recreation* was added to the title in 1938, creating AAHPER. In the mid-1960s, the NEA began to feel pressure, because of a challenge from the American Federation of Teachers, to become more active in the welfare movement for teachers. This challenge made the NEA look more closely at its focus. It was supporting thirty departments that had members of their own, most of which were not members of the NEA (Anderson, 1985). In 1968, the NEA changed its "bylaws regarding their departments: to remain a department, all its members had to join the NEA: one alternative was to become an affiliated organization, still identified with NEA and paying a small fee for rent and services; another choice was to become an autonomous associated organization paying the full costs of services rendered by NEA" (Anderson, 1985, p. 95). In 1968, AAHPER chose the former. "This status continued until September 1, 1975, when another NEA bylaws change discontinued this affiliated relationship and AAHPER became completely disassociated from NEA" (Anderson, 1985, p. 95). AAHPER added *dance* to its title in 1979 (Anderson, 1985).

Though all the associations in AAHPERD are associated with the promotion of healthy lifestyles, the one most directly related to the discipline of health education is the American Association for Health Education. Therefore, it will be the only one discussed here.

Table 8.2   Information about Key Professional Associations/Organizations

THE AMERICAN ACADEMY OF HEALTH BEHAVIOR

Address:
P.O. Box 31264
Charlotte, NC 28231
Telephone: 704/330-6592
Facsimile: 704/896-0580
Internet: http://www.aahb.org

AMERICAN ALLIANCE FOR HEALTH, PHYSICAL EDUCATION, RECREATION AND DANCE (AAHPERD)

Address:
1900 Association Drive
Reston, VA 20191
Telephone: 800/213-7193; 703/476-3400
Facsimile: 703/476-9527
Internet: http://www.aahperd.org

AMERICAN ASSOCIATION FOR HEALTH EDUCATION (AAHE)

Address:
1900 Association Drive
Reston, VA 20191
Telephone: 703/476-3437
Facsimile: 703/476-6638
Internet: http://www.aahperd.org/aahe

AMERICAN COLLEGE HEALTH ASSOCIATION (ACHA)

Address:
P.O. Box 28937
Baltimore, MD 21240
Telephone: 410/859-1500
Facsimile: 410/859-1510
Internet: http://www.acha.org

AMERICAN PUBLIC HEALTH ASSOCIATION (APHA)

Address:
800 I Street, NW
Washington, DC 20001
Telephone: 202/777-APHA (2742)
           202/777-2500 (TTY)
Facsimile: 202/777-2534
Internet: http://www.apha.org

(Table 8.2 *continues*)

The **American Association for Health Education (AAHE)** is a relatively new name (since July 1, 1996) for an older organization, the Association for the Advancement of Health Education (also AAHE). The Association for the Advancement of Health Education evolved from the School Health Division of AAHPER when the AAHPER was reorganized in 1973 (Nolte, 1985). Membership in AAHE is open to current, retired, and student (preparing for careers as) health educators and health promotion specialists regardless of their work setting. Current membership is at

(Table 8.2 *continued*)

AMERICAN SCHOOL HEALTH ASSOCIATION (ASHA)

Address:
7263 State Route 43
P.O. Box 708
Kent, OH 44240
Telephone: 330/678-1601
Facsimile: 330/678-4526
Internet: http://www.ashaweb.org

ETA SIGMA GAMMA (ESG)

Address:
2000 University Avenue
Muncie, IN 47306
Telephone: 800/715-2559; 765/285-2258
Facsimile: 765/285-3210
Internet: http://www.bsu.edu/web/esg

INTERNATIONAL UNION FOR HEALTH PROMOTION AND EDUCATION (IUHPE)

Address:
42 Boulevard de la Liberation
93103 Saint-Denis Cedex, France
Telephone: (33) (01) 48 13 71 20
Facsimile: (33) (01) 48 09 17 67
Internet: http://iuhpe.org

SOCIETY FOR PUBLIC HEALTH EDUCATION, INC. (SOPHE)

Address:
750 First Street NE, Suite 910
Washington, DC 20002
Telephone: 202/408-9804
Facsimile: 202/408-9815
Internet: http://www.sophe.org

NATIONAL WELLNESS INSTITUTE, INC. (NWI)

Address:
1300 College Court
PO Box 827
Stevens Point, WI 54481
Telephone: 800/243-8694
Facsimile: 715/342-2979
Internet: http://www.nationalwellness.org

---

approximately 7,500 members. The mission of AAHE is to advance "the profession while serving health educators and other professionals who strive to promote the health of all people. The leaders and members of the organization attain the organizational mission through a comprehensive approach which encourages, supports, and assists health professionals concerned with health promotion through education and other systematic strategies. "AAHE serves professionals in a variety of settings: healthcare, community/public agencies, businesses, schools (Pre-K–12), and institutions of higher learning" (AAHE, 2004b, ¶ 2). In working toward this mission AAHE seeks to reach these goals:

- Develop and promulgate standards, resources, and services regarding health education to professionals and nonprofessionals
- Foster the development of national research priorities in health education and promotion and provide mechanisms for the translation and interaction between theory, research, and practice
- Facilitate communication among members of the profession, the lay public, and other national and international organizations with respect to the philosophic basis and current application of health education principles and practices
- Provide technical assistance to legislative and professional bodies engaged in drafting pertinent legislation and related guidelines
- Provide leadership in promoting policies and evaluative procedures that will result in effective health education programs
- Assist in the development and mobilization of resources for effective health education and promotion (AAHE, 2004b, ¶ 3)

The AAHE produces several publications that health educators find very useful. AAHE has two peer-reviewed journals (a journal in which other professionals in the field decide what is published and what is not). The *American Journal of Health Education* is a bimonthly print publication. It "provides penetrating articles on research findings, teaching ideas, community learning strategies, industry trends, and recent resource materials. Many articles are designed as self-study courses, with continuing education questions and response forms built right in" (AAHPERD, no date, p. 2). The second AAHE journal is the *International Electronic Journal of Health Education*. It "is the first peer-reviewed electronic journal to service the health education/health promotion field in the world. The journal creates global outreach and uses technology to reach health practitioners all over the world" (AAHE, 2004b, ¶ 5). AAHE's newsletter is called "HE-XTRA." It is published four times per year and updates members on health issues, sample curricula, continuing education programs, association activities, advocacy issues, case studies about ethical issues, and career opportunities. In addition, AAHE publishes a biannual directory of undergraduate and graduate professional programs in school, community, and public health education (AAHE, 2003).

In recent years, AAHE has been involved in several activities of note:

- As part of the AAHPERD Advocacy Legislative Center, AAHE coordinates the Health Education Action Link (HEAL) network. This Web-based advocacy network is "designed to provide AAHE members and all health educators the resources to conduct online advocacy with Congress, the Federal Government, and the media on behalf of AAHE and the profession" (AAHPERD, 2004, ¶ 1).
- AAHE is recognized as a multiple event provider of health education continuing education contact hours (CECHs) by the National Commission for Health Education Credentialing (NCHEC). This designation allows AAHE to offer CECHs for Certified Health Education Specialists (CHESs) through the *American Journal of Health Education* and other special publications, and for participation in the annual AAHPERD/AAHE National Convention (AAHE, 2004a).

- The SOPHE/AAHE Baccalaureate Program Approval Committee (SABPAC) is a joint committee of SOPHE and AAHE "responsible for directing and carrying out the undergraduate program approval process for eligible college and university programs preparing undergraduate preservice health education specialists" (AAHE, no date, p. 1).

- AAHE/ASHA Committee on Health Education Preparation Responsibilities and Competencies for Elementary Teachers. In January 1990, AAHE and ASHA formed a joint committee to establish guidelines to prepare elementary teachers in health education. The resulting guidelines were titled "Health Instruction Responsibilities and Competencies for Elementary (K–6) Classroom Teachers" (AAHE, no date).

- The National Council for Accreditation of Teacher Education (NCATE) has allowed AAHE to be the professional health education association/organization responsible for reviewing folios submitted to NCATE by colleges and universities when they are seeking NCATE accreditation for their teacher education programs.

- In an effort to improve the quality of health educators and, in turn, health education, in 2001 AAHE and SOPHE created a joint National Task Force on Accreditation in Health Education to develop a plan for a unified system of accreditation for undergraduate and graduate professional preparation programs in health education. The report of the Task Force was completed in 2004. At the time this book was being written, plans were under way for a national meeting to determine how the system could be implemented.

American Public Health Association.   The **American Public Health Association (APHA)** "is the oldest and largest organization of public health professionals in the world" (APHA, 2004a, ¶ 2). The APHA was founded in 1872 "as a result of the public health movement to combat yellow fever and other diseases in the 1870s" (APHA, no date, p. 3). The purposes of the APHA are "to protect and promote personal and environmental health; to exercise leadership with health professionals and the general public in health policy development and action, with particular focus on the interrelationship between health and the quality of life and on developing a national policy for health care and services and on solving technical problems" (Cauffman, 1982, p. 93).

Membership in the APHA is open to professional, student/trainee, and retired health workers, as well as consumers who are interested in supporting the mission of the association. Currently, the more than 50,000 members come from over 50 occupations in public health (APHA, 2004). Once individuals become members, they have the opportunity to select one or more of the subgroups of the organization. "Sections are the basic organizational unit of APHA's membership. The 24 discipline-based Sections and 7 Special Primary Interest Groups (SPIGs) enable members to share knowledge and experience with peers, develop new techniques and contribute to the growing body of scientific knowledge within those respective fields" (APHA, 2004b, ¶ 1). More specifically, these subgroups propose policy statements, advise on publications, provide testimony and reports, help develop the content and structure of annual meetings, and assist in APHA governance

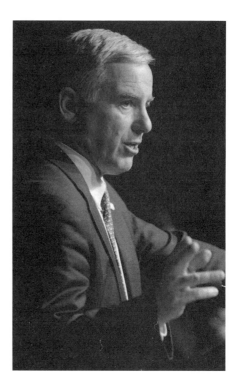

Former Vermont Governor and presidential candidate Howard Dean addressed the membership at the APHA meeting in 2002. Annual professional conventions are an important benefit of membership in a professional organization. (AP/Worldwide Photos)

(APHA, no date). The sections most closely related to health education are (1) Public Health Education Section, which formed in 1922 and in 1991 changed its name to Public Health Education and Health Promotion Section, and (2) School Health Education Section, which formed in 1942 and in 1980 changed its name to School Health Education and Services Section.

The mission of the Public Health Education and Health Promotion Section (PHEHP, 2004, ¶ 1–2) is twofold:

1. To be a strong advocate for health education, disease prevention and health promotion directed to individuals, groups, and communities in all activities of the Association
2. To set, maintain, and exemplify the highest ethical principles and standards of practice on the part of all professionals and disciplines whose primary purpose is health education, disease prevention, and/or health promotion

To achieve this mission, the Section's key activities include the following:

1. To recruit and involve a large and diverse group of professionals representative of the nation's populations and of the disciplines whose primary purpose is health education, disease prevention, and health promotion
2. To encourage the inclusion of health education, disease prevention, and health promotion activities in all of the nation's health programs
3. To stimulate thought, discussion, research, and programmatic applications aimed at improving the public's health

4. To improve the quality of research and practice in all public health programs of health education, disease prevention, and health promotion

5. To provide the Association with expertise and leadership in regard to health education, disease prevention, and health promotion

6. To provide networking opportunities for persons whose professional interests and training include, but are not limited to, the disciplines of health education, health communication, health promotion, social marketing, behavioral and social sciences, and public relations

7. To provide Section members with opportunities to become informed and engaged in all of the activities and matters of concern to the Association

8. To facilitate collaboration with all of the Association's boards, committees, sections, SPIGs, caucuses, and affiliates

9. To provide Section members with such benefits as the annual meeting program, continuing education opportunities, newsletters, and a structure for exercising Association leadership

10. To identify and recognize individuals who make outstanding and substantial contributions to health education, disease prevention, health promotion and the operation of the Section

The purpose of the School Health Education and Services Section (CNHEO, 2004c, ¶ 1) is:

- To provide a section within the association that works independently, with other association substructures, and with external organizations toward the improvement of early childhood, school, and college health programs

- To interpret the functions and responsibilities of health agencies to daycare, preschool, school, and college personnel

- To interpret early childhood, school, and college health education and service objectives to other public health personnel and assist them in integrating the objectives in their community

- To provide a forum for discussion of practices and research in early childhood, school, and college health

- To encourage the provision of health promotion programs within the school and college settings that address the needs of children and school personnel

- To encourage among interested association members the study and discussion of procedures and problems in early childhood, school, and college health services, health education, and environmental health programs

The primary publication of APHA is the *American Journal of Public Health (AJPH)*. This peer-reviewed journal is published monthly. A typical issue of the *AJPH* includes editorials, commentaries, book reviews, job announcements, notification of upcoming meetings, and authoritative articles in both general and specialized areas of research, policy analysis, and program evaluation of public health. Areas covered in the articles include the environment, maternal and child health, health promotion, epidemiology, administration, occupational health, education, international health, statistics, and more. The association also publishes *The Nation's Health* twelve times per year. This newspaper includes reporting on current and proposed legislation, policy issues, news of actions within the federal agencies and

Congress, and special features. The publication also includes association news, job openings, and information on upcoming conferences. In addition to the *AJPH* and *The Nation's Health,* the APHA also publishes books and other media on a variety of public health topics. Examples include the best-selling titles *Control of Communicable Disease Manual* (Heymann, 2004) and *Communicating Public Health Information Effectively* (Nelson, Brownson, Remington, & Parvanta, 2002).

There are other professional health associations that have a more focused mission. Some of those include the American College Health Association (ACHA), the American School Health Association (ASHA), the National Wellness Institute, Inc. (NWI), the Society for Public Health Education, Inc. (SOPHE), and the American Academy of Health Behavior.

American College Health Association. The **American College Health Association (ACHA)** was founded originally as the American Student Health Association in 1920. In 1948, the name of the association was changed to its current name. ACHA's mission is to "be the principal advocate and leadership organization for college and university health. The association will provide advocacy, education, communications, products, and services, as well as promote research and culturally competent practices to enhance its members' ability to advance the health of all students and the campus community" (ACHA, 2004d, ¶ 2). The association has three distinct types of memberships. One is for institutions of higher education. Currently, there are more than 900 such members. ACHA also serves more than 2,400 individual members who are interested in college health—that is, the health of college students. Included in the members are administrators, physicians and physicians' assistants, nurses and nurse practitioners, health educators, pharmacists, dentists, support staff who care for this special group of young adults, and students who are dedicated to health promotion on their campus. Most of these individual members are associated with the health service facilities on their respective campuses. The third type of membership is called sustaining members. This group is made up of nonprofit and for-profit associations, organizations, and corporations that are interested in being more connected with the college health field (ACHA, 2004c).

Like some of the other associations/organizations, the ACHA also has subgroups. "ACHA recognizes a total of 11 affiliate organizations arrayed across six regions of the United States. Each of these affiliate organizations is governed by its own elected affiliate officers, who provide guidance and leadership to members and help forge strong partnerships with colleagues on the state or regional level, including conducting their own annual educational meetings" (ACHA, 2004a, ¶ 1). In addition, ACHA has eight membership sections, which are defined by the disciplines of college health. The Health Education Section, now called the Health Promotion Section, was formed in 1958.

ACHA publishes several newsletters, numerous health information brochures, and other special publications. It has a members-only newsletter that is available online at the Association's Web site. The professional journal of the ACHA is the *Journal of American College Health.* It is published bimonthly and is the only journal devoted entirely to the health of college students. The journal publishes articles encompassing many areas of college health, "including clinical and preventive medicine, environmental health and safety, nursing assessment, interventions, and

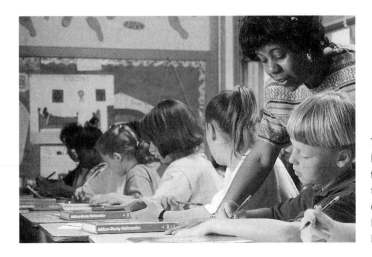

The American School Health Association focuses on the health of the school-aged child. (Will & Deni McIntyre/Photo Researchers)

management, pharmacy, and sports medicine. The journal regularly publishes major articles on student behaviors, mental health and healthcare policies, and includes a section for discussion of controversial issues" (ACHA, 2004b, ¶ 1).

American School Health Association.   The **American School Health Association (ASHA)** began on October 27, 1927, as the American Association of School Physicians. It began to use its current name in 1936 (ASHA, 1976). The mission of the ASHA "is to protect and promote the health of children and youth by supporting coordinated school health programs as a foundation for school success" (ASHA, 2004a, ¶ 5).

Membership in the association "is open to any individual or school system with an interest in the health and well-being of school-aged children and youth" (ASHA, 2004c, ¶ 1). The ASHA is a multidisciplinary organization with more than 2,000 members. Included in its membership are administrators, counselors, dentists, health educators, physical educators, school nurses, and school physicians who advocate for high-quality coordinated school health programs. With membership in the ASHA comes the opportunity to join subgroups of the association called sections and councils. These subgroups allow members to interact with others who have the same school health interests. Examples of a few of the councils are health behaviors, international and cross-cultural health, school health instruction and curriculum, food and nutrition education, and sexuality education.

The ASHA has several publications. They include the *Journal of School Health,* which is published ten times per year; "The Pulse," a newsletter that is published four times per year and provides the latest news and analysis of the ASHA; a variety of other resources for school health personnel, such as *Guidelines for Protecting Confidential Student Health Information,* and *Health Is Academic: A Guide to Coordinated School Health Programs;* and *Health in Action,* ASHA's newest publication. *Health in Action,* which is published four times a year, "is a focused, informative and practical publication specifically for health and education professionals at the middle and high school levels" (ASHA, 2004b, ¶¶ 1, 3–4). Each issue has a specific focus and includes items such as handouts for students and their families, suggestions for policy makers, suggestions for classroom activities and working with individual students, and other valuable resources.

The *Journal of School Health* is recognized widely and includes in-depth articles, results of professional research, case studies of successful school health programs and practices, school health service applications, teaching techniques, book reviews, commentaries, and other current information such as job and workshop announcements. The *Journal* publishes material related to health promotion in school settings. The readership of the *Journal* includes administrators, educators, nurses, physicians, dentists, dental hygienists, counselors, social workers, nutritionists, dietitians, and other health professionals. These individuals work cooperatively with parents and the community to achieve the common goal of providing children and adolescents with a coordinated school health program to promote health and to improve learning.

National Wellness Institute, Inc.   The National Wellness Institute (NWI), founded in 1977, "was formed to realize the mission of providing health promotion and wellness professionals unparalleled resources and services that promote professional and personal growth. Sharing a mutual commitment to promoting wellness, NWI's founders sought to bring together a group of professionals to share their knowledge, research, expertise, and to build a network of friends dedicated to wellness and health promotion" (NWI, 2004a, ¶ 1). The mission of NWI "is to serve the professionals and organizations that promote optimal health and wellness in individuals and communities" (NWI, 2004c, ¶ 1). The mission is accomplished by:

- Identifying quality resources for health promotion and wellness professionals
- Providing quality education resources and continuing education
- Promoting opportunities for life-long learning in health and wellness
- Providing new and innovative professional development programs
- Developing effective educational lifestyle assessments
- Serving professionals and organizations that promote health and wellness (NWI, 2004c, ¶ 2)

There are two types of membership in NWI, individual and organizational. The organizational membership is for entities like corporations or institutions such as colleges and universities. Within the individual membership category, one can have a student, core, or core plus membership. With membership comes a number of publications. They include four online publications: *Wellness Management,* a quarterly newsletter, the monthly *Wellness News You Can Use,* bimonthly reproducible articles for newsletters in the *Health Promotion Practitioner,* and the bimonthly *HEALTH ISSUES Update/RESOURCE News* newsletter, published by Health Enhancement Systems. For those who are core plus members, the peer-reviewed *American Journal of Health Promotion* is also provided bimonthly (NWI, 2004b).

One of the most visible components of the NWI is its National Wellness Conference, held each July in Stevens Point, WI. It is open to members and nonmembers alike, and is a unique conference because it is a week of immersion into a wellness experience (see Box 8.2).

Box 8.2 Practitioner's Perspective: Professional Association (NWI)

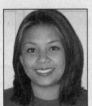

NAME: Cheryl Castillejos, B.A., CHES

CURRENT POSITION/TITLE: Assistant Wellness Director

EMPLOYER: Health Solutions, Inc.

DEGREE/INSTITUTION/YEAR: B.A., Purdue University, 2002

MAJOR: Health Promotion

MINOR: Psychology

Job responsibilities: As Assistant Wellness Director, I maintain operations for the Sears, Roebuck and Co. Health Center by coordinating health promotion and disease prevention events and screenings. I create, manage, and market all health promotion programs. I also research, guide, and present educational lectures to the Sears community. In addition, I continually update the wellness Web site and educational materials for staff development and associate awareness.

How I obtained my job: I was fortunate to be hired as a health educator following my successful internship at Sears. During my first year while working as health educator, I was promoted to my current position following a change in management.

What I like most about my job: I am able to work with a diverse group of health professionals. The Sears Health Center incorporates both a fitness and a wellness center. The fitness facility houses a variety of cardiovascular exercise equipment, a full line of weight machines and free weights, and a group exercise room staffed by fitness specialists. The wellness facility offers health education and promotion as well as walk-in medical treatment with a full-time nursing staff. Exposure to both the clinical and fitness sides of wellness enhances my experience as a health educator. My position has also enabled me to work hand in hand with those in the Sears community and assist in the development of their benefits and wellness offerings.

What I like least about my job: We have recently integrated our fitness and wellness services in order to offer a comprehensive wellness program. To date the full potential of integrating the services has not been reached because our teams are housed in separate locations and overseen by two different departments.

The impact of the National Wellness Institute (NWI): My membership in the National Wellness Institute has impacted my professional experience in many ways. The NWI is the clearinghouse of information for new wellness initiatives and current news. It provides monthly updates that are easily accessible via e-mail and the Internet. As a member, I have been able to network with other health educators and professionals in the field, which is very helpful in an entry-level position. It allows one to share ideas and learn from others in the same profession. Most importantly, the NWI offers comprehensive continuing education opportunities as well as encouragement, inspiration, and support for the development of my career.

Recommendations for those preparing to be health educators: My recommendation to those preparing to be health educators is to get involved in the profession as early as possible. Networking through professional organizations, volunteer opportunities, and service learning experiences will enable preservice professionals to develop relationships with those in the field and gain a better understanding of the career opportunities for the future.

Society for Public Health Education, Inc.   The Society of Public Health Educators (SOPHE), founded in 1950, is the only professional organization devoted exclusively to public health education and health promotion. In 1969, the organization changed its name to the **Society for Public Health Education, Inc. (SOPHE).** The purpose of SOPHE is "to provide leadership to the profession and to promote the health of all people by: stimulating research on the theory and practice of health education; supporting high quality performance standards for the practice of health education and health promotion; advocating policy and legislation affecting health education and health promotion; and developing and promoting standards for professional preparation of health education professionals" (SOPHE, 2004a, ¶ 3). Membership in SOPHE is open to individuals with formal training and/or interest in health education and health promotion. At the national level, SOPHE's membership includes more than 4,000 professionals from throughout the United States and twenty-five foreign countries. Members work in a variety of places, including K–12 schools, universities, medical/managed care settings, corporations, voluntary health agencies, international organizations, and federal, state, and local government. There are currently twenty-four SOPHE chapters covering thirty-three states and several others under development (SOPHE, 2004b). Like several of the other associations/organizations, SOPHE members have the opportunity to associate with one or more of its nine special-interest groups within the larger organization.

SOPHE has four primary publications. They include two peer-reviewed journals, *Health Education and Behavior* and *Health Promotion Practice,* a newsletter called "News & Views," and an annual membership directory and buyer's guide. *Health Education and Behavior,* published bimonthly, is a well-respected journal that is aimed primarily at the dissemination of research findings, but a typical issue also includes perspective papers, practice notes, book reviews, and SOPHE-related information. *Health Promotion Practice,* the newest publication of SOPHE, is published quarterly and "seeks to advance the application of health promotion and education through the stimulation and publication of articles detailing the applied work of health promotion practice and policy" (Schwartz & Goodman, 2000, p. 5). "News & Views" is published bimonthly and includes information on the latest trends, public policies, meetings, and resources (SOPHE, 2004c).

Over the years, SOPHE has had a good working relationship with the APHA. SOPHE holds its annual meeting the weekend prior to the APHA annual meeting in the same city as the APHA. Like several of the other associations/organizations, the annual meeting of SOPHE provides opportunities to share and receive the most recent research findings, to earn continuing education contact hours, to participate in its job bank service, and to network with other professionals.

In addition to the above-mentioned items, SOPHE has been involved in some other special project. Some examples include:

- An annual health education advocacy summit at which health educators receive training in advocacy techniques and get to apply their new knowledge on a trip to Capitol Hill in Washington, DC, to discuss health-related issues with staffers from key legislative subcommittees and representatives of their congressional districts

- An annual mid-year scientific conference in the spring, which focuses on a topic of special interest to those in the health education and health promotion disciplines
- Partnership in the SOPHE/AAHE Baccalaureate Program Approval Committee (SABPAC) (see p. 235).

International Union for Health Promotion and Education.   Though all of the professional associations/organizations noted already in this chapter have members from countries other than the United States, there is one professional association that is truly worldwide: the **International Union for Health Promotion and Education (IUHPE).** The IUHPE, founded in 1951 in Paris, is a global association with a mission "to promote global health and to contribute to the achievement of equity in health between and within countries of the world" (IUHPE, 2004a, ¶ 1). More specifically, the IUHPE has four major goals:

a. Advocate for health—to advocate for actions that promote the health of populations throughout the world
b. Build knowledge of effective health promotion and health education—to develop the knowledge base for health promotion and health education
c. Improve effectiveness of policy and practice—to improve and advance the quality and effectiveness of health promotion and health education practice and knowledge
d. Build capacity for health promotion and health education—to contribute to the development of capacity in countries to undertake health promotion and health education activities (IUHPE, 2004a, ¶ 3)

Because IUHPE is a worldwide organization, it is organized through six regional offices (Europe [IUHPE/EURO], Latin America [IUHPE/ORLA], North America [IUHPE/NARO], Northern Part of the Western Pacific [IUHPE/NPWP], Southeast Asia [IUHPE/SEARO], and Southwest Pacific [IUHPE/SWP]) and has a total international conference only once every three years. The most recent one was in Melbourne, Australia, in April 2004. The IUHPE has four peer-reviewed journals, *Promotion & Education, Health Education Research, Health Promotion International,* and *Reviews of Health Promotion and Education Online. Promotion & Education* is a multilingual quarterly journal that publishes authoritative articles and practical information that reflect the three strategic priorities of the IUHPE, namely: advancing knowledge, advocacy, and networking. *Health Education Research,* published bimonthly, is the official research journal of the IUHPE and "deals with all the vital issues involved in health education and promotion worldwide—providing a valuable link between the researcher and the results obtained by practising [sic] health educators and communications" (IUHPE, 2004b, ¶ 4). *Health Promotion International* is a "quarterly journal published in association with the World Health Organization. It contains refereed original articles, reviews and debate articles on major themes from various sectors including education, health services, employment, government, the media, industry, environmental agencies and community networks" (IUHPE, 2004b, ¶ 3). The former *Internet Journal of Health Promotion* has been transformed into *Reviews of Health Promotion and Education Online* and has become the official electronic journal of the IUHPE (IUHPE, 2004b).

American Academy of Health Behavior. The **American Academy of Health Behavior (AAHB)** is a professional organization unlike those presented so far in this chapter. Founded in 1997, the AAHB, or just *The Academy,* as it is referred to, is a society of researchers and scholars in the areas of health behavior, health education, and health promotion. *The Academy* "was created to improve the stature of health educators by supporting and promoting quality health behavior, health education, and health promotion research conducted by health educators" (Werch, 2000, p. 3). The mission of *The Academy* "is to advance the practice of health education and health promotion through health behavior research" (AAHB, 2004, ¶ 1). More specifically, *The Academy's* objectives are to:

- Foster and disseminate findings of health behavior, health education, and health promotion research through sponsorship of scientific meetings, symposia, and publications

- Recognize outstanding achievements in the areas of health behavior, health education, and health promotion research

- Facilitate collaborative research efforts by bringing *The Academy* members in contact with each other through a membership directory, professional meetings, professional publications, and electronic media

- Advance health education and health promotion by influencing health policy and allocation of resources (government agencies, private foundations, universities, etc.) by developing and disseminating a cohesive body of knowledge in the area of health behavior research (AAHB, 2004 ¶ 2)

Individuals must apply for membership in *The Academy* and acceptance is based upon one's area of academic preparation and level of scholarly activity. The specific qualifications for membership are listed on *The Academy's* Web site (see Table 8.2). The official journal of *The Academy* is the *American Journal of Health Behavior.* In a typical copy of this bimonthy publication, readers will find a number of data-based research articles along with articles on research techniques, uses of technology for research, biographical sketches of members of *The Academy,* and book reviews.

Eta Sigma Gamma. Founded in 1967, **Eta Sigma Gamma (ESG)** is the national health education honorary. The idea for the organization was born when three professors from Ball State University, Drs. William Bock, Warren E. Schaller, and Robert Synovitz, were on their way to a professional conference and were talking about the need for an honorary for the discipline. Their discussion led to the formation of the organization, which has had, from its very beginning, the primary purpose of furthering the professional competence and dedication of individual members of the health education profession (ESG, 1991). The ideals of the honorary are symbolized in its seal. The seal (see Figure 8.1) "is divided into four equilateral triangles, each carrying a symbol. A lamp of learning is in the center triangle, surrounded by an open book representing teaching, a microscope signifying research, and an outstretched hand representing service. These three elements form the basic purposes of the organization and profession; teaching, research, and service. The unifying element of these purposes is symbolized by the lamp of learning, since it is through the learning process that each purpose is achieved" (ESG, 1991, p. 2).

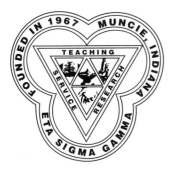

Figure 8.1 Seal of Eta Sigma Gamma

Source: National Office of Eta Sigma Gamma, 2000 University Ave., Muncie, IN 47306.

As noted in Table 8.2, the national office of Eta Sigma Gamma is located in Muncie, Indiana, on the campus of Ball State University in the Department of Physiology and Health Science. This is also where the Alpha Chapter (the first chapter of the honorary) is located. As of June 2004, there have been 112 chapters installed on university/college campuses throughout the United States (see Appendix C). Chapters are awarded to colleges/universities based on a review and vote by the National Executive Committee of Eta Sigma Gamma on an application prepared by personnel at the petitioning college/university. From its beginnings, Eta Sigma Gamma has focused on the student members. It is while individuals are either undergraduate or graduate students that most people join the honorary. Membership is open to those who have a major or minor in health education and a grade point average equivalent to at least a *B–*. In fact, students can achieve membership only by affiliating through a collegiate chapter. Through their affiliation with the collegiate chapters they are eligible to apply for the awards and scholarships of the honorary. Professionals active in the discipline of health education and holding a degree can affiliate through the Chapter-At-Large (ESG, 1991).

Eta Sigma Gamma regularly produces three publications: its journal, *The Health Educator; The Health Education Monograph Series;* and "The Vision," a newsletter. Each of these publications is distributed twice a year. Like the publications of the other associations/organizations, these publications include the current works of the professionals in the field. However, unlike the others, only individuals who are current members of Eta Sigma Gamma can write articles for *The Health Educator* and *The Health Education Monograph Series.* Another unusual characteristic of the publications of Eta Sigma Gamma is that one entire issue of the *Monograph Series* each year is comprised of articles written only by student members. This is another indication that the honorary is very concerned about the preservice professional.

Associations for Directors.   There are two other professional groups that have ties to health education. They are the (1) Directors of Health Promotion and Education and (2) Society of State Directors of Health, Physical Education, and Recreation. Unlike all the other professional groups discussed, membership in these organizations is determined by the professional position held, not by application for membership. The individuals who belong to these organizations are employees of their respective state/territorial departments of health or education. The primary functions of the **Directors of Health Promotion and Education**

Box 8.3 Practitioner's Perspective: Professional Association (ESG)

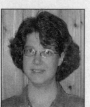

NAME: Suzanne Batdorff
CURRENT POSITION/TITLE: Health Educator
EMPLOYER: Delaware County (IN) Health Department
DEGREE/INSTITUTION/YEAR: B.S., Ball State University, 1995
MAJOR: Health Science
MINOR(S): Gerontology and Public Health

Job responsibilities: My primary responsibility is to promote health, wellness, and safety to the Delaware County community through educational presentations, services, and written materials. Therefore, a good portion of my work includes planning, developing, implementing, and evaluating community health education services. Examples of these services include making presentations and working at events for the "Safe Kids Coalition of Delaware County," teaching CPR classes to city high school students and the public, teaching Universal Precautions classes, conducting the American Cancer Society's FreshStart smoking cessation classes, and providing a Tobacco Education Group to students as a positive alternative to school suspension. I also spend time collaborating with other health professionals and agencies to promote wellness. As part of my responsibilities I have worked with the American Stroke Association, the American Diabetes Association (now planning a "Kiss the Pig" fund raiser), TEAMwork for Quality Living (a local organization to improve the quality of life in the community), and the AIDS Task Force in each of the area high schools. I also spend time providing educational presentations to area schools, daycare centers, adult centers, and the public on topics including such things as nutrition, physical fitness, dangers of smoking, heart health, stroke, diabetes, seasonal safety (heat, winter and falls, Halloween, etc.), bicycle safety, poison prevention, and fire safety.

How I obtained my job: While not working in the health education field, I maintained contact with professional health educators to keep abreast of the issues and of any position opening. One of the persons I kept a friendship with is

(Box 8.3 *continues*)

(DHPE), which was formed in 1946, are to work to enhance the health education standards in public health agencies and to provide a means by which its members have an opportunity to network with one another. More specifically, DHPE has the following purposes (DHPE, 2004, ¶ 2):

- To serve as a channel through which directors of health promotion and public health education programs of states and territories may exchange and share methods, techniques, and information for the enrichment and improvement of health promotion and public health education programs

- To establish position statements that increase public awareness of the necessity of health promotion and public health education

(Box 8.3 *continued*)

also a health educator for the Delaware County Health Department, and she let me know about the position I now hold. By the way, she is someone I first met through the Eta Sigma Gamma chapter where I went to school.

What I like most about my job: The variety of our daily activities. No two days are the same. There are new programs and activities being planned and implemented all the time. I also really like being able to promote a positive way of living to the public.

What I like least about my job: My position within the Delaware County Health Department is grant funded. The grant was received to carry out a statewide Hepatitis B program. However, my position is funded with the overhead dollars from the grant and thus I have no direct responsibilities with the grant project. Thus, I have nothing to do with the success of the program or the renewal of the grant funding. My position can be dissolved at any time, based upon the work of others.

The impact of Eta Sigma Gamma on my preparation to become a health educator: Eta Sigma Gamma is a great organization to belong to. As a student member of the organization, I was able to meet and interact with other people wanting to be health educators. It also provided me with great opportunities to meet and network with many practicing health educators. Eta Sigma Gamma also provided me with the opportunity to participate in health education community services, which in turn allowed me to learn more about how health education programs are implemented. It helped me create a bridge between the theory of the classroom and the practice in the field. In addition I served as my chapter's secretary, which helped me learn what is involved with being on a committee board.

Recommendations for those preparing to be health educators: Become as involved as possible in your classes and Eta Sigma Gamma. The more you network with professionals, the better. Volunteer or do extra shadowing with professionals in a variety of health education settings (i.e., health care, volunteer health organization, governmental agency) to gain an understanding of how different programs are implemented and organizations are run.

- To participate with the Association of State and Territorial Health Officials (ASTHO) in promoting health and preventing disease
- To identify methods of improving the quality and practice of health promotion and public health education
- To elicit the cooperation of and coordination with national, public, private, and voluntary agencies related to public health programs
- To provide a forum for continuing education opportunities in health promotion and public health education

This association is also an affiliate of the Association of State and Territorial Health Officials (ASTHO) (see the URL for this Web site in the Web Links at the end of the chapter), which is the association for those who oversee state and territorial health departments. You can obtain more information about DHPE by contacting any state or territorial department of health, or by logging on to the DHPE Web site (see the URL for this Web site in the Web Links at the end of the chapter).

The Conference of State Directors of Health, Physical Education, and Recreation, which later changed its name to **Society of State Directors of Health, Physical Education, and Recreation (SSDHPER),** was founded in 1926 and is "a professional association whose members supervise and coordinate programs in health, physical education, and related fields within state departments of education. Associate members are those who are interested in the goals and programs of the Society who do not work within a state education agency" (SSDHPER, 2004, ¶ 1). The mission of the SSDHPER "is to provide leadership in facilitating and promoting initiatives to achieve health and education goals and objectives. The Society promotes effective school programs and practices that involve collaboration with parents and community groups to positively impact a healthy and active lifestyle. The Society maintains a network for professional development and a forum for sharing knowledge, ideas, and strategies for implementing quality programs at the national, state, and local levels" (SSDHPER, 2004, ¶ 12). The purposes of the SSDHPER are:

- To promote sound programs of health, physical education, and recreation in educational settings throughout the United States

- To consider critical issues relevant to the Society's mission and take appropriate actions

- To provide a basis for exchange of ideas and programs among members of the organization

- To cooperate with governmental agencies, postsecondary institutions, and professional, voluntary, and civic organizations in furthering the development of programs in health, physical education, and recreation (SSDHPER, 2004, ¶ 13)

You can obtain more information about SSDHPER by contacting any state department of education or the SSDHPER Web site at (see the Web Links at the end of the chapter).

Coalitions.   Because of the large number of professional health education associations, there are times when there is a need to have a common voice for the profession. To help provide such a voice, coalitions of health associations/organizations have been created. The most prominent coalition is the Coalition of National Health Education Organizations, USA.

The **Coalition of National Health Education Organizations, USA (CNHEO)** is a nonprofit federation of organizations dedicated to advancing the health education profession (CNHEO, 2004b). It is comprised of representatives (delegates and alternates) from ten national associations/organizations that have identifiable health educator memberships and ongoing health education programs. The associations/organizations included are the American Academy of Health Behavior; the American College Health Association, Health Education Section; the American Public Health Association, Public Health Education and Health Promotion Section; the American Public Health Association, School Health Education and

Services Section; the American School Health Association; the American Association for Health Education; Directors of Health Promotion and Education; Eta Sigma Gamma; the Society for Public Health Education, Inc.; and the Society of State Directors of Health, Physical Education, and Recreation. For many years there were only eight members of the CNHEO. The two most recent additions to CNHEO were Eta Sigma Gamma in 1999 and the American Academy of Health Behavior in 2003 (Capwell, 2004).

The CNHEO was formed on March 1, 1972, after a series of three meetings in 1971 and 1972 to determine the feasibility of such an organization. The primary mission of the coalition is "the mobilization of the resources of the Health Education Profession in order to expand and improve health education, regardless of the setting" (CNHEO, 2004a, ¶ 1). The work of the CNHEO is financed by funds obtained from coalition member organizations, public and private agencies, and contributions and gifts from individuals. Over the years, the working relationship of the member organizations has been outlined in the *Working Agreement of the CNHEO.* Also included in this document are the purposes of the coalition (CNHEO, 2004a):

1. Facilitate national-level communication, collaboration, and coordination, among the member organizations

2. Provide a forum for the identification and discussion of health education issues

3. Formulate recommendations and take appropriate action on issues affecting member interests

4. Serve as a communication and advisory resource for agencies, organizations, and persons in the public and private sectors concerning health education issues

5. Serve as a focus for the exploration and resolution of issues pertinent to professional health educators

Unlike the other organizations and groups discussed in this chapter, the CNHEO functions with no paid staff members or permanent location. "The CNHEO carries on business by means of e-mail communication, monthly conference calls, and periodic face-to-face meetings during member organization conferences. Through these means it has made significant progress in addressing its purposes and priorities" (Capwell, 2004, p. 13). Since its inception, the CNHEO has operationalized its purposes in a number of ways, contributing to the growth of the profession. Below is a list of some of the recent activities and accomplishments in which the CNHEO has been involved. (Note: Some items in this list are discussed in greater detail in other chapters of this book when they apply to the content of that chapter.)

- Creation of position papers on topics of importance to the profession, e.g., preparation of elementary school teachers in the area of health education, and the strengthening of health education in the public health arena

- Mobilization of health education professionals seeking to add the Standard Occupation Classification (SOC) of *health educator* to the "List of Community and Social Service Occupations" by the United States Department of Labor, Bureau of Labor Statistics (USDOL, 2001) (see Chapter 2)

- Cosponsoring two invitational conferences in 1995 (NCHEC & CNHEO, 1996) and 2002 (CNHEO, 2003) to examine the status and future of the health education profession. These conferences led to the creation of goals and recommendations for the profession for the twenty-first century, and commitments by member organizations to lead or assist in addressing the recommendations (CNHEO, 2003). (See Chapter 10 for more on the future of health education.)

- Creation of a unified "Code of Ethics for the Health Education Profession" (see Chapter 5 and Appendix A)

- Cosponsoring the annual National Health Education Advocacy Summit that began in 1998. The purpose of the Summit is to increase the capacity of health educators to engage in effective advocacy for a common health education agenda. At the Summit attendees receive policy advocacy training and make legislative visits to educate congresspersons on priority issues in health education (CNHEO, 2004b)

- Support of the *Health Education Advocate* Web site. "The mission of the *Health Education Advocate* is to provide a central, timely source of advocacy information related to the field of health education and health promotion" (CNHEO, 2004b, ¶ 1). (See Web Links at the end of this chapter for the URL of the Web site.)

More information about CNHEO can be obtained by contacting the office of any of the member organizations or by logging on to the CNHEO Web site. The URL for this site is presented in the Web Links at the end of the chapter.

Joining a Professional Health Association/Organization

Becoming a member of a professional organization is not difficult. With the exception of a few of the associations/organizations previously noted (the coalition, the American Academy of Health Behavior, Eta Sigma Gamma, and DHPE and SSDHPER), membership in a professional organization can be obtained by completing an application form (available from any of the organizations, included in many of the official publications, or found at the organization's Web site [see Table 8.2]) and sending the money with the desired length and category of membership (different rates apply to different types of membership—for example, student, professional, retired) to the association/organization of choice. Most individuals join a professional association/organization for a year at a time. Some associations, however, provide multiple-year memberships at a reduced rate or even a lifetime membership. In general, the cost of a membership in a state or regional association/organization is separate from and less than a membership in a national association/organization. If you are interested in joining a state or local association/organization, you can usually contact its national office to find out whom to contact locally.

SUMMARY

This chapter discussed the various health agencies, associations, and organizations with which the profession of health education interacts. The agencies/associations/organizations were presented within three major categories: governmental, quasi-governmental, and nongovernmental. The primary emphasis of the chapter was to present information about a subcategory of the nongovernmental associations/

organizations, the professional associations/organizations. Those discussed included the American Academy of Health Behavior; the American Alliance for Health, Physical Education, Recreation and Dance; the American Association for Health Education; the American Public Health Association; the American College Health Association; the American School Health Association; the National Wellness Institute, Inc.; the Society for Public Health Education, Inc.; the International Union for Health Promotion and Education; Eta Sigma Gamma; and associations for directors (Directors of Health Promotion and Education, and the Society of State Directors of Health, Physical Education, and Recreation). Also, information about a coalition—the Coalition of National Health Education Organizations, USA—was presented. The chapter concluded with information on how to become a member of a professional association/organization.

REVIEW QUESTIONS

1. Define and explain the differences among the following types of agencies: governmental health agency, quasi-governmental health agency, nongovernmental health agency.

2. At what levels do governmental agencies exist? Provide an example of an agency at each level.

3. What are the four primary activities of most voluntary health agencies? Give an example of each.

4. What are the purposes of a professional association/organization?

5. What are the benefits derived from membership in a professional association/organization? Why should students become members?

6. What is the oldest and largest professional health association in the United States?

7. Name three professional health associations/organizations that focus their efforts on work settings for health educators. Name two other professional health associations/organizations that are not as focused on a work setting.

8. What is the name of the health education honorary? Where was it founded and where is the national office located? In general, where are the chapters of the honorary found?

9. What makes the American Academy of Health Behavior different from the other professional organizations/associations presented in this chapter?

10. What is a coalition? Name one health education coalition. What is the primary purpose of this coalition? What are some of the recent activities of the coalition?

11. How does a person become a member of a professional organization?

CRITICAL THINKING QUESTIONS

1. For a number of years, many practicing health educators have pushed for a single professional health education association that would bring together many of the existing associations (i.e., AAHE, ACHA, ASHA, SOPHE) so that health education would have a single professional association voice. Would you be in favor of or against combining all the health education professional associations into a single association? Defend your response. As part of your response, indicate what you think are the strengths and weaknesses of your position.

2. In this chapter you have read about a number of different professional health education associations. Upon graduating from college few new professionals have enough money to join several different professional groups. Assuming that you have enough money to join one professional group upon graduation, what association/organization would it be? Explain the reasoning you would use to select the one organization to join.

3. One of the major issues facing many professional health education associations is retaining members from year to year. Some members do not renew their membership because of cost. Others do not renew because they do not feel that they receive enough benefits. After conducting a membership survey, a professional health association has decided to revamp the benefits provided to members. Assume that you have been appointed as a student member to the executive committee of the professional association and that the president of the association has charged the committee with revamping the membership benefits package. Each member of the executive committee has been asked to create a list of benefits. What would be on your list? Explain why you selected each item.

ACTIVITIES

1. Closely examine one professional health association/organization and write a two-page paper on the history of that association/organization.

2. Interview two health education faculty members at your school and ask them the following:

   • Do they belong to any professional health education associations/organizations?

   • If they belong, why?

   • What benefits do they see in belonging to them?

   • What association/organization would they recommend that you join?

3. Does your school have a chapter of Eta Sigma Gamma? If not, make an appointment with the department head/chairperson to inquire about the possibility of starting one on your campus.

4. Write a one-page paper using the following two sentences to start the paper:

   "If I could join one professional health association/organization, it would be _____. My reasons for choosing that association/organization are _____."

5. Visit the Web site of the Coalition of National Health Education Organizations (CNHEO) (http://www.hsc.usf.edu/CFH/cnheo/index.html). Once at the site, read the three "21st Century" reports (note that the executive summaries provide a nice overview of these: (1) *The Health Education Profession in the Twenty-First Century: Setting the Stage*, (2) *The Health Education Profession in the Twenty-First Century Progress Report 1995–2001*, and (3) *Coalition of National Health Education Organization's 2nd Invitational Conference: Improving the Nation's Health Through Health Education—A Vision for the 21st Century*. After reading the reports, create your own list of five activities that you feel the profession should engage in during the next ten years to move the profession forward. Provide a brief (i.e., a couple of paragraphs) rationale for why you included each activity on your list.

WEBLINKS

1. **http://www.astho.org**

   The Association for State and Territorial Health Officers (ASTHO)

   This is the Web site for the ASTHO, which is the national nonprofit organization representing the state and territorial public health agencies of the United States, the U.S. Territories, and the District of Columbia. Among other items, this site includes links to each of the state and territorial health departments.

2. **http://www.astdhpphe.org**

   Directors of Health Promotion and Education (DHPE)

   This is the home page for DHPE. This association is comprised of the 55 directors of health education/promotion units of state health departments and U.S. possessions as well as the 11 directors of the health education units of Indian Health Service Area Offices. In addition, the DHPE also has approximately 300 associate and emeritus members. This site provides the latest news on topics appropriate to its membership and those interested in public health education/promotion.

3. **http://www.thesociety.org**

   Society of State Directors of Health, Physical Education, and Recreation (SSDHPER)

   This is the Web site for the SSDHPER. The Society is open to professionals in state departments of education who are leaders of programs in comprehensive school health and physical education, and categorically funded programs such as HIV/AIDS prevention, safe and drug-free schools and communities, and nutrition education. Professionals who have duties or interests in health, physical education, recreation, or related fields and others who support the mission of the Society may become associate members. This site provides information about school health, physical education, and recreation programs.

4. **http://www.cancer.org/**

   American Cancer Society (ACS)

   This is the home page for ACS. The site presents the most up-to-date information on cancer, including treatment and prevention. The site also provides information about the ACS and the resources it can provide for cancer survivors and program planners.

5. **http://www.hsc.usf.edu/CFH/cnheo/index.html**

   Coalition of National Health Education Organizations (CNHEO)

   This is the home page for CNHEO. At the site, you will find information about all the member organizations, as well as the Coalition's mission, goals, *Working Agreement*, the Code of Ethics for the Health Education Profession, and the three "21st Century" reports.

6. **http://www.americanheart.org**

   American Heart Association (AHA)

   This is the home page for the AHA. It provides health educators with a wealth of information and materials about many of the cardiovascular diseases and stroke.

7. **http://www.lungusa.org**

   American Lung Association (ALA)

   This is the home page for the ALA. It provides a variety of information about various lung diseases, including asthma, chronic obstructive pulmonary disease (COPD), and lung cancer.

8. **http://www.welcoa.org**

   The Wellness Councils of America (WELCOA)

   This is the home page for the WELCOA. This site provides a variety of resources for those interested in worksite wellness programs.

9. **http://www.cdc.gov/**

   Centers for Disease Control and Prevention (CDC)

   This is the home page of the CDC. It includes information for the lay public (i.e., traveler's health and emergency preparedness) as well as information to assist health educators (i.e., health topics A–Z, CDC recommendations, *MMWR,* and special funded initiatives).

10. **http://www.healtheducationadvocate.org/**

    Health Education Advocate

    This is the homepage of the Health Education Advocate that is sponsored by the Coalition of National Health Education Organizations. This site provides up-to-date advocacy information for health educators, as well as links to other advocacy sites.

    (Note: See Table 8.2 for the URLs of the various professional associations/organizations discussed in this chapter.)

CASE STUDY

Hilary has been employed by the XYZ voluntary health organization for almost a year now. The job has really gone well. She enjoys the work, likes her coworkers, and has been able to use much of what she learned during her health education professional preparation program. Just recently the organization received word that it had been awarded a $15,000 grant to conduct a health education program for a local senior citizens group on living a healthier life. Her supervisor, Ms. Denison, has given Hilary the responsibility to take the leadership for the project. One restriction on the use of the money is that the program must be planned by a representative group from local voluntary and governmental health education organizations. Therefore, Hilary's first task is to invite local groups to send a representative to the initial planning meeting. Hilary has set the goal of having seven different health voluntary and governmental agencies involved. If you were Hilary, which organizations would you invite to the initial meeting? Justify why you would select these seven.

REFERENCES

American Academy of Health Behavior (AAHB). (2004). *Mission statement and objectives.* Retrieved June 5, 2004, from http://www.aahb.org/
American Alliance for Health, Physical Education, Recreation and Dance (AAHPERD). (no date). *Give yourself a healthy promotion.* Reston, VA: Author.

American Alliance for Health, Physical Education, Recreation, and Dance (AAHPERD). (2004). *AAHE's focus on advocacy.* Retrieved June 5, 2004, from http://capwiz. com/aahe/home/

American Association for Health Education (AAHE). (2003). Directory of institutions offering undergraduate and graduate degree programs in health education. *American Journal of Health Education, 34* (1), 219–235.

American Association for Health Education (AAHE). (2004a). *Continuing education.* Retrieved June 5, 2004, from http://www.aahperd.org/aahe/template.cfm?template= development-continuing.html

American Association for Health Education (AAHE). (2004b). *General overview.* Retrieved June 5, 2004, from http://www.aahperd.org/aahe/template.cfm?template= aahe-about.html

American College Health Association (ACHA). (2004a). *Affiliates.* Retrieved June 5, 2004, from http://www.acha.org/about_acha/affiliates.cfm

American College Health Association (ACHA). (2004b). *Publications and periodicals.* Retrieved June 5, 2004, from http://www.acha.org/info_resources/journal_intro.cfm

American College Health Association (ACHA). (2004c). *Membership.* Retrieved June 5, 2004, from http://www.acha.org/about_acha/membership.cfm

American College Health Association (ACHA). (2004d). *Mission and goals.* Retrieved June 5, 2004, from http://www.acha.org/about_acha/mission.cfm

American Public Health Association (APHA). *About APHA.* (2004a). Retrieved June 5, 2004, from http://www.apha.org/about/.

American Public Health Association (APHA). (no date). *The American Public Health Association: Keeping public health in the public eye for more than a century.* Washington, DC: Author.

American Public Health Association (APHA). (2004b). *Sections SPIGS and Caucuses.* Retrieved June 5, 2004 from http://www.apha.org/sections/

American School Health Association (ASHA). (1976). *History of the American School Health Association, 1926–1976.* Kent, OH: Author.

American School Health Association (ASHA). (2004a). *About ASHA.* Retrieved June 5, 2004, from http://www.ashaweb.org/profile.html

American School Health Association (ASHA). (2004b). *Health in action.* Retrieved June 5, 2004, from http://www.ashaweb.org/healthinaction.html

American School Health Association (ASHA). (2004c). *Membership.* Retrieved June 5, 2004, from http://www.ashaweb.org/newmembers.html

Anderson, G. (1985). AAHPERD from the beginning. *Journal of Physical Education, Recreation and Dance, 56*(4), 94–96.

Association for the Advancement of Health Education (AAHE). (no date). *The Association for the Advancement of Health Education introduces ProNet.* Reston, VA: Author.

Capwell, E. M. (2004). Coalition of national health education organizations. *California Journal of Health Promotion, 2* (1), 12–15.

Coalition of National Health Education Organizations (CNHEO). (2004a). *Coalition of National Health Education Organizations.* Retrieved June 5, 2004, from http://www.hsc. usf.edu/CFH/cnheo/index.html

Coalition of National Health Education Organizations (CNHEO). (2004b). *Health Education Advocate.* Retrieved June 5, 2004, from http://www.healtheducationadvocate. org/

Coalition of National Health Education Organizations (CNHEO). (2004c). *School Health Education and Services Section.* Retrieved June 5, 2004, from http://www.hsc.usf.edu/ CFH/cnheo/apha-shes.htm

Directors of Health Promotion and Education (DHPE). (2004). *Overview.* Retrieved June 5, 2004, from http://www.astdhpphe.org/about.asp#Mission

Eta Sigma Gamma (ESG). (1991, November). *Eta Sigma Gamma.* Muncie, IN: Author.

Green, L. W., & Ottoson, J. M. (1999). *Community and population health* (8th ed.). Boston: WCB/McGraw-Hill.

Heymann, D. L. (Ed.). (2004). *Control of communicable diseases manual.* (18th ed.). Washington, DC: American Public Health Association.

International Union for Health Promotion and Education (IUHPE). (2004a). *About us.* Retrieved June 5, 2004, from http://www.iuhpe.org

International Union for Health Promotion and Education (IUHPE). (2004b). *Publications.* Retrieved June 5, 2004, from http://www.iuhpe.org

McKenzie, J. F., Pinger, R. R., & Kotecki, J. E. (2005). *An introduction to community health* (5th ed.). Sudbury, MA: Jones & Bartlett Publishers.

Miller, D. F., & Price, J. H. (1998). *Dimensions of community health* (5th ed.). Boston, MA: WCB/McGraw-Hill.

National Commission for Health Education Credentialing, Inc., & Coalition of National Health Education Organizations, USA (NCHEC & CNHEO), (1996). The health education profession in the 21st century: Setting the stage. *Journal of School Health, 66* (8), 291–298.

National Wellness Institute (NWI). (2004a). *History.* Retrieved June 5, 2004, from http://www.nationalwellness.org/index2.php

National Wellness Institute (NWI). (2004b). *Member benefits.* Retrieved June 5, 2004, from http://www.nationalwellness.org/nwi_home/NWI.asp?id=32&Year=2002&Tier=5

National Wellness Institute (NWI). (2004c). *Mission.* Retrieved June 5, 2004, from http://www.nationalwellness.org/index2.php?id=165&id_tier=1

Nelson, D. E., Brownson, R. C., Remington, P. L., & Parvanta, C. (Eds.). (2002). Communicating public health information effectively: A guide for practitioners. Washington, DC: American Public Health Association.

Nolte, A. E. (1985). Health education: An alliance commitment. *Journal of Physical Education, Recreation and Dance, 56* (4), 107–108.

Pritchard, D. R. (Ed.). (2001). *The American heritage dic•tion•ary,* (4th ed.). New York: A Dell Book.

The Public Health Education and Health Promotion Section (PHEHP). (2004). *The Public Health Education and Health Promotion Section of the American Public Health Association!* Retrieved June 5, 2004, from http://www.jhsph.edu/hao/phehp/mission.htm

Reagan, P. A., & Brookins-Fisher, J. (2002). *Community health in the 21st century* (2nd ed.). San Francisco: Benjamin Cummings.

Schwartz, R., & Goodman, R. M. (2000). Health promotion practice: Advancing the state of health promotion and education practice. *Health Promotion Practice, 1* (1), 5–9.

Society for Public Health Education (SOPHE). (2004a). *About SOPHE.* Retrieved June 5, 2004, from http://www.sophe.org/

Society for Public Health Education, Inc. (n.d.). *Health education professional organizations and you* (a handout). Washington, DC: Author.

Society for Public Health Education (SOPHE). (2004b). *Membership benefits at a glance.* Retrieved June 5, 2004, from http://www.sophe.org/

Society for Public Health Education (SOPHE). (2004c). *SOPHE publications and journals.* Retrieved June 5, 2004, from http://www.sophe.org/

Society of State Directors of Health, Physical Education, and Recreation (SSDHPER). (2004). *A statement of basic beliefs.* Retrieved June 5, 2004, from http://www.thesociety.org/beliefs.html

U.S. Department of Labor, Bureau of Labor Statistics (USDOL). (2001). *Health educators.* Retrieved June 7, 2004, from http://www.bls.gov/soc/soc_f1j1.htm

Werch, C. E. (2000). Editorial: What use, the American Academy of Health Behavior? *American Journal of Health Behavior, 24* (1), 3–5.

Young, K. J., & Boling, W. (2004). Improving the quality of professional life: Benefits of health education and promotion association membership. *California Journal of Health Promotion, 2* (1), 39–44.

CHAPTER 9

The Literature of Health Education

Chapter Objectives

After reading this chapter and answering the questions at the end, you should be able to:

1. Describe the difference between a *primary,* a *secondary,* a *tertiary,* and a *popular press* literature source.
2. Write an abstract or a summary of an article from a refereed journal.
3. Use appropriate questions to critique a journal article.
4. Name the most commonly used journals in the field of health education.
5. Locate an article related to some aspect of health education, using an index or an abstract.
6. Identify the most commonly used online computerized databases for finding health education information.
7. Conduct an Internet search for information about a health-related topic, using one of the World Wide Web sites listed in the chapter.
8. Critique the validity of the information obtained from searching a site on the Internet.

Key Terms

abstracts	hypertext transfer protocol	search engine
browser	indexes	secondary sources
computerized databases	Internet	tertiary sources
home page	popular press publications	Uniform Resource Locators
hypertext	primary sources	World Wide Web
hypertext markup language	refereed journal	

It is no secret that the amount of information about any given topic is growing at almost an exponential rate. Terms such as *information overload* and *information burnout* are being heard more and more. Arguably, the area in which

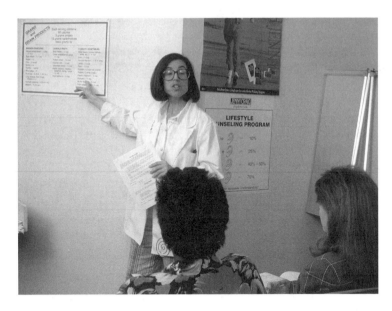

Health educators often make presentations to community groups. (Michael Newman/ PhotoEdit)

information is growing fastest and in which there is tremendous public interest is health. People today seem almost obsessed with the need to gather information about such health topics as diet, exercise, stress management, vitamins, drugs, sexuality, depression, safety, disease, violence prevention, health care policies, and health insurance options.

The fact that there is an increasing demand for information, coupled with the fact that information is being produced at an ever greater rate, creates added need for health educators. Two of the major responsibilities of a health educator as discussed in Chapter 6 involve being a resource person for health information (Responsibility 6) and communicating to others health education needs, concerns, and resources (Responsibility 7). In order to perform these tasks, the health educator must have the skills to find information, evaluate the source of the information to determine its credibility, disseminate the information to consumers through the appropriate channels, and explain the meaning of the information in an understandable manner. This chapter introduces prospective health education students to the most common sources of health-related information used by health educators. It also describes how to access the information from these sources.

Types of Information Sources

When accessing information, it is important to note whether the source is primary, secondary, or tertiary. **Primary sources** of data or information are published studies or eyewitness accounts written by the people who actually conducted the experiments or observed the events in question. A journal that publishes original manuscripts only after they have been read by a panel of experts in the field (referees) and recommended for publication is termed a **refereed journal.** Examples of primary sources are research articles written by the researcher(s), personal records (autobiographies), official records of legislative sessions or minutes of community meetings, newspaper eyewitness accounts, and annual reports.

Secondary sources, on the other hand, are usually written by someone who was not present at the event or did not participate as part of the study team. The value of these sources is that they often provide a summary of several related studies or chronicle a history or sequence of events. The writers of secondary sources may also provide editorial comments or alternative interpretations of the study or event. Secondary sources often provide a bibliography of primary sources. Examples of secondary sources are journal review articles, editorials, and noneyewitness accounts of events occurring in the community, region, or nation.

Although refereed journals most often have primary source articles published in them, they occasionally contain secondary source articles. The types of secondary source articles most likely to be found in a refereed journal are articles summarizing the results of several studies, editorials, or positions deemed important enough (by the panel of expert reviewers) to be of interest and utility to those who read the journal.

Tertiary sources contain information that has been distilled and collected from primary and secondary sources. Examples include handbooks, informational pamphlets/brochures from governmental organizations (or from organizations like hospitals or national nongovernmental agencies such as the American Cancer Society or March of Dimes), almanacs, encyclopedias, fact books, dictionaries, abstracts, and other reference tools. At this stage, information from such sources is accepted as fact by the scientific community. The operative word in the preceding sentence is "fact." Information that has no documentation and contains material laced with opinion or intended for marketing a service or product is not considered a tertiary source; publications of that type are classified as popular press sources. A fourth source of health information, and probably the most difficult to check for credibility, is the **popular press publications**. Popular press publications range from weekly summary-type magazines (e.g., *Time, Newsweek, U.S. News & World Report*) and newspaper supplements (e.g., *Parade*) to monthly magazines (e.g., *Reader's Digest, Better Homes and Gardens, Esquire*) and tabloids (e.g., *The Star*). At times, any of these may be a primary source of information (as in an interview). Most often, however, they are secondary sources at best. Often, articles in the popular press include opinions or editorials that contain the bias of the author or the editor of the publication. Popular press articles should be heavily scrutinized as to the source of the information before being cited as authentic and accurate.

Before concluding this discussion, it is important to note that no Web site references were included in the literature types described above. This is because Web sites are generally not refereed. Just about anyone can publish an article on the Web without an impartial reader or group of readers reviewing it beforehand. To be sure, Web pages are often wonderful sources of information, but they can just as often be replete with bad information. A discussion of methods to determine the accuracy of information on the Web is included later in this chapter. Sorting through the maze of health information can be a daunting task, even for the most skilled health educator. In order to equip the health educator for assuming the responsibilities of providing and disseminating information, several tasks need to be mastered. The next several sections of this chapter are designed to provide background for the student in:

(1) identifying the components of a research article; (2) critically reading a research article; (3) ascertaining the accuracy of the information in articles that are nonresearch based or are from secondary or popular press sources; (4) writing an abstract or a summary of a journal article; (5) identifying and locating primary and secondary sources most commonly used by health educators using indexes, abstracts, and computerized databases; and (6) retrieving health-related information on the Internet.

Identifying the Components of a Research Article

A research article usually begins with an abstract, which is a brief description of the study's results. The abstract describes the research questions that were tested, outlines the study design, and lists one or two major findings from the study. The abstract is meant to communicate essential information, so that readers will know whether the study has information related to the topic they are interested in. An example of an abstract (Seo & Torabi, 2004) follows:

> This study examined emotional and perceptional changes American people had experienced 10 to 12 months after the September 11 (9/11) terrorist attacks. A nationally representative sample of 807 U.S. adults ages 18 or older was interviewed using random-digit dialing that included unpublished numbers and new listings. The results indicated that 5 to 8 percent of the respondents had probable posttraumatic stress disorder symptoms such as angry outbursts, trouble falling asleep, difficulty concentrating, and experiencing nightmares even 10 to 12 months after the attacks. Twenty-two percent reported more frequently life-threatening perceptions and 50 percent more concerns about personal safety than before the 9/11 attacks. Chi-square and logistic regression analyses indicated that gender, age, race/ethnicity, geographic region, and employment status were significant predictors for experiencing differential emotional and perceptional changes (p. 37).

The introduction section follows the abstract. Its purpose is usually threefold: (1) to give readers a more detailed description of the research question(s) or hypotheses being tested; (2) to review related literature; and (3) to explain the need for or the significance of the study. This section communicates the rationale behind the researchers' decision to conduct the study.

The methodology section comes directly after the introductory material. In this section, there is usually a description of (1) the research design used, (2) the subjects who took part in the research, (3) the instruments used to gather the information necessary to answer the research questions, and (4) any administrative procedures involved in conducting the research, such as methods used to select the subject, gather the data, or protect the rights of the subjects.

Following the methodology section are the results and discussion sections. The results section gives the research findings by describing the results of the statistical procedures used in analyzing the data (in the case of studies involving quantitative methods—methods involving the analyses of numerical data) and provides an overall answer to the research questions or hypotheses that were described in the introductory section. The discussion section provides a forum for the researcher to interpret the conclusions and meanings and to comment on the implications of the data analyses. In addition, the researcher often includes a narrative about the limitations of the study and makes recommendations for further research on the topic.

Critically Reading a Research Article

The volume of articles on any one health topic continues to escalate. It is important to be able to evaluate the information found in any source for accuracy and saliency. Beginning students in the field of health education are not expected to be able to immediately understand every nuance in a research article. It is essential, however, to begin to frequently read scientific reports and journal articles to become familiar with their style. Often, preformulating generic questions suitable for critiquing any study can help when evaluating study results. Following is a list of hints that have been found to be of help when such an evaluation is necessary. The list is adapted from information found in *Studying a Study and Testing a Test: How to Read Medical Evidence* (Riegelman, 2000).

1. Were the aims of the study defined in a clear manner?
2. Were the research questions/hypotheses clearly stated?
3. Was the description of the subjects clear? Did the article state how the subjects were recruited?
4. Were the design and location of the study described clearly?
5. Were the data collection instruments described?
6. Did the results directly address the research questions/hypotheses?
7. Were the conclusions logical in terms of the research design and data analyses performed?
8. Were the study implications meaningful to the population you serve?

The final test comes when students can read an article and begin to view themselves in the position of a reporter who has the task of describing the study, its findings, and its limitations to an audience in no more than five minutes. People who can restate study findings and limitations in their own words have accomplished much in becoming critical consumers of scientific and nonscientific literature, as well as better resources for others.

Evaluating the Accuracy of Nonresearch-Based Sources

As with journal articles that are research based, it is important to be able to evaluate whether or not the information presented is reliable, regardless of the source. Cottrell (1997) conducted a search for instruments that could assist him in teaching his students to assess the accuracy of information found in almost any type of journal or magazine. A compilation of the questions that emanated from the results of his search include the following:

1. What are the author's qualifications? Does the person have an academic degree in the field being written about? A note of caution—a degree does not make someone absolutely qualified, but it provides evidence to suggest that the person is qualified.
2. What is the style of presentation? Look for health information written in a scientific style of writing, not a style that uses generalities or testimonials.

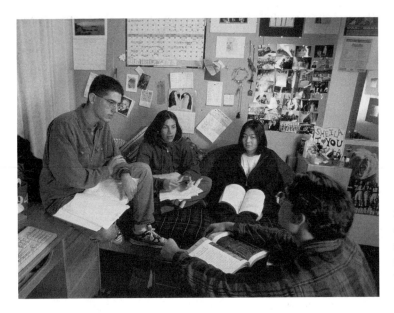

Summarizing research articles in small group settings sharpens the ability to correctly interpret research findings. (Mark Richards/ PhotoEdit)

3. Are references included? A well-written article provides references to the primary sources used. Be aware when someone is writing about another person's research, as that individual may be interpreting the results in a different way than the author did.

4. What is the purpose of the publication? Be aware of news publications and publications that contain advertisements designed to sell items being discussed in the articles.

5. What is the reputation of the publication? Is it refereed? Professional journals are good sources of information. Popular press publications can sometimes have poor information related to health issues.

6. Is the information new? When reading for the first time, be skeptical. Information must be validated over time. New information is newsworthy but may not be valid.

It is important to realize that acquiring the skill of becoming a skeptical, critical consumer of printed health information is an important first step in being seen by others as credible. In order for the public to use the expertise and training of health educators to a greater degree, the health educators must develop a reputation for providing accurate and current information.

Writing an Abstract or a Summary

Another valuable skill when reading and interpreting health-related literature of any kind (primary, secondary, tertiary, or popular press) involves learning to write an abstract or a summary of an article. Although abstracts and summaries are both short forms of describing a research study, the major differences lie in the extent of the content. Abstracts are short (usually 150–250 words). They are written to identify the purpose of the research, the study questions, the methods used by the researcher, and one or two major findings. Summaries, on the other hand, may be two to three pages in length and include all of the elements of the abstract. In addition, summaries are meant to reveal any secondary findings, to describe study limitations, and to provide for a more detailed review of the researcher's conclusions and recommendations from the viewpoint of the summary's author.

It is recommended that beginning health educators practice writing both abstracts and summaries of the articles they read. Using this technique sharpens the ability of the health educator to discriminate between health-related articles that are of substance and meaning for health promotion and those that contain erroneous or misleading claims or information.

Locating Health-Related Information

Health educators serve as major health information resource persons for many constituencies. It does not matter if they are employed in the school, the clinic, the worksite, or the community setting. In all cases, inquiries from a variety of people wanting to know about a health topic or wanting interpretation of the latest research findings are directed to health educators. Therefore, it is essential that the latter be knowledgeable about how to find the information requested. The next section identifies resources that health educators can use to locate information on health education and health promotion, and explains how the information can be accessed.

Journals

As has been previously mentioned, much of the information that health educators use to make decisions when planning, implementing, and evaluating health promotion programs can be found in journals that publish primary research articles and position papers about health topics and health programs. Featured below are examples of journals commonly used by health professionals. The list is by no means inclusive of all journals of benefit to the health educator. For a more exhaustive listing of journals that publish articles relating to the health education competencies (as discussed in Chapter 6), consult the article by Donohue et al. (2002) referenced at the end of this chapter.

1. *AIDS Education and Prevention.* An international journal designed to support the efforts of professionals working to prevent HIV and AIDS, *AIDS Education and Prevention* includes scientific articles by leading authorities from many disciplines, research reports on the effectiveness of new strategies and programs, debates about key issues, and reviews of book and video resources. In addition to discussing models of AIDS education and prevention, the journal covers a wide range of public health, psychosocial, ethical, and public policy concerns related to HIV and AIDS.

2. *American Journal of Health Behavior* (formerly *Health Values*). Articles accepted for publication feature research about the impact of personal behavior patterns, practices, and characteristics on health promotion. Examples of successful multidisciplinary approaches to improving health at the community level are also included.

3. *American Journal of Health Education.* This journal is published by the American Association for Health Education. Most articles have broad application to the field of health education. Readers might find articles concerning opinions, original research on health issues and policies related to schools, communities, or worksites, and methods and strategies for health instructional programs.

4. *American Journal of Health Promotion.* Original research articles, the testing of health behavioral theory on selected populations, and program evaluation are prominent. It is an excellent source of articles related to worksite health promotion.

5. *American Journal of Health Studies* (**formerly** *Wellness Perspectives*). Articles target health promotion and wellness in the broadest sense. Readers will find selections on social and environmental support for health, health program planning strategies and evaluation methods, testing of health behavioral theory, and opinions on the implications of health policy.

6. *American Journal of Public Health.* Published by the American Public Health Association, this journal features reports related to health research, program evaluations, and health policy analysis, as well as articles on special topics on the health of selected groups and communities.

7. *Evaluation and the Health Professions.* Articles generally focus on research related to the development, implementation, and evaluation of community-based health programs. Philosophical and innovative aspects of evaluation are also covered.

8. *Family and Community Health.* Articles contain information and research on nutrition, exercise, health-risk appraisals, and the physical and emotional development of a variety of age groups. The overall goal of this journal is to publish articles that foster the role of self-care in health promotion.

9. *The Health Educator: The Journal of Eta Sigma Gamma.* Published by Eta Sigma Gamma, the health education honor society, users will find articles related to most health education or health promotion topics in a variety of settings. Many of the studies and commentaries are submitted by undergraduate and graduate students in health education/public health programs.

10. *The Hastings Center Report.* This journal focuses on the ethical, social, legal, moral, economic, and religious tenets of health policy and health decisions.

11. *Health Education & Behavior* (**formerly** *Health Education Quarterly*). The official publication of the Society for Public Health Education, Inc. (SOPHE), its articles center on health behavior and education, case studies in health, and program evaluation. Each submission includes a commentary on the application of findings to the practice setting.

12. *Health Education Research* (**formerly** *Health Education Research: Theory and Practice*). It features articles concerning health promotion program planning, implementation, and evaluation. An effort is made to publish articles that may assist those in the field to apply the results of the studies.

13. *Health Promotion International.* The majority of research studies and commentaries are on issues related to health promotion in schools, clinics, worksites, and communities located outside of the United States.

14. *Health Promotion Practice.* This journal publishes articles devoted to the practical application of health promotion and education in a variety of settings, including community, health care, educational, worksite, and international. Articles featuring the best practices and their application to health policies that promote health and prevent disease are also a focal point.

15. *The International Electronic Journal of Health Education.* This journal published its first edition in January 1998. It features articles on nearly every aspect of health education, including school health, community health, worksite health promotion, the ethical implications of health education, and the philosophy of health education.

16. *The Journal of American College Health.* Published by the American College Health Association, its articles are limited to those that relate to health promotion or health service provision in the college or university environment.

17. *Journal of Community Health.* This is an all-inclusive journal, with articles relating to all aspects of community health, preventive medicine, and socioeconomic, biocultural, and ethical issues in public health.

18. *Journal of Health Communication.* This peer-reviewed journal is published bimonthly. It presents the latest development in the field of health communication, including research in risk communication, health literacy, social marketing, communication (from interpersonal to mass media), psychology, government, policy making, and health education around the world.

19. *Journal of Nutrition Education.* A journal devoted to original research on factors influencing food behavior and how these factors can be modified to promote sustainable dietary change, it contains articles on nutrition education and best practices and policies.

20. *Journal of Rural Health.* Published by the Rural Health Association, this journal's articles focus on professional practice, research, theory development, and policy issues related to health in the rural setting.

21. *Journal of School Health.* Published by the American School Health Association, all material is related to the public or private school setting at the preschool through twelfth-grade levels. Articles generally focus on children's health issues but may include information related to other aspects of coordinated school health programs, such as employee wellness.

22. *Promotion and Education.* This journal is affiliated with the World Health Organization and the International Union for Health Promotion and Education. Most issues are topical in nature (e.g., environmental health, population health, infectious disease prevention) and feature articles related to the application of public health and health promotion in countries around the globe. Articles are published in several languages.

23. ***Public Health Reports.*** The official publication of the Public Health Service, this journal reports findings from many avenues of research related to health services acquisition, health policy development, and health promotion at the community level.

Indexes

Indexes are books that provide a link to articles from many refereed journals, books, and research reports. Each index references articles from journals, books, and reports pertaining to topics that fall under the subject headings for which the index was created. For example, *Index Medicus* lists articles relating to clinical and preventive medicine and does not include references to articles in the social sciences.

The procedures for locating references in an index and the list of journals that are included in the index are found in the front pages of each volume. Many of the indexes are now also found on CD-ROM (or in an online format in academic libraries), but the method of locating an article or a topic is the same. Generally, there are many similarities in how references can be located from one index to the next. Users begin by looking up the topic of interest in the index (e.g., health behavior). Using a volume of the 2004 *Index Medicus* as an example, two samples of citations from the topic "health behaviors" are listed:

> Assessment of selected patient education materials of various chain pharmacies. Kirksey, et al. *J Health Commun* 2004 9(2): 91–93.

> Physical activity, dietary practices, and other health behaviors of at-risk youth attending alternative high schools. Kubik, M.Y., et al. *J Sch Health* 2004 Apr; 74(4): 119–24.

When reading the citation, the parts are as follows: the title of the article in the journal, the authors' names, the abbreviated title of the journal, the year and month of publication, the volume number, and the page numbers.

Health educators then need to go to the journal listed and find the article of interest. Indexes most used by health educators are:

1. ***Index Medicus.*** This index includes references to more than three thousand biomedical journals. It is updated monthly and cumulated annually.

2. ***Cumulative Index to Nursing and Allied Health Literature (CINAHL).*** Included are references to more than three hundred nursing, allied health, and health-related journals. It is updated bimonthly and cumulated annually.

3. ***Education Index.*** This index references more than four hundred journals on topics related to education. The index is updated monthly and cumulated annually.

4. ***Physical Education Index.*** This index includes references to more than four hundred periodicals on physical education, health education, dance, physical therapy, and sports medicine. It is published six times a year and cumulated annually.

5. ***Current Index to Journals in Education (CIJE).*** *CIJE* includes references to more than 775 journals related to education. The index citations correspond to Educational Resources Information Center (ERIC) reference numbers. (See the "Computerized Databases" section later in this chapter for more information.) It is updated monthly and cumulated annually.

Abstracts

Abstracts are book volumes that include short summaries of research studies that have appeared in other journals. An abstract is usually more valuable than an index in that it provides both a reference and a summary for each article included, whereas an index provides only the title of the article. An abstract allows the user to decide whether or not the article has information worth pursuing further.

To use an abstract, locate the index at the end of each volume. The index is organized so you can search by subject or author. Find the subject or author you are interested in, and look at the titles of the articles listed under that subject/author heading. At the end of each article reference there is a number. Go to the volume of the abstract that includes that number (the numbers included in each volume are listed on the outside binding of the volume), turn to the number of the article you are interested in (the numbers are listed consecutively), and locate the desired article abstract. A sample abstract (number 10963) from *Psychological Abstracts* (2004) under the subject area "health behavior" follows:

> 2003-10963-006. O'Connell, Meghan L. et al. (Yale-Griffin Prevention Research Center, New Haven, CT). Smoking cessation for high school students: impact evaluation of a novel program. *Behavior Modification,* Jan 2004, Vol 28(1), 133–146. This pilot study was designed to evaluate the feasibility and the impact of a smoking-cessation program that would meet the specific needs of high school students. Feedback from focus groups conducted with adolescent smokers at a Connecticut high school was used to develop a tailored intervention. Intervention components included commonly used behavioral strategies, with additional options to assist students to quit smoking, including use of bupropion, concomitant support for parent smoking cessation, stress management, and physician counseling. On completion, 20 of the 22 enrolled students remained committed to quitting. Twenty-seven percent of students quit smoking and 69% of those who continued to smoke reduced the number of cigarettes smoked per day by an average of 13. Providing additional options to students and additional support for concomitant parental cessation may enhance the appeal of adolescent smoking-cessation programs. Further investigation into efficacy of bupropion use for adolescent cessation is warranted.

The abstracts most commonly used by health educators are:

1. *Psychological Abstracts.* This abstract includes abstracts of journal articles and books in psychology and other social and behavioral sciences.

2. *Sociological Abstracts.* It includes a collection of abstracts of the literature in sociology and related disciplines. It is published six times a year and cumulated annually.

3. *Biological Abstracts.* Indexed by author, subject, biosystem, and generic heading, this resource includes articles from more than five hundred biology-related publications. It is published bimonthly and cumulated annually.

4. *Resources in Education.* It includes abstracts on hundreds of studies and papers related to education and provides information on how a copy of an article or a speech can be obtained (e.g., request from the publisher, microfilm).

Government Documents

The U.S. Government Printing Office (GPO) publishes volumes of materials of use to health educators/health promotion specialists. This section (adapted from the University of Akron library Web site) is meant to provide a generic description of the types of documents that can be accessed in the government documents section of an academic library. Because each library has slightly different procedures for finding these documents, students are encouraged to communicate with the government documents librarian at their university for the specifics on locating documents.

Government publications range from official documents including laws, court decisions, and records of congressional actions to the results of government-sponsored technical and scientific studies. Information on topics such as obesity, water treatment, or exercise can also be found in a government documents section.

Government documents are not organized under the same classification scheme as a traditional general collection. Instead, they are organized and shelved according to SuDocs (Superintendent of Documents) numbers. The SuDocs number is unique in that it has a colon. For example, A1:1 is an annual report from the Agriculture Department. Numbers of the documents are arranged alphabetically by agency, and the numbers are whole numbers, not decimals (e.g., HE 1.6: comes before HE 1.9:). The letter that begins the SuDocs number signifies the publishing agency, as noted below:

A   Agriculture Department

C   Census Bureau

D   Department of Defense

E   Department of Energy

HE   Health and Human Services

X-Y   Congress

Government documents contain a storehouse of valuable and current information and should not be overlooked when seeking information on a health topic of interest. Most libraries have online search capabilities for government documents, so—as with many "traditional sources of information"—accessing them has become much less labor intensive.

Computerized Databases

Computerized databases often provide a preferred alternative to manually searching indexes or abstracts in that they store large compilations of reference information on a computer CD-ROM or server. Most, if not all, of the publishers of the hard-copy abstracts and indexes discussed earlier either have converted or are converting their documents to this form of storage. Much like an index or abstract, each database has a general subject area (e.g., medicine, education, psychology, community health). The computerized or electronic database provides access to the cumulative information found in several books of index or abstract sources. Computer searches using databases are generally faster than manual searches, and they have the advantage of enabling the user to link several concepts together to provide focus for a search.

For example, if a person wanted to search for articles about "health behavior" and the influence of "health communication" on behavior, a computerized database would allow the user to enter both terms into the computer and connect them by placing the word "and" between them. The result will be to eliminate articles not containing both "health behavior" and "health communication" as key terms. Other terms can also be inserted to make the search as specific as desired. The main concern the computer database user faces is to accurately specify the key terms associated with the information desired so the resulting list of references will be of use. Computerized searches require very little computer background; however, it is advisable to seek the assistance of a reference librarian when starting. The databases most used by health educators are:

1. *Educational Resources Information Center (ERIC).* It includes the previously mentioned *Current Index to Journals in Education (CIJE)* and *Resources in Education (RIE)*. ERIC is an information clearinghouse that collects, sorts, classifies, and stores thousands of documents on topics pertaining to education and allied fields of study. An advantage to using ERIC is that many types of documents are contained in the database that are not journal articles—for example, proceedings of meetings, teaching strategies, lesson plans, commentaries, and policy documents.

2. *MEDLINE.* This is the premier biomedicine database indexing more than 3,000 journals. It covers the fields of medicine, nursing, dentistry, veterinary medicine, and preclinical sciences.

3. *Cumulative Index to Nursing and Allied Health Literature (CINAHL).* It contains more than 300,000 citations from 1983 until the present. It references journal articles and book chapters, pamphlets, audiovisuals, educational software, and conference proceedings in the areas of nursing, health education, health services, and health care administration.

4. *BIOETHICSLINE.* This database covers ethical, legal, and public policy issues surrounding health care and biomedical research. Citations are derived from the literature of law, religion, ethics, social sciences, philosophy, the popular media, and the health sciences.

5. *Psychological Abstracts (PsycInfo).* This database is the analog of *Psychological Abstracts* in computerized form. As with all computer databases, narrowing a search to a specific topic can be accomplished more easily using *PsycInfo*.

6. *Ovid Healthstar.* Ovid Healthstar is comprised of data from the National Library of Medicine's (NLM) MEDLINE and former HealthSTAR databases. As such, it contains citations of the published literature in health services, technology, administration, health policy, health economics, and research. It focuses on both the clinical and nonclinical aspects of health care delivery.

The Internet and the World Wide Web

Until a few years ago, it was only possible to dream about the day when health information would be readily available at home or at the office at the "touch of a button." Today, of course, that dream is a reality through the use of the Internet and

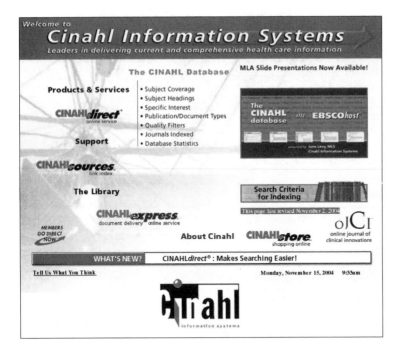

Computerized databases provide ready access to information on a particular topic.

the World Wide Web. The **World Wide Web** is an interactive information delivery service that includes a repository of resources about almost any subject imaginable. In "the Web," documents that are related by subject area or place of origin are linked to each other, thus creating a web, or network, of materials. The Web relies mainly on **hypertext** as its means of interaction with users. Hypertext is nearly the same as regular text in that it can be searched, edited, and stored, but hypertext contains connections within the text to documents (in the form of printed matter, pictures, graphics, and/or sound) found on computers connected to each other around the globe. This integrated network of computers is known as the **Internet**.

In order to use the Web, a person must have access to a **browser**. The browser is a software package that can be installed on any computer with a graphical interface and can greatly simplify the ability to access information on the Web. Examples of commonly available browsers include Netscape and Internet Explorer. Use of the browser involves entering a Web address, which usually starts with the characters "http://" (http stands for **hypertext transfer protocol**). Web addresses are known as URLs, or **Uniform Resource Locators**, which are unique identifiers for a location on the global Internet much as the mailing address of your home is unique to where you live. The URL is composed of the Internet access protocol, the location, and the file—for example, http://www.cdc.gov/mmwr/ is the URL for the **home page** of the CDC publication Morbidity and Mortality Weekly Report (MMWR). A home page is analogous to a combination of a cover and a table of contents in a book, in that it names the site and directs the user to a list of information options available within the site. In the example, the "http://" is the Internet access protocol; the "www.cdc.gov" is the location; and "mmwr/" is the file.

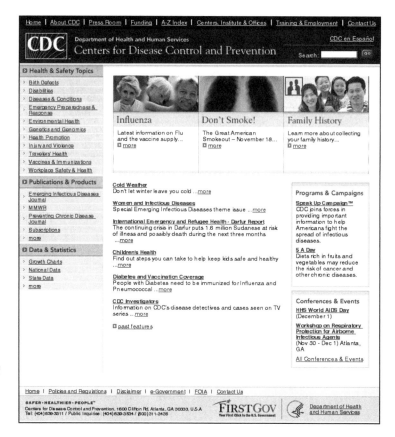

Figure 9.1   Home page of the Centers for Disease Control and Prevention as found on the Internet.

Assume you are looking for times, dates, and locations of some training sessions on certain aspects of health promotion that will be conducted by the Centers for Disease Control and Prevention (CDC). In order to find the information at the CDC Web site, you might open the Internet Explorer (or Netscape) browser by double-clicking on its icon on the desktop of your computer. Once the browser opens, you can get to the desired Web page in one of the following two ways:

- You can place the cursor on the column labeled "File" at the top left-hand side of the screen. Click and hold down the mouse to reveal the menu that cascades down below "File." Move the cursor to "Open" and release. A dialogue box will appear on the screen that asks you to type in the address (URL) of the location you are seeking.

- You may also type the desired Web address (URL) into the horizontal space marked "Address" that is located on the left side of your screen just below the term "File."

In either case, type in http://www.cdc.gov (the URL of the Centers for Disease Control and Prevention) and the home page of the CDC will appear (as shown in Figure 9.1).

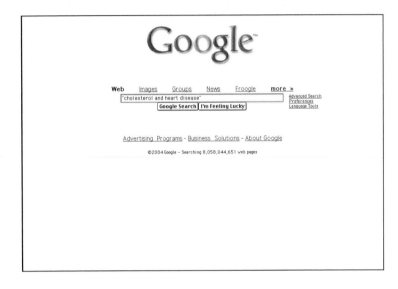

Figure 9.2   Google search engine page with "cholesterol and heart disease" entered in the "search" box.

On the home page will be some buttons to click to direct you to find the information you are looking for. In addition, any blue wording on an organization's home page can be double-clicked with the mouse, and information that relates to the word or phrase that is clicked will be provided. The blue wording denotes a topic or name that has been linked to another site to help the user access additional information about that topic.

Another method for locating information on the Internet involves using a **search engine**. Various search engines are available (e.g., Google, Yahoo, AltaVista, Excite, Infoseek, Webcrawler, Lycos, PubMed, Hotbot). The advantage of using a search engine over typing in a URL (which is specific to one site) is that the search engine allows you to type in the name of the topic you want to find information about, and after a few seconds identifies and lists several sites related to that topic. All the user needs to do to access the information from any of the sites listed is to click the pointer on the name of the site and it will appear. The search engines are usually located on the main search page of the browser or may be accessed by typing in their URL.

An example of the page for the Google search engine can be found in Figure 9.2. Note that in this example the topic being searched for is "cholesterol and heart disease." After entering that phrase in the search box and clicking on "search" or pressing "enter" on the keyboard, a list of sites related to "cholesterol and heart disease" will appear (see Figure 9.3). Click on any one of the sites and you will be transported to the page and information corresponding to that site.

Sometimes you may want to use a specific search engine. Because all of the search engines have nearly the same URL, the home page for any of the search engines can be readily accessed by typing in the specific Web address (URL) from the Internet Explorer "File" menu, as was demonstrated in the example using the Centers for Disease Control. For example, the URL for the Google search engine

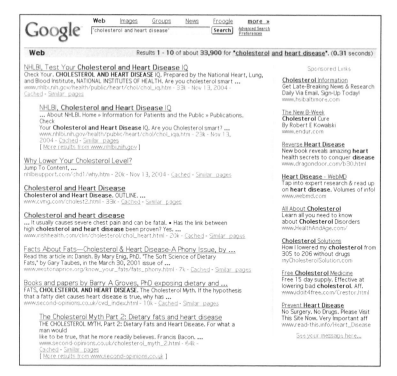

Figure 9.3 Google page with site matches to the search query for the term "cholesterol and heart disease."

is http://www. google.com; for Yahoo, it is http://www.yahoo.com; for Lycos, it is http://www. lycos.com; for AltaVista, it is http://www.altavista.com.

If the term you are searching for has more than one word (such as "sexually transmitted diseases"), it is wise to use quotation marks around the term when it is entered into the box marked "search." This will let the search engine know that the exact phrase, as contained in the quotation marks, is to be used when seeking sites that match. If the quotation marks are not used, the search engine will find sites that contain all of the words in the query. However, at least some of the sites might not be relevant to the topic of interest (sexually transmitted diseases in this case), as the words can appear in any order and any place on the sites searched.

Evaluating Information on the Internet

Earlier in the chapter, directions were given for evaluating the accuracy and validity of information from journal and popular press sources. Because of the massive amount of information available on the Internet and because nearly anyone who has a knowledge of "html" (**hypertext markup language**, the programming language used on the Internet) can publish on the World Wide Web, it is equally imperative that the health educator know how to evaluate information obtained via an Internet search. Kotecki and Chamness (1999) published an excellent article in the *Journal of Health Education* that featured a tool for evaluating a health-related Internet site. The information included in their article corresponds closely with that provided by Strong (2004), a reference specialist in the Albertson Library, at Boise State University. Both of these expert sources mention that the most important areas to consider when evaluating information retrieved on the Internet are:

1. **Content.** Material included has been verified or has survived a minimal screening or refereeing process. Sources are cited. Frequently, the addresses end in ".edu," ".gov," or ".org" if from a known professional organization.

2. **Authority.** The credentials of the authors are clearly presented. The authors' e-mail addresses and/or phone numbers are provided for contact.

3. **Publisher source.** This information should be unambiguous and clearly identifiable. It should be readily apparent who is sponsoring or otherwise representing the page.

4. **References.** Have other pages used this site as a link to their own page?

5. **Documentation.** Documentation is consistently provided. The sources are important, because a source that lacks documentation often falls in the opinion or editorial category.

6. **Facts.** Are the facts consistent with information obtained from other sources? Be cautious of sites that have an address ending in ".com," as they are commercial sites and may be selling a product.

SUMMARY

This chapter has presented an overview on accessing and evaluating health-related information. The fact that there is an increasing demand for health information, coupled with the fact that the information is being produced at an ever greater rate, creates added responsibility for health educators. Two of the major roles of health educators as discussed in Chapter 6 involve being resource people for health information and communicating to others health education needs, concerns, and resources. In order to perform these tasks, the health educator must have the skills to find information, must evaluate the source of the information to determine its credibility, and must disseminate the information through the appropriate channels to consumers. In addition, the health educator must be able to explain the information effectively. Becoming familiar with the tools found in this chapter is a necessity for all students wanting to enter the field of health education.

REVIEW QUESTIONS

1. Describe the difference between a primary, a secondary, a tertiary, and a popular press source.

2. How do an article abstract and an article summary differ in content?

3. What are the questions you should ask yourself when critiquing a journal article? What are the differences between the questions asked when evaluating a primary research article and those asked when evaluating a secondary source or popular press article?

4. What are five of the most commonly used journals in the field of health education? What types of information would you expect to find in each of the journals you named?

5. What is the difference between using an abstract and using an index to find health-related information?

6. What is the Internet and how does it enable one to access so much information?

7. How does one go about evaluating information retrieved from the Internet?

8. In your own words, describe how to access information concerning "breast cancer" on the World Wide Web.

CRITICAL THINKING QUESTIONS

1. Assume that all information about any topic is available on the Web. If that were true, would there be any need for health educators? Defend your answer.

2. Make a list of the five greatest advantages and the five greatest disadvantages of the Internet from your perspective. If your lists reflected universal truths about the Internet, how might you persuade a noncomputer user to adopt computer use?

3. How does the availability of so much material online affect the use of a library?

4. Several health agencies have begun conducting workshops online designed to help practicing health professionals update their skills. Is there a type of health professional this training would best suit? Provide rationale for your answer.

5. If the Internet had been developed in the early 1900s, how might the U.S. health care system and the role of health educators differ from what they are today?

ACTIVITIES

1. You are employed as a health educator in a district health department and have just received a call from a member of a local coalition wanting to know where to find an article that summarizes the content and effectiveness of available school-based sexuality education curricula. Use an index and find a reference to an article that meets those criteria.

2. Was the article you located in activity #1 a primary or secondary source of information? Provide rationale for your answer.

3. Using a database (CINAHL, MEDLINE, or ERIC), find a primary research article relating to traffic safety (e.g., the use of seat belts, air bags, road surfaces). Critique the article by applying the questions found in the Critically Reading a Research Article section of this chapter.

4. As a newly employed health educator in a hospital outpatient clinic, one of your jobs is to provide information to patients after they have seen the physician. Ms. X has just been diagnosed with coronary artery disease, and the physician has sent her to you to discuss the role of lifestyle on her condition. Using the World Wide Web, find several sources of information that you could give her to read that might assist you with the education process. Evaluate the accuracy of the information you retrieve.

5. Make a list of the health education journals described in this chapter that are available at your college/university library. For those journals not in your library's holdings, check with a librarian to determine if they are available through interlibrary loan or another exchange service.

WEBLINKS

Epidemiological and Statistical Information

1. **http://wonder.cdc.gov**

   CDC Wonder

   This site offers wide-ranging online data for epidemiologic research in an easy-to-use, menu-driven system that makes the information resources of the Centers for Disease Control and Prevention (CDC) available to public health professionals and the public at large. It provides access to a wide array of public health information.

2. **http://www.cdc.gov/nchs/**

   National Center for Health Statistics

   NCHS is the nation's principal health statistics agency. Its Web site offers access to an extensive collection of health statistics intended to guide those working to improve public health.

3. **http://www.cdc.gov/mmwr/**

   Morbidity and Mortality Weekly Report (MMWR)

   MMWR is a weekly report prepared by the Centers for Disease Control and Prevention. State health departments report their findings to MMWR. The site offers access to studies and reports, and also provides useful information on a wide range of diseases.

4. **http://www.cdc.gov/ncidod/**

   U.S. Statistical Data from the U.S. Bureau of the Census

   The Web site of the U.S. Census Bureau allows the user to access specific data for his or her state, county, or city. View results from Census 2000 and access analytical reports on population change, race, age, family structure, and more.

Infectious Diseases

5. **http://www.cdc.gov/ncidod/**

   National Center for Infectious Disease Statistics

   With the mission of preventing illness, disability, and death caused by infectious diseases, the NCID conducts epidemic investigations, laboratory research, and public education programs to attempt to prevent and control infectious diseases.

Chronic Diseases

6. **http://www.cdc.gov/genomics/activities/chronic.htm**

   CDC Genomics and Disease Prevention—Chronic Diseases

   This section of the CDC is dedicated to chronic diseases and provides links to a variety of helpful sites, including a diabetes public health resource and sites discussing heart disease, nutrition, and physical activity.

7. **http://www.nci.nih.gov**

   National Cancer Institute

   The National Cancer Institute's Web site covers information on a variety of cancer topics, discussing treatment, prevention, research, and much more. The NCI supports prevention and treatment of cancer, rehabilitation, and continued care of cancer patients and their families.

8. **http://www.diabetes.org**

   American Diabetes Association

   The ADA provides diabetes research, scientific findings, information, and advocacy. The site contains helpful information for people with diabetes, their families, health professionals, and the public.

Disease Control and Prevention

9. **http://www.phppo.cdc.gov/CDCRecommends/AdvSearchV.asp**

   CDC Recommends: The Prevention Guidelines System

   CDC Recommends is a searchable storehouse of documents containing recommendations approved by the CDC for the prevention and control of disease, injuries, and disabilities.

10. **http://www.health.org**

    The National Clearinghouse for Alcohol and Drug Information (NCADI)

    NCADI is a clearinghouse for alcohol and drug and information. The clearinghouse provides free educational material to help combat the misuse and abuse of alcohol, tobacco, and other drugs.

11. **http://www.samhsa.gov/centers/csap/csap.html**

    Center for Substance Abuse Prevention (CSAP)

    CSAP is funded by the Substance Abuse and Mental Health Services Administration (SAMHSA) and is responsible for improving the access to and quality of substance abuse prevention services to the public. CSAP provides national leadership in the development of policies, programs, and services to prevent the onset of illegal drug use and underage alcohol and tobacco use, and to reduce the negative consequences of using substances.

12. **http://www.whitehousedrugpolicy.gov**

    Office of National Drug Control Policy (ONDCP)

    With the goal of reducing illicit drug use, substance abuse-related crimes, drug trafficking, and drug-related health problems, the ONDCP is working to establish a national strategy to fight these dilemmas. The site contains national priorities, annual reports, and a tremendous amount of drug information.

13. **http://www.cdc.gov/hiv/dhap.htm**

    CDC's Division of HIV/AIDS Prevention

    With a mission to prevent HIV infection and reduce the incidence of HIV-related illness, the CDC's Division of HIV/AIDS Prevention Web site provides useful information for those working in the health field. The site includes such topics as prevention tools, research, brochures, and fact sheets.

14. **http://www.medmatrix.org**

    Medical Matrix

    Medical Matrix is a peer-reviewed site that offers continually updated clinical medicine resources. The information is organized in such a way as to make searching for information more timely and efficient. Over 6,000 medical Web sites are listed.

15. **http://www.childrenssafetynetwork.org**

    Children's Safety Network

    The Children's Safety Network, funded by the Maternal & Child Health Bureau and the U.S. Department of Health and Human Services, provides technical assistance, training, and resources to MCH and other injury prevention professionals in an extensive effort to reduce the burden of injury and violence to our nation's children.

16. **http://vm.cfsan.fda.gov/list.html**

    FDA Center for Food Safety and Applied Nutrition

    The site not only outlines national programs intended to increase food safety awareness, but it also contains information concerning the laws enforced by the FDA and provides helpful tips on preventing food-related illness.

17. **http://oncolink.com**

    OncoLink

    OncoLink, provided by the Abramson Cancer Center of the University of Pennsylvania, is the Web's first cancer resource. The site provides up-to-date cancer news and research. Locate information on the causes of cancer, screening and prevention, clinical trials, and other resources of cancer information.

18. **http://www.cdc.gov/travel/**

    Traveler's Health

    Locate health information for specific destinations, stay up to date on outbreaks throughout the world, and learn how to avoid illness from food and water.

19. **http://www.cdc.gov/nchstp/tb/**

    CDC's Division of Tuberculosis Elimination

    With the mission of "preventing, controlling and eventually eliminating tuberculosis from the United States," the Web site of the CDC's Division of Tuberculosis Elimination contains useful information to aid that mission. Learn all there is to know about TB, locate statistics on the occurrence of TB, and obtain education and training materials on TB.

20. **http://www.4women.gov**

    National Women's Health Information Center

    The National Women's Health Information Center, sponsored by the Department of Health and Human Services Office on Women's Health, provides health information for women across the country. It offers information on heart disease, body image, breastfeeding, screening and immunizations schedules, and more.

21. **http://www.menshealthnetwork.org**

    Men's Health Network

    The Men's Health Network is an informational and educational organization recognizing men's health as a specific social concern.

22. **http://www.kidshealth.org**

    KidsHealth

    KidsHealth is the largest and most visited site on the Web, providing doctor-approved health information about children from before birth through adolescence. Created by The Nemours Foundation's Center for Children's Health Media, the award-winning KidsHealth provides families with accurate, up-to-date, and jargon-free health information.

23. **http://www.nsc.org**

National Safety Council

The National Safety Council is focused on providing safety and health information in order to reduce the number of injuries and deaths from preventable accidents. Its Web site contains information on new policies and laws enacted to prevent unintentional injuries. Readers can also locate statistics and helpful tips regarding safety.

24. **http://ctb.ku.edu**

Community Tool Box

The goal of the Community Tool Box is to support work in community health promotion and development. The Tool Box provides multiple pages of practical skill-building information on over 250 different topics related to community development. Topic sections include step-by-step instruction, examples, checklists, and related resources.

National Agencies

25. **http://www.cdc.gov**

CDC—Centers for Disease Control and Prevention

The Centers for Disease Control and Prevention is recognized as the leading federal agency for protecting the health and safety of the public, providing credible information to enhance health decisions and promote health. The Web site of the CDC includes a variety of helpful health and safety topics. The information covers everything from health promotion to vaccines to traveler's health. Data, statistics, publications, and products are also available.

26. **http://www.os.dhhs.gov**

DHHS—Department of Health and Human Services

The Department of Health and Human Services is the U.S. government's principal agency for health protection and the provision of human services. Its site is divided into health topics such as Safety & Wellness, Diseases & Conditions, and Families & Children. Readers can also use the Resource Locator and Reference Collections to find such things as health care facilities and publications.

27. **http://www.epa.gov**

EPA—Environmental Protection Agency

The EPA is focused on protecting human health and the environment by working for a cleaner, healthier environment. The site provides air quality reports, current environmental news stories, and tips on how the public can make the environment healthier. The QuickFinder allows fast and easy access to a variety of environmental topics.

28. **http://www.ihs.gov**

HIS—Indian Health Services

Indian Health Services is the federal health program for American Indians and Alaska Natives. IHS is focused on improving the health of these groups while attempting to ensure they have access to culturally acceptable health services.

29. **http://www.ama-assn.org**

    American Medical Association

    The Web site is divided into a section for physicians and medical students and a section for patients. The Patient section allows the user to search for a doctor and obtain health information and resources. The physician section provides information on such topics as medical education, legal issues, and advocacy.

30. **http://www.nih.gov**

    NIH—National Institutes of Health

    The Web site of the National Institutes of Health is loaded with a wide variety of great health information. It contains an A–Z index of health resources, a wealth of grant information, and a section dedicated to scientific resources.

International Agencies

31. **http://www.who.int/en**

    WHO—World Health Organization

    The Web site of the World Health Organization is an incredible resource. The site includes a tremendous listing of pages organized by health and development topics that contain links to WHO projects, initiatives, activities, information products, and contacts.

32. **http://www.paho.org**

    PAHO—Pan American Health Organization

    The Pan American Health Organization, affiliated with the World Health Organization, focuses on a multitude of public health topics, with the mission of promoting health in the Americas.

Web-Based MEDLINE Search Systems

33. **http://www.ncbi.nlm.nih.gov/pubmed**

    PubMed

    PubMed is a service of the National Library of Medicine. It includes literally millions of citations for biomedical articles going back to the 1950s. The citations are from MEDLINE and additional life science journals. PubMed includes links to many sites providing full-text articles and other related resources.

34. **http://www.medscape.com/px/urlinfo**

    Medscape from WebMD (free access to MEDLINE)

    Medscape allows the user to register for free access to MEDLINE, CME courses, medical journals, medical news, and more. MEDLINE's database of medical abstracts may be searched by title or author.

35. **http://www.nlm.nih.gov**

    National Library of Medicine

    The National Library of Medicine (NLM), on the campus of the National Institutes of Health in Bethesda, Maryland, is the world's largest medical library. The Library collects materials and provides information and research services in all areas of biomedicine and health care.

36. **http://medlineplus.gov**

MedlinePlus

Health professionals and the general public alike can easily access information on MedlinePlus that is accurate and up to date. MedlinePlus has extensive information from the National Institutes of Health and other trusted sources on over 650 diseases and conditions.

Public Health Practice

37. **http://www.phppo.cdc.gov**

CDC—Public Health Practice Program Office

The Public Health Practice Program Office focuses on "four elements essential to an effective, vibrant and strong community public health presence: the public health workforce, organizational effectiveness, the scientific capacity of public health laboratories, and the systems that manage public health information and knowledge."

38. **http://www.apha.org**

American Public Health Association

The APHA is the world's largest and oldest organization of public health professionals. Useful sections include Continuing Education, Newsroom, and Science and Programs.

State and Local Public Health Departments

39. **http://www.statepublichealth.org/index.php**

StatePublicHealth.org

StatePublicHealth.org is a product of the Association of State and Territorial Health Officials (ASTHO) and ASTHO affiliates. It is designed to facilitate the dissemination of basic state-based public health information.

40. **http://www.healthguideusa.com/index.htm**

Health Guide USA

Health Guide USA provides quick reference to a tremendous listing of health care-related resources throughout the United States. State and local health departments, as well medical schools and medical licenses are listed.

General Health Information

41. **http://www.altavista.com**

AltaVista

AltaVista is an excellent keyword search engine. With advanced settings and helpful tools, users can refine their searches and quickly access the most pertinent and useful health information.

42. **www.google.com**

Google

Google's keyword search engine is pop-up free and a great tool for finding anything on the Web. Visit "Google Help Central" to locate advice on advanced searches, access the Web Search Features, and check out the Google Services and Tools.

43. **http://www.HealthAtoZ.com**

    Health A to Z

    Health A to Z is a Web site directory and search engine that has been cataloged by medical professionals who have a strong background in health and medicine.

44. **http://www.yahoo.com/Health/**

    Yahoo! Health

    Get in-depth coverage on a variety of health issues, including a directory of the most popular Web sites related to a particular health topic.

45. **http://netbook.miph.org**

    The Netbook

    This guide offers clear, concise information about the Internet and how it can be utilized to advance substance abuse prevention efforts.

46. **http://www.mayoclinic.com**

    Mayo Clinic

    The Mayo Clinic offers a wealth of health information developed and reviewed by more than 2,000 physicians and scientists. The site also allows access to healthy living tools, such as a personal health card, and a first-aid and self-care guide.

47. **http://www.berkeleywellness.com**

    Cal Berkeley Wellness Letter

    The Wellness Letter relies on the expertise of the School of Public Health and other researchers at UC Berkeley, as well as other top scientists from around the world. It translates this leading-edge research into practical advice for daily living—at home, at work, while exercising, and in the market or health-food store.

48. **http://www.healthfinder.gov**

    healthfinder®

    Healthfinder, developed by the Department of Health and Human Services, directs the user to various health resources depending on his or her needs. Resources include such things as online publications, clearinghouses, support groups, government agencies, and Web sites.

49. **http://www.noah-health.org**

    NOAH: New York Online Access to Health (Bilingual Site)

    NOAH provides access to full-text consumer health information in English and Spanish. Listing a multitude of health topics and a comprehensive subject index, the user can easily obtain information of interest.

50. **http://www.chid.nih.gov**

    CHID—Combined Health Info Database

    CHID is a bibliographic database updated four times a year that is produced by health-related agencies of the federal government. This database provides titles, abstracts, and availability information for health information and health education resources.

51. **http://firstgov.gov/Citizen/Topics/Health.shtml**

    FirstGov.gov-Citizen Gateway

    The Health section of the U.S. Government's Official Web Portal is filled with great health information. The Get It Done Online! section allows the user to assess his or her weight, take part in online checkups, and compare nursing homes. The site also features health topics for population groups and helps the user locate health services in his or her area.

52. **http://www.grantproposal.com**

    GrantProposal.com

    GrantProposal.com provides free resources for both advanced grant-writing consultants and inexperienced nonprofit staff. Many "helpful hints" are included that are proven to bring positive results in obtaining grants.

53. **http://www.goaskalice.columbia.edu**

    Go Ask Alice!

    Go Ask Alice's Q&A database houses numerous health-related questions and answers. The site is produced by Columbia University's Health Education Program.

54. **http://www.health.gov/nhic**

    National Health Information Center

    The National Health Information Center (NHIC) is a health information referral service. NHIC puts health professionals and consumers who have health questions in touch with organizations that are best able to provide answers.

News Stories

55. **http://www.reutershealth.com**

    Reuters Health Information Service

    Reuter's is the premier supplier of health and medical news on the Internet. The Health eLine is a wonderful section for the general public.

56. **http://www.usatoday.com/news/health/front.htm**

    USA Today Health

    This section of *USA Today* provides some of the most current news stories related to health.

57. **http://www.nlm.nih.gov/medlineplus/newsbydate.html**

    Medline Plus—News

    The news section of MedlinePlus provides current health-related articles from the past 30 days from the New York Times Syndicate, Reuters Health Information, and others.

Health Education/Health Promotion Jobs

58. **http://www.hpcareer.net**

    Health Promotion Career Network

    This is the official career resource site for the American Kinesiotherapy Association (AKTA), the Medical-Fitness Association (MFA), and the National

Commission for Health Education Credentialing (NCHEC). The site is divided into the following sections: Jobs, Academic Faculty Jobs, Graduate School Programs, CHES Fellowships, and Internships.

59. **http://www.sph.emory.edu/studentservice/career.html**

   Rollins School of Public Health at Emory—Career Action Center

   This site includes sections entitled Public Health Employment Connection and Public Health Candidate Connection. Career Action Tip Sheets are also available.

60. **http://member.aahperd.org/careercenter**

   American Alliance for Health, Physical Education, Recreation, and Dance (AAH-PERD) CareerLink

   CareerLink is AAHPERD's chief online employment resource for health and physical education, recreation, dance, and sport professionals. The site has sections meant for the job seeker and the employer.

Health Policy

61. **http://www.nashp.org**

   National Academy for State Health Policy

   The National Academy for State Health Policy conducts policy analysis; provides training and technical assistance to states; produces informational resources; and convenes state, regional, and national forums. This site enables the user to access these services and the results of policy studies that have been completed.

62. **http://www.heritage.org**

   The Heritage Foundation

   This site provides access to well-written and well-documented health policy research and analysis papers in which the conclusions often reflect a more conservative perspective.

63. **http://rwjf.org/index.jsp**

   The Robert Wood Johnson Foundation

   The Robert Wood Johnson Foundation has a goal of funding projects that improve the health and health care of all Americans. This site features many of the foundation's policy papers, current and future studies, and projects the foundation is or will consider funding. The organization is considered nonpartisan.

64. **http://kff.org**

   The Henry J. Kaiser Family Foundation

   The Henry J. Kaiser Family Foundation is a nonprofit, privately operating foundation focusing on the major health care issues facing the nation. The foundation is an independent voice and source of facts and analysis for policy makers, the media, the health care community, and the general public.

65. **http://www.cmwf.org**

   The Commonwealth Fund

   This site contains policy briefs and full-text health policy papers that are well written and well documented and are often from a more liberal perspective.

66. **http://statecoverage.net/index.htm**

State Coverage Initiatives

The State Coverage Initiatives (SCI) program is a national initiative of The Robert Wood Johnson Foundation that works with states to plan, execute, and maintain health insurance expansions, as well as to improve the availability and affordability of health care coverage. The site includes the results of many states' initiatives to increase health insurance coverage for their residents.

CASE STUDY

As a health education major, you have just finished studying about the Responsibilities and Competencies for Entry-Level Health Educators (found in Appendix B of this text). During this unit the instructor invited a group of practicing health educators to the class to participate in a panel discussion on the validity of the various roles in the real-life practice of health education.

Following the presentation, each of the panelists offered to host two to three students from the class for four hours per week for three weeks at her/his place of work. This opportunity resulted from student questions to the panelists concerning their desire to transfer the classroom learning to the work setting. Several of the students expressed frustration at what they perceived to be the emphasis on theory and the lack of application in their courses and coursework. The panelists readily conceded that the twelve-hour block of time each student would spend at the worksite with them would not totally solve theory-practical application problems, but they hoped it might help the students to see that, at least in the case of the majority of the responsibilities and competencies, what they studied about in class was what the health educator was doing.

After a quick meeting between the instructor and the panel members, placement assignments were made for the students. Because of your interest in becoming a health promotion specialist in a clinical setting, you were assigned to a community health clinic to shadow a physician to see what kind of health education is given to patients.

On your first day the physician to whom you are assigned requests that you accompany him into the examination room as he sees patients. During the first two hours he sees three patients for colds/influenza, two patients for hypertension, one patient for diabetes, and two patients (teenagers) for sports physicals. After these appointments, he takes some time to visit with you and discuss your initial perceptions. During the conversation, he asks if you are aware of any good health education information sites for teens on the Internet. You promise to do some research on this question and bring the information on your next visit. What information do you think would be of benefit to teens? What two or three sites would you choose and why?

REFERENCES

American Psychological Association. (2004). *PsycINFO_1897 Database Record, 2003-10963-006.* Washington, DC: American Psychological Association.

Cottrell, R. R. (1997). *A guide to evaluating a journal article.* Unpublished manuscript.

Cozby, P. C. (1993). *Methods in behavioral research* (5th ed.). Mountain View: Mayfield.

Daniel, E. L. (1997). *Jump start with weblinks: A guidebook for fitness/wellness/personal health.* Englewood, CO: Morton.

Kennedy, G. E., & Montgomery, T. T. (1993). *Solving problems through technical and professional writing.* (pp. 1–82). Boston: McGraw-Hill.

Kittleson, M. J. (1997). *Web sites for health professionals.* Sudbury, MA: Jones and Bartlett.

Kotecki, J. E., & Chamness, B. E. (1999). A valid tool for evaluating health-related WWW websites. *Journal of Health Education, 30*(1), 56–59.

Larsson, L. (1996, November). *Internet demonstration for public health practitioners.* American Public Health Association Convention, New York.

Levene, L. A. (1990). Health educators and library resources. *Health Education, 21*(5), 25–29.

O'Connell, M. L. et al. (2004). Smoking cessation for high school students: Impact evaluation of a novel program. *Behavior Modification, 28*(1), 133–146.

Riegelman, R. K. (2000). *Studying a study and testing a test: How to read medical evidence,* (4th ed., pp. 5–100). Philadelphia: Lippincott Williams & Wilkins.

Rivard, J. D., & Olpin, M. (1997). *Quick guide to the Internet for health.* Boston: Allyn and Bacon.

Seo, D. C., & Torabi, M. R. (2004). National study of emotional and perceptional changes since September 11. *American Journal of Health Education, 35*(1), 37–45.

Strong, J. (2004). Personal communication, Albertson Library, Boise State University, February.

University of Akron (2004). How to access government documents. Available at: http://www3.uakron.edu/ul/instruct/govdocs-access.html

CHAPTER 10

Future Trends in Health Education

Chapter Objectives

After reading this chapter and answering the questions at the end, you should be able to:

1. Identify two settings in which health educators will practice to a greater degree than they do today.
2. Describe four major societal changes that will influence the practice of health education in the twenty-first century.
3. Explain how demographic changes will impact health education delivery into the future.
4. Delineate the major implications of credentialing for future health educators.
5. Compare and contrast the roles of health educators in the four practice settings.
6. Identify several reasons that health educators should be optimistic about future employment opportunities.
7. Describe the need for health educators in two alternative settings.

Key Terms

conservative	microlevel	postsecondary institution
demographic profile	moderate	technology
liberal	postmodern family	traditional family
macrolevel		

It has been said that one of the few constants is change. Clark (1994) notes that large trends in society are acting on the profession of health education as never before. Health seems to be the current watchword of the populace in the United States. With increasing numbers of citizens interested in health information, spiraling health care costs, a reliance on technology for information delivery and acquisition, rapidly changing demographic patterns, a heightened skepticism of the medical establishment, and a more interconnected world, the environment that will confront health educators in the future is vastly different from that of only a decade ago. These changes present the health educator with enormous opportunities. The focus of this chapter will be to explore future developments in the discipline of health education/promotion and, hopefully, to create a sense of excitement and anticipation about the challenges that lie ahead.

Picture yourself as having just arrived in the United States from another planet. The year is 1970. Assume that the first thing you see is a one-hour television news program. Based solely on that program and the commercial messages during the station breaks, how would you describe the lives of people on the planet you are visiting? Now, transport yourself ahead to the year 2000, and repeat the exercise. Although the purpose of this chapter is not to dwell on comparative history, it is noteworthy that, in a brief, thirty-year span, the United States and many other countries have changed so dramatically as to be almost unrecognizable. Certainly, some of the problems faced by individuals, communities, and local, state, and federal governments are the same and the dress styles and modes of transportation have not changed much, but demographic and societal changes, some subtle and others not so subtle, have altered the landscape forever. Several of these changes have profound implications for the way health education will be practiced in the twenty-first century.

The first chapter section will discuss changing demographic patterns. Societal trends that are predicted to play a role in the practice of health education in future decades will be featured. Issues related to credentialing and preparation will be covered next. Using this information as a foundation, the chapter will conclude by postulating about the impact of these changes for the health educator in the school, community/public health, worksite, and medical care settings. One caveat is in order prior to this discussion: Obviously, no one knows exactly what the future will hold. The information presented is meant to stimulate thinking about the role health educators will play from now until the years 2020–2030.

Demographic Changes

Over the past thirty years, the population growth rate in the United States has increased at about 1 percent per year. Although this stable growth pattern is probably manageable for the long term, a more in-depth study of the **demographic profile**, the breakdown of the United States population by age group, sex, race, and ethnicity, shows a dramatically altered picture from that of just ten years ago. It is this consistently changing demographic profile—specifically, a greater percentage of minority residents and an ever aging population—that has important implications for the future practice of health educators.

Minority Population Changes

Clark (1994) states, "We are undergoing a massive change in culture in our society. We are literally looking different as a nation and the conventional majority values and norms are being challenged as we become a more diverse, more ethnic, more

Table 10.1   Projected U.S. Population Percentages of African Americans, Hispanics, American Indians, and Asians or Pacific Islanders: 2010, 2020, 2030, and 2040

Race	Year			
	2010	**2020**	**2030**	**2040**
African American	13.5%	14.0%	14.4%	13.7%
Hispanic	13.8%	16.3%	18.9%	21.7%
American Indian	0.8%	0.8%	0.8%	1.1%
Asian/Pacific Islander	4.8%	5.7%	6.6%	7.9%

integrated culture. Health educators have long prided themselves with working across cultures. . . . The cultural changes are . . . greater than we have experienced previously" (p. 137).

It seems that the increased racial and ethnic diversity in the United States has several major causes. In the 1800s and early to mid-1900s, the bulk of immigrants to the United States came from Western Europe. Hale (2000) mentions that worsening economic conditions in Mexico and Central America over the past decade are largely responsible for the large number of immigrants from those areas. Gheisar and Clark (2000) write that the refugee populations streaming to America from war-ravaged regions of Asia, Africa, and Eastern Europe are presenting new challenges (and opportunities) for the public health community. This wave of new immigration, coupled with the fact that, regardless of country of origin, immigrants have higher rates of fertility than native-born peoples, means that the shifts in culture and the challenges to majority norms alluded to by Clark are likely here to stay.

Statistics from the U.S. Bureau of the Census (2002) indicate that in 2004 the U.S. minority population was 13.0 percent African American, 12.2 percent Hispanic, 4.0 percent Asian or Pacific Islander, and 0.9 percent Native American. Table 10.1 shows the projected percentage figures for each of these population groups for the years 2010, 2020, 2030, 2040 (U.S. Bureau of the Census, 2004).

From Table 10.1 it is readily apparent that the greatest percentage increase over the next thirty years will come from the Hispanic and Asian/Pacific Islander groups. The percentage increase of Hispanics and Asians from 2000 until 2040 is 54 percent and 61 percent, respectively. During this same time period, the percentage of non-Hispanic whites in the population will fall from 71.4 percent in the year 2000 to about 56.7 percent in the year 2040, a decrease of about 20 percent.

Clark (1994) mentions that at least one ramification of these changes, increasing numbers of ethnic minority students in public school, is already being felt in the classrooms of our nation. In 2000, approximately 35 percent of the children in public schools in the United States were minorities. Additionally, in New York City in the next decade, 35 to 40 percent of the residents will be Hispanic, 25 percent African American, and 25 percent white. The escalating minority population makes an already diverse nation even more so and presents health educators with an ever widening array of opportunities and challenges as we race into the twenty-first century.

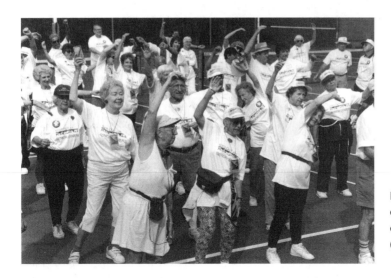

Health promotion for the elderly will be in increasing demand in the next century. (Spencer Grant/Stock, Boston)

Aging

Another demographic factor that will impact the practice of health education in the future is the aging population. The U.S. Bureau of the Census (2002) lists persons age sixty-five or older as representing 12.8 percent of the U.S. population. Between the years 2010 and 2030, the population over sixty-five is expected to grow to equal 20.5 percent of the total. To further illustrate this trend, the median age of the U.S. population in 2000 was 35.5 years. In the year 2010, it will be 37.2; in 2020, it will be 37.6; in 2030, it will be 38.5.

One of the major reasons for the aging trend relates to the fact that older Americans are living longer than ever before. Other causative factors accentuating changes in age demographics are that married couples in the United States are having fewer children, and the baby boomer cohort (those born between 1946 and 1964) is now reaching middle age. This group's massive size causes it to have a dominant effect on U.S. population statistics. "Clearly the aging of the American population creates an increased need for health-related programs for older adults" (Schuster, 1995, p. 338).

Societal Trends

There probably has not been a time when societal change has been as rapid as in the latter three or four decades of the twentieth century. For example, since 1960, there have been changes in societal mores and practices, such as more openness to cohabitation, a greater tolerance for premarital sex, more vocal and open gay relationships, a greater number of single-parent households, an increase in child abuse, more violence, an increase in the amount and availability of pornographic materials, massive changes in the number of ethical issues related to medicine, alterations in the way the medical establishment is organized and medical care is delivered, a decreasing respect for authority of any kind, declining support for public schools, an infusion of and a reliance on technology, and a distrust of the political process in general. All of these factors play a big role in shaping the structure of society in the future. This section will discuss several of the major societal trends that experts agree will impact health education in the new millennium.

Technology

Certainly it is no secret that the boom in **technology** has impacted, if not transformed, the lives of most people around the globe. It can be argued that many of the advances in communication, medicine, transportation, engineering, and ease of access to information have created an enhanced quality of life for many citizens on Earth. The increased availability and use of technology also creates a myriad of opportunities for the prospective health educator in the planning, design, implementation, and evaluation of programs and materials.

One would be hard pressed to find a campus today that did not feature student computer labs in numerous locations. Access to a computer is almost a prerequisite for taking a class in any discipline. Many courses are conducted using fiber optics and satellites to beam "real-time" lessons to a different part of campus or to remote locations. Some entire degree programs are available on "the Web," eliminating the need for students to travel to campus. Students can acquire the information needed to complete assignments using technological advances such as the online search services on the Internet, computerized reference databases, CD-ROMs, and videodiscs. Several journals are published only in electronic form; no printed hard copy is available. This knowledge explosion, fueled by new innovations in educational technology, shows no sign of diminishing.

What does this mean for health educators? As a baseline in preparing for the delivery of health education, health educators must be competent in using a variety of software programs, including but not limited to presentation software, statistical software, word-processing software, and publication software. Butler (1997) declares that future health educators must be able to access information, select and use the data obtained, make sound decisions about the appropriateness of the data, and create solutions that meet the needs of the audience with whom they are working. Clark (1994) believes that, though technology will be central to the future use of health education, the emphasis will need to be on user-friendly technology. In short, health educators will need to help others learn how to learn. This means that the health educator's role will not only include serving as a resource for health information but also helping the public develop skills in finding valid sources of health information and teaching them to evaluate the accuracy of that information.

Family Structure

The American family structure has changed dramatically since the 1960s. The **traditional family** (two parents and their children) is becoming less and less common because of factors such as high rates of divorce, smaller families, postponed marriage and childbearing, teenage and nonmarital childbearing, stepfamilies, homosexual couples, and dual-earner marriages (Acock & Demo, 1994). These changes have spawned a new sociological family descriptor, the **postmodern family** (Cheal, 1991; Stacy, 1991).

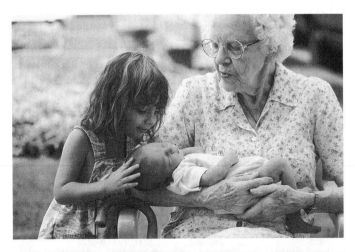

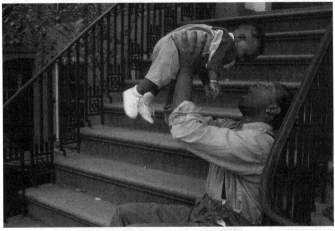

An awareness of different family structures, such as extended families or single parents, is an important consideration when planning prevention messages. (Sue Ann Miller/Stone; Richard Lord/The Image Works)

Hale (2000) summarizes the "new paradigm" in family structure in the United States when she states:

> About 30% of Americans live alone or in non-family combinations, such as with housemates, friends, or partnerships outside legal marriage. Even if we restrict families to the standard definition, 43% are married couples without children younger than 18, and 35% are married couples with children. Another 10% are female-headed families with children, 3% are male-headed families with children, and 10% are other family types (p. 1).

When comparing statistics for African American families with statistics for all races combined, the picture is different. In 1960, 67 percent of children under eighteen lived with both parents, and 19.9 percent lived with the mother only. In 1992, 35.6 percent lived with both parents and 53.8 percent lived with the mother only (U.S. Bureau of the Census, 1992).

The impact caused by these new structures is being felt throughout our society. Children are the most affected. Many parents today provide less guidance and support, and many seem to lack the commitment needed to be parents.

Simons-Morton, Greene, and Gottlieb (1995) document other stressful changes in the family. They mention that the high costs of providing for a family today have almost necessitated that a family have two incomes. This places a strain even on nuclear families with two parents; affordable daycare services for the children must be obtained. For many low-income and single-parent families, the choice is no care or supervision at all—a situation that puts children at risk. In addition, fewer employers are offering health insurance, particularly in service-oriented positions that often pay minimum wage and are a major source of employment for many low-skilled workers. As a result, nearly 22 percent of children in the United States are living in poverty. This is the highest rate in the industrialized world (*Kids Count* data book, 2003). The linkage between these factors may be a predisposing condition leading to an increased rate of child abuse (McKenzie, Kotecki, & Pinger, 2002).

The changes previously noted have massive implications for health educators. Family structures will likely remain diverse in the coming years and will probably operate on a new set of norms. Clark (1994) emphasizes that family structures of the future "will demand new laws, new policies, new procedures, and new health education in recognition of these new types of family" (p. 137). In other words, new methods of reaching individuals, families, and communities will need to be created in order to improve the health of all family members in accordance with their needs.

Political Climate

As was mentioned earlier, there remains little doubt that today there is an increasing frustration with politics and politicians in general. Whether a person is a **conservative**, one who generally distrusts governmental regulations and tax-supported programs for addressing social or economic problems; a **moderate,** one who usually acts in a more situationally specific manner in regard to using tax-supported programs to solve societal problems; or a **liberal,** one who generally desires more government programs to attack social and economic problems, there seems to be no end to the bickering and infighting that goes on among members of various political parties. Many of the political issues considered in Congress relate to health. The landmark agreement between the tobacco industry and the states over the sale and marketing of tobacco products to minors, the addition of prescription drug benefits to Medicare, the repeal of a motorcycle helmet law in Texas, the development of a Department of Homeland Security after September 11, 2001, the passage of a physician-assisted suicide law in Oregon, and the settlement of a lawsuit related to the storage of nuclear waste in Idaho are examples of legislation that directly impacts the health of the populace.

Politics and health seem to be inextricably linked. Some governmental officials and legislators claim that public health programs infringe on personal autonomy by advocating for seat belt laws, tobacco laws, air bags, healthier options in fast foods, gun control laws, and health insurance for all. Others believe legislation fostering an environment that enhances the health of the population as a whole is worth the sacrifice of some personal choice.

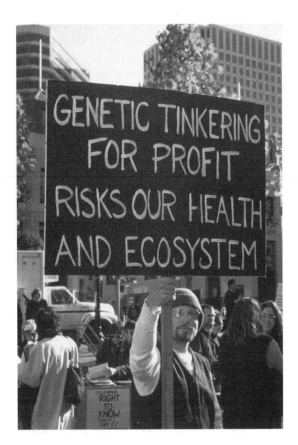

An awareness of political issues that affect
health will be even more crucial in the future.
(Rachel Epstein/PhotoEdit)

As citizens and professionals, the involvement of health educators in the political process is important. O'Rourke (1989) states, "Health education not only
seeks to change lifestyles, but to create public understanding of the political issues
involved in public health programs" (p. 9). He goes on to challenge all health educators to assume a **macrolevel** view of health problems. Using this approach, health
educators move from a position of assisting behavior change one person at a time
to community-based interventions. In implementing the community-based programs, success often depends on the health educator having a working knowledge
of the political process and how it impacts every decision. As a further indicator of
the importance of political competence to the career of a health educator, at a conference held in 2002 in Atlanta, Georgia, representatives from groups making up the
Coalition of National Health Education Organizations listed advocacy as one their
major focal areas. Conference participants agreed that advocacy efforts must occur
at all levels (institutional, local, tribal, state, regional, national, and international)
in order for the health education profession to grow and for health education messages to have the greatest impact on the health of populations and individuals.

The time has arrived for health educators to be politically active. To paraphrase Clark (1994), there is a great need for health educators to capture the energy and power of all in order that health promotion/education agendas are realized in the coming years. Clark goes on to say, "We need governments that are operating on the basis of healthful policies, regulations, and programs. We need organizations that enact healthful policies, maintain healthful facilities, implement healthful programs. We need individuals who are healthful in their behavior, and in the physical and psychological aspects of their life. All these levels must be involved to engender improved health status in society" (p. 140).

To that end, a method for health educators to increase their visibility and political clout is advanced by Warner (1996) and McDermott (2000) when they challenge present and future health educators to consider the importance of research in the practice of health education. The effectiveness of interventions requires that health educators use tested best practices when these practices are known. Future gains in the effectiveness and scope of prevention programs will most likely be made only when health educators insist on pushing the research envelope to determine factors that: affect health and cause health disparities in populations; are components of effective intervention programs; and allow for dissemination of these programs across a variety of settings. Legislators and others in a policy-making capacity will most likely be more open to prevention interventions that are research based.

Medical Care Establishment

In her article on future directions in health education, Clark (1994) lists several societal trends that are powerful forces for change. One of these is the erosion of the power base of the medical care establishment. No longer are physicians' decisions going unquestioned by either patients or insurance providers. There is a strong desire on the part of citizens to be participants in their own care and to be provided with options. Clark (1994) also notes that the health goals of the public are slowly shifting from a "longevity mentality" to one focusing on quality of life.

There are several reasons for this trend. Though few would question the fact that our medical care system has been responsible for saving countless lives, it has become apparent to many that health is largely a reflection of personal lifestyle choices and living standards and not a medical care system. Medical care tends to concentrate on secondary and tertiary care and to ignore the value of primary prevention.

These points are substantiated in a landmark study done by McGinnis and Foege (1993), who changed the paradigm by analyzing the factors responsible for the leading causes of death. They concluded that the majority of the factors are lifestyle related and not readily amenable to medical intervention.

Mokdad, Marks, Stroup, and Gerberding (2004) updated and extended the findings of Foege and McGinnis by using the causes of death reported to the Centers for Disease Control and Prevention (CDC) for 2000, relative risks and prevalence estimates from governmental reports, and published literature to determine the actual causes of death. They found that the use of tobacco, poor diet and lack of exercise, and alcohol consumption led the list as causes. As these factors are largely lifestyle related, the authors urge the rapid movement toward a health care system climate that fosters a prevention-oriented approach.

The public is receptive to the notion that health education can make a difference in disease management (Butler, 1997; Clark, 1994). In addition to the reasons previously discussed, several other factors bode well for enhanced opportunities for health educators in future years: the advent of managed care, the fact that almost 44 million Americans have no health insurance, the restructuring of both the Medicare and Medicaid systems, and the growing influence of insurers. Given these circumstances, health educators can facilitate patient choice by helping patients understand their options regarding physician choice, health care insurance plans, type of care, and intensity of services. In addition, they can assist medical organizations by increasing patient satisfaction through contributing to more one-on-one contact, improving patterns of communication between patient and provider, and enhancing patient compliance with treatment regimens (Butler, 1997; Epperly, 2004, 1997; Lorig, Manzonson, & Holman, 1993).

Professional Preparation and Credentialing

Although the issues of professional preparation and credentialing were extensively covered in Chapter 6, both have implications for the future practice of health education. Thus, highlighting the reasons health education practice might be impacted by these issues is of some importance.

Professional Preparation

In this discussion, it is not our intent to provide a list of courses that must be taken to become a "better" health educator. Coursework is by nature specific to the institution you are attending. Course titles and descriptions vary widely from one program to another. As you are aware, the coursework you will take in your degree program is interdisciplinary. We will attempt to provide some ideas, concepts, and objectives for you to consider as you enter your preparation program.

The social changes previously discussed in this chapter are the driving force behind challenging the health educator of the future to be proactive in meeting the demands placed on her. What tasks will a health educator need to be able to perform to be effective in the decades ahead? Clark (1994) helps answer this question by making several salient points in speaking about health education in the future:

1. The mission will be less providing factual information and more helping people become more analytical thinkers—thus enabling them to deal better with complex issues and uncertainty.

2. There will be newer, stronger partnerships with the medical establishment. This collaboration will give a new power to health education and will capitalize on the idea that health education makes a difference in disease management.

3. Educators will need to analyze situations and examine past and future trends to see the threats to quality of life. Long-term, not short-term, thinking will be a must.

4. A greater emphasis will be placed on values clarification. Health educators must learn to account for the effects of culture and then find processes that reach people with different values.

5. Mechanisms need to be perfected for designing and delivering multilevel approaches to optimize health education in addressing priority health problems. Education at the community level will be the focus of most health interventions.

6. There will be an enhanced need for quality research, so that the effectiveness of health education methodologies can be ascertained. The need for cost-effective, efficient strategies will remain.

7. Health educators must determine how to use technology to help people learn.

8. The need to integrate education, health, and social services within the schools will become more recognized. The gap between school and community services will close.

9. Environmental activism will continue to emerge, and health educators can play an important role in facilitating multidimensional programs that cross all socioeconomic and political boundaries.

10. In the final analysis, people will judge the success of health education by whether or not their quality of life has improved.

Several of Clark's thoughts echo those of O'Rourke (1989), who challenges health educators to be more macrolevel-oriented. In other words, there is an ever growing need to facilitate health education interventions at the community level (as opposed to the individual level, or **microlevel**). Inherent in this charge is that those who reside in the community where the intervention occurs will be totally involved in the planning from the outset. English and Videto (1997) affirm these observations when they state, "Regardless of our place of practice, our ability to identify and meet the needs of our local communities and neighborhoods is likely to be the measure that will determine our success as health educators . . . successful programs use community involvement" (p. 4).

Three additional documents that discuss some of the competencies and/or skills the health educator of the future needs to be successful must also be noted. The first, Conference Proceedings from the Coalition of National Health Education Organizations' Second Invitational Conference: Improving the Nation's Health Through Health Education—A Vision for the 21st Century (2002), lists and discusses what experienced health educators and health education organizations in general need to emphasize in order for health education to have a major role in assisting the United States to reach many of the objectives of *Healthy People 2010*. The entire report can be found in the Web Links section near the end of this chapter.

The second article summarizes the deliberations by members of the Committee on Educating Public Health Professionals for the 21st Century (this report can also be found in the Web Links section of this chapter). The participants attending the workshop from which the article "Who Will Keep the Public Healthy? Workshop Summary" (2003) was written identify eight new content areas that should be added to the curricula of individuals studying to practice public health: informatics, genomics, communication, community-based participatory research, global health, health policy, health law, and public health ethics. Although the report is largely directed at universities offering graduate programs, even a cursory glance at the suggested content areas finds several that are very relevant to the practice of health education and health promotion. The list also points out the rapidly expanding knowledge base the future health educator will need to have to successfully inter-act with health professionals from a variety of other fields. The more understand-ing a health educator has about the vocabulary and nature of the work of other health providers, the more likely she or he is to be an accepted and valued mem-ber of the health care community.

The third document, a cogent paper written by McKenzie (2004), cautions that those in charge of health education preparation programs must not assume that it is possible or even advisable to prepare "generic" health educators. The four prac-tice settings to which he refers in the quote that follows are discussed later in this chapter. McKenzie states, ". . .even though the responsibilities and competencies of health educators are similar regardless of the settings, the work is indeed different and the preparation cannot be the same..." (p. 48).

It is apparent that tomorrow's health educators must be able to respond rapidly to changes in all avenues of society. When planning, implementing, and evaluating programs and working in multidimensional settings, they must enter into collabo-rative relationships with health care professionals from other disciplines in a spirit of cooperation. Health educators who are not afraid to be innovative, who respect but do not fear change, who are not just purveyors of information but community builders and facilitators of learning, who continue to be curious and learn them-selves, who have a sense of adventure, and who seek the truth through thought-ful research, study, and dialogue are the individuals who will lead our profession into the next several decades.

Credentialing

The history of and reasons for credentialing were thoroughly covered in Chapter 6, yet there are several facets of credentialing that need reemphasis, as they have pro-found implications for the future practice of health education.

The credentialing process as it now stands begins with the candidate's submit-ting a transcript of coursework in health education to the National Commission for Health Education Credentialing (NCHEC). Upon verification by NCHEC that the candidate has completed coursework leading to a degree in health education and the coursework has focused on the responsibilities and competencies of an entry-level health educator, the applicant is given permission to sit for the certification exam. Exam questions are based on the seven responsibilities and competencies for entry-level health educators. An individual who passes the exam is awarded a Cer-tified Health Education Specialist (CHES) credential.

This process is not without its detractors. The major reason for disagreement stems from the fact that all individuals who are seeking a CHES certification must complete the same process. This tends to skew the credential in favor of creating a generic health educator (see McKenzie, 2004 in the reference section). Many practicing health educators argue that the skills needed to teach health in a school setting differ from those needed to conduct a community program at a local Amer-ican Cancer Society office or to direct health promotion programs at a worksite. For example, school health educators often see the need to be content specialists, whereas community health educators are more process and skills oriented.

Simons-Morton, Greene, and Gottlieb (1995) accurately mention that health education is a diverse profession. Health educators practice in a variety of settings (e.g., school, worksite, community, health care); they may work with different populations (e.g., adults, the aged, children, minorities); they may be process specialists (e.g., program planners, program implementers, program evaluators); or they may be content specialists (e.g., specialists in HIV/AIDS, chronic diseases, injury or violence prevention, nutrition). Should there be a generic credential? Perhaps in the future there will be "practice-specific" credentials. At any rate, it is important to be aware of this issue, as it probably will be debated for years to come.

An important consequence of having a CHES credential is that of eligibility for reimbursement for services rendered. As managed care sweeps the country, there is a growing tendency on the part of insurers to limit the types of providers eligible for reimbursement. Without some external credential or license, it is highly unlikely that any health education services rendered in a medical care setting will be reimbursed (personal conversation with Idaho Blue Shield Human Resources Department representative, 2004).

Another issue related to credentialing was raised by Butler (1997). He states, "The CHES credential places much more emphasis on the acquisition of skills than on health content. This concept is somewhat in conflict with many of the textbooks written for content areas such as human sexuality or substance abuse. . . . It also conflicts with the philosophies of many institutions that continue to emphasize courses in health content" (p. 334). In this manner, professional preparation programs are affected by the credentialing process.

Though doubtless discussions related to this issue will continue, the credentialing process is "here to stay." The bottom line is that this certification program does "establish a national standard for individual health education practitioners. It differs from state and local certifications and registries in that the requirements do not vary from one locale to another" (NCHEC, 2004).

As the profession of health education continues to evolve and as health educators become more visible partners in the delivery of health services, students considering careers in this field would be wise to seriously consider obtaining CHES certification. The CHES credential assists employers in identifying practitioners who have met national standards, and it serves as a tangible assurance to the consumers of health education services that the health educator with whom they are working is deemed a competent professional.

Implications for Practice Settings

Chapter 7 detailed the variety of settings in which health educators can choose to practice: the worksite, school, health care, or community/public health. Each setting has unique characteristics. The content areas covered, the population characteristics, and the competencies required differ according to the organization's mission and structure (Simons-Morton, Greene, & Gottlieb, 1995, p. 425). However, they are also similar in that the goal of health education is to create a climate that facilitates the improvement of health status for every member of the population served by the setting. The first part of this chapter described various influences

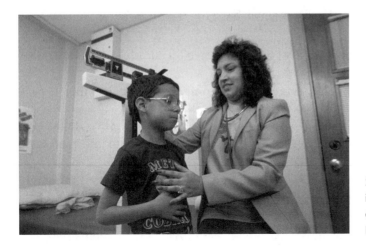

Schools can serve as sites for offering preventive health services and education. (Bob Daemmrich/The Image Works)

destined to impact the health of the populace into the next century. This section briefly summarizes the future role of the health educator in each setting.

School Setting

"Children don't learn as well when they are not healthy" (Seffrin, 1994, p. 397). "Schools in the future will be a key in collaboration to serve kids' health and social service needs" (Clark, 1994, p. 140). These statements characterize the goal of school health education and provide direction for school health educators. If children's well-being is to be maintained or enhanced, a comprehensive approach (sometimes called a coordinated approach) to providing health education is needed (Allensworth & Kolbe, 1987). The comprehensive approach referred to consists of eight components that are integrated to provide for all of the health needs of the children and adolescents attending the school: classroom school health education lessons, the school lunch program, health screenings, physical education, a healthy and safe school environment, the availability of trained school counselors, faculty and staff health promotion, and family and community support for education and health. Actually implementing this model is a tall order. In their discussion summarizing a study on school health policies and programs, Kolbe and colleagues (1995) said,

> School health policies and programs, particularly at the school level, may not adequately address several of the most serious public health problems today such as violence, unintentional injuries such as motor vehicle crashes, and unintended pregnancies. School health services that do not respond to these problems, classroom instruction that is inadequate in scope and depth, and school health policies that only include punitive rather than remedial responses to violations must be replaced with more responsive programs. (p. 343)

Should you choose to practice health education in a school setting, what skills and abilities must you possess if schools are really going to incorporate a comprehensive health education program to address the health needs of children and adolescents, both now and in the future? Given the information on influences on health in this chapter and incorporating information from Chapter 7 on settings for health education, following is a list of skills that we think are imperative. You must be able to:

1. Read and interpret the findings of health research on effective health programs and practices

2. Create a logical scope and sequence to health content units that incorporate age-appropriate information

3. Prepare and deliver lessons that are participatory in nature, stress skill development, and foster attitudes necessary for problem solving and informed decision making

4. Use both qualitative and quantitative strategies to evaluate your lessons, your units, and the district health education program

5. Assess the health needs of the students, faculty, and staff

6. Assure that health and counseling services are provided for students

7. Create or coordinate a parent/community health education advisory council

8. Actively participate in local, state, regional, and national professional organizations

9. Use technology to assist in both updating your own skills and delivering health education messages to your school and community

10. Learn about, cultivate a sensitivity toward, and instill in your teaching an awareness of the influence of culture on health

11. Assist teachers at all grade levels in obtaining age-appropriate health education materials and help coordinate a classroom scope and sequence for all grade levels in your district

12. Serve as resource person and liaison between the school health setting and other settings in which health education might occur

13. Acquire sound oral and written communication techniques

14. Work both independently and as a member of a team

15. Apply behavior-change strategies and what is known about environmental influences on behavior to the classroom setting

16. Collaborate with health educators practicing in the community, worksite, or health care setting to coordinate the delivery of disease prevention and health promotion messages and programs

School health educators who possess these skills will be well prepared to lead programs that enhance the health of the students and teachers in their schools.

Worksite Setting

It is no secret that the workplace of today bears little resemblance to that of only twenty years ago. Because many employers want to attract the top employees and because the employers realize that employee satisfaction is a key ingredient in productivity and retention, worksites have introduced an array of programs for employees and their families that provide continuing education, recreational opportunities, health promotion, and financial planning. In particular, worksites have become an increasingly important setting for health education/health promotion programs. The 1992 National Survey of Worksite Health Promotion Activities (US-DHHS, 1993) found that 81 percent of worksites with fifty or more employees offered at least one health promotion activity, compared with 66 percent in 1985. Typically, the health promotion programs address injury prevention, exercise, the control of smoking, stress management, and alcohol and other drug abuse (Simons-Morton, Greene, & Gottlieb, 1995). An increasing number of sites are expanding their programs to include occupational safety and health issues such as the influences of physical, chemical, and psychosocial work exposures on employee health (Glasgow, McCaul, & Fisher, 1993).

Earlier in this chapter, the influence of changing demographic patterns on health education was discussed. However, there is another factor that must be taken into account when anticipating the future direction of worksite health promotion. According to the U.S. Bureau of Labor Statistics (2004), between 2000 and the year 2010, 17 million people will join the U.S. workforce, but only 30 percent will be white males. The rest will be women and minorities (Fullerton & Toossi, 2001).

The expansion of worksite health promotion programs bodes well for the future of health education and the concurrent need for an increasing number of trained health educators. Reasons for this growth have been chronicled by Green and Kreuter (1991), who state that the growth

> has been influenced by four phenomena: 1) changing demographic profiles in most workplaces, 2) growing concern for the burden on industry of medical care costs, health insurance premiums, [and] the costs of lost productivity in unhealthy workers, 3) the recognition of the greater influence of behavior and environment on health, and 4) emerging evidence that health education and health promotion strategies have been effective in altering the behavioral and environmental precursors of health. (p. 308)

These trends have broad implications for the practice of worksite health education/promotion into the future. Keeping in mind the information presented both in this chapter and in Chapter 7, the following competencies are baseline for the future practice of health education in worksite settings:

1. Recognize the importance of cultural and demographic influences on individual and group health behavioral choices

2. Coordinate needs assessments of worksite populace and conduct evaluations of program components

3. Identify and work with aspects of the corporate organizational climate that facilitate or impede participation

4. Prepare and conduct prevention presentations to worksite subgroups

5. Conduct fitness assessments and participate in health screenings

6. Use up-to-date technology to market programs to worksite supervisors, employees, and their families through newsletters, brochures, Internet chat groups, and other media

7. Plan and manage a budget

8. Coordinate employee coalitions/steering committees to maximize employee input into program components

9. Function as a resource person for health information for employees and their families

10. Be able to apply behavior-change strategies and what is known about environmental influences on behavior to the worksite setting

11. Implement programs in a consistent manner with management philosophy

12. Attain a working knowledge of epidemiological and statistical principles and applications

13. Acquire sound oral and written communication techniques

14. Work both independently and as a member of a team

15. Design and employ evaluation strategies that are outcomes based to assess program effectiveness

16. Gain a thorough understanding of current, relevant literature and well-designed research studies that influence practice in the worksite setting

Incorporation of these competencies into the professional preparation program will help ensure that the student is ready to begin practice as a worksite health educator.

Community/Public Health Setting

The community setting has the greatest variety of options for the practice of health education. For example, health educators are employed in many local, city, state, and federal health departments; in many federal agencies; in county extension agencies; in volunteer health organizations (e.g., American Cancer Society, American Heart Association, American Red Cross); in churches; in homeless shelters; in grassroots community organizations; and in prisons. One of the reasons for the diversity of opportunities is that the mission, goals, and objectives of one community agency may differ dramatically from those of another. Some of the agencies might have a health educator serving in the role of coordinator of services or as fund-raiser, while in another agency the educator plans, conducts, and evaluates programs. Another, more obvious reason for increased opportunity for employment is that almost every locale in the United States has one of the aforementioned groups.

The purpose of community health organizations is to both monitor and improve the health of the public they serve. Mullen and colleagues (1995) affirm the notion of the importance of community health promotion by making the point that the setting allows the educator to focus on reaching defined populations. Forming coalitions of key groups and community organizations has been shown to increase peoples' participation and mobilize residents to take action to enhance the health of all community members (Clark & McLeroy, 1995, p. 277). Goodman (2000) adds that when health educators combine forces with people from other professional disciplines (e.g., ecologists, economists, anthropologists, communication specialists), the possibility exists that the outcome of reducing the health risks of populations is heightened. Consequently, collaboration with community organizations and with other professionals to address population health is a skill that must be fostered by all health educators. In this era of using health education/promotion to help reduce health care costs, and with an increasing need for community-level programs, community health educators are well positioned to participate in improving the health of citizens from all regions of the United States.

With employment opportunities for community health educators on the rise, what skills will the community health educator of the future need in order to function effectively? Following is a list of competencies or attributes that will be critical to the effective practice of community health education. They are not in any specific order of importance.

1. Recognize the importance of cultural and demographic influences on individual and group health behavioral choices

2. Maintain competence in the use of technology to access and deliver health-related information

3. Learn and use strategies to seek information, guidance, and support from community members regarding their health needs

4. Assess strengths of communities in building a plan to assist them in meeting their health needs

5. Be able to apply behavior-change strategies and what is known about environmental influences on behavior to the community setting

6. Learn coalition-building strategies

7. Actively participate in local, state, regional, and national professional organizations

8. Study and apply the fundamentals of obtaining extramural funding

9. Use a variety of marketing strategies to reach diverse community constituencies

10. Learn to be flexible, as the job probably will involve changing and varied responsibilities

11. Learn another language

12. Advocate policies that enhance the role of prevention and provide for universal access to health services when needed

13. Foster the ability to work in a multidisciplinary environment

14. Attain a working knowledge of epidemiological and statistical principles and applications

15. Acquire excellent oral and written communication techniques

16. Work independently and as a member of a team

17. Design and employ evaluation strategies that are outcomes based to assess program effectiveness

18. Gain a thorough understanding of current, relevant literature and well-designed research studies that influence practice in the community setting, i.e., community-based participatory research

A well-trained community health educator will undoubtedly have an increased role in contributing to the health of populations. With the increasing health awareness of U.S. citizens and the multitude of cultural changes in society, community health educators have a bright and exciting future.

Health Care Setting

Health care settings employ health educators in a variety of institutions and in a multitude of ways. Health educators can be employed in for-profit and public hospitals, health maintenance organizations (HMOs), medical care clinics, and home health agencies. They might be involved in conducting one-on-one patient education; planning and implementing education programs for enrollees or other medical providers; coordinating community education programs on a variety of health topics; conducting program evaluations; marketing the health services available through the hospital, clinic, or HMO; conducting health promotion activities for the employees; or serving as a member of a community health promotion team.

Clark (1994) mentions that there is an ever increasing receptivity among medical providers, insurance companies, and the public to the idea that health education can make a positive contribution to the prevention and management of disease. Clark predicts that medicine will be a partner with health education, partly due to the erosion of influence among the medical establishment, the changes in the structure of the health care delivery system toward managed care, and the fact that prevention is more cost effective than treatment.

Redman (1993) and Rankin and Stallings (1996) echo these thoughts. Both researchers note that in the past 20 years patient education in the health care setting has moved from an interesting innovation to a required service. This change has prompted a huge shift in practice norms by most clinical health care professionals, resulting in the need for trained personnel to assure that the education that occurs in the health care setting meets the needs of both the patient and the provider and motivates the patient to both adopt a healthier lifestyle and comply with any treatment regimen.

With the advent of medical acceptance of the value of health education in patient care, the outlook is positive for more employment opportunities in health care settings for health educators. What skills, competencies, and attributes will be absolutely necessary for the health educator of the future who seeks employment in a health care setting? Following is a list (not in any significant order):

1. Obtain a working knowledge of epidemiological and statistical principles and applications

2. Maintain competence in the use of technology to access and deliver health-related information

3. Be able to apply behavior-change strategies and what is known about environmental influences on behavior to the health care setting

4. Recognize the importance of cultural and demographic influences on individual and group health behavioral choices

5. Use up-to-date technology to market programs to patients, employees, and their families through newsletters, brochures, Internet chat groups, and other media

6. Provide training in health education theory to other members of the health care team

7. Become familiar with the clinical disease process and with the terminology used in a clinical facility

8. Advocate policies that enhance the role of prevention and provide for universal access to health services when needed

9. Prepare and deliver lessons that are participatory in nature, research based, that stress skill development, and that foster attitudes necessary for problem solving and informed decision making

10. Coordinate interdisciplinary teams/steering committees to maximize input into program components

11. Learn to be flexible, as the job probably will involve changing and varied responsibilities

12. Serve as a liaison between the health care setting and other settings in which health education might occur

13. Function as a resource person for health information for patients and their families

14. Learn another language

15. Acquire sound oral and written communication techniques

16. Work independently and as a member of a team

17. Obtain a working knowledge of the role of informatics in assisting in prevention at all vulnerable points in the causal chains leading to disease, injury, or disability (Davies, Smith, & Gustafson, 2001)

With rapid changes occurring in medical care delivery today, there is much reason for health educators to be optimistic about employment opportunities. As the public demands health education/promotion and disease prevention as a part of medical care treatment plans, health educators will increasingly be identified as the best prepared to assist individuals in adopting healthy lifestyles.

Alternative Settings

Besides the four traditional practice settings previously discussed, there are several other viable alternatives for the practice of health education into the next century. The purpose of this section is to very briefly introduce these choices, so that individuals who are interested can research these areas further.

The first alternative is to teach health education in a **postsecondary institution**, usually defined as an institution that educates people after they graduate from high school. There will continue to be a need for qualified instructors. Minimum standards for obtaining one of these positions is usually a master's degree in health education and two to five years of experience for a community college or vocational school position, and a doctorate and two to five years of experience for a college or university position.

For students who are interested in combining the fields of health education and journalism, positions can be found in both the print and TV media as reporters for newspapers, magazines, and TV stations, researching stories on health. A broad-based knowledge of health issues and a passion for writing and/or speaking are necessary qualifications.

Because of the increasing interdependence among nations and because there are many areas of the world in which health assistance is badly needed, there will continue to be health educator positions available in foreign countries. Examples include positions with organizations such as the Peace Corps, Project Hope, the United Nations, the Pan American Health Organization, and the World Health Organization. Many national church organizations also send interdisciplinary health teams to international locations to improve the health of the populace. Often, the health educator must have a college degree, some experience, and ability to speak a foreign language.

Medical supply companies, pharmaceutical companies, sports equipment manufacturers, health food stores, and textbook publishers often employ health educators in sales positions. A college degree is required. In addition, a willingness to travel, excellent oral and written communication skills, and an ability to work with all types of people are necessary prerequisites.

Because of the aging of the U.S. population, there is an escalating demand for health educators in long-term care institutions and retirement communities. Usually, a college degree is required. Excellent oral and written communication skills are essential, as is a desire to listen and learn from the wisdom of individuals residing in these communities.

There continues to be an increasing number of opportunities for health educators in entrepreneurial and consultant roles. As self-employed persons, these individuals are free to set up their own practice, hiring out as consultants to organizations that temporarily need someone with expertise in grant writing, program planning and evaluation, software development, professional speaking, or technical writing. Other possibilities include contracting with several small businesses to conduct worksite health promotion, freelancing with HMOs and other insurance providers to offer health education services (reimbursement will be an issue), serving as a content specialist (e.g., stress management, eating disorders, substance abuse) to businesses and corporations, becoming a certified personal trainer, and teaching part-time in colleges, community colleges, or evening community education programs.

Now that the differences in the various practice settings have been explored, it is important to reemphasize the fact that there are common tasks for health educators that transcend the individual practice setting. Dr. John Seffrin, director of the American Cancer Society, eloquently reminds us of the direction health education must take, no matter where the practice setting, if it is to realize its potential. In his scholar's address, given to members of the American Association for Health Education (AAHE) in St. Louis in March 1997, he describes four actions for present and future health educators:

1. Look at ourselves as major players in keeping Americans healthy; to that end, work with policy makers to affect legislation that truly promotes health.

2. Collaborate with other health professionals in both the for-profit and the not-for-profit sectors.

3. Strive to exhibit greater professional solidarity; be an advocate for the profession of health education and the role trained health educators can contribute as part of the health care team.

4. Advocate for those who do not have a voice; be a spokesperson in the political arena, and work to assure that health services and health education/promotion are available for all.

Summary

This chapter began with the notion of change as a constant. Although no one can actually "see" into the future, it is obvious that the need to be flexible in order to adapt to ongoing change is imperative. This is an exciting time to become a health educator. Opportunities have never been greater and the future has never looked brighter. There is little doubt that health education will continue to expand in all of the more traditional as well as some of the nontraditional settings. Health educators have the training and expertise to make a positive difference in enhancing the quality of life for all people.

In conclusion, a quote from Dr. Bob Gold's (1997) address at the American Public Health Association meeting in Indianapolis succinctly and eloquently sums up both the present and future roles of the health educator: "As for the future, your task is not to foresee, but to enable it." In many ways you have the opportunity to make the practice of health education have an ever-widening influence in enhancing the health of the populace. We wish you every success as you begin your journey.

Review Questions

1. Identify three worksite settings in which health educators will practice to a greater degree than they do today.

2. How will each of the societal changes discussed in the chapter impact the practice of health education in the worksite setting? the medical care setting? the school setting? the community/public health setting?

3. What are the implications of CHES credentialing in each of the four major practice settings?

4. How will changing demographic patterns affect the practice of health education in nontraditional settings?

5. List three reasons health educators should be optimistic about the future and provide reasons for your choices.

6. What is meant by the statement "health educators need to become advocates for the profession"?

Critical Thinking Questions

1. What two or three major demographic trends will most impact the delivery of health education in the next several decades? Given your answer, describe the health educator in the year 2020.

2. Compare and contrast the lists of competencies noted in the chapter for the four major practice settings in which a health educator might practice. Use your findings to support or refute the claim made by some professionals that health educators will

be much more effective if their preparation programs include coursework specific to the setting in which they will practice.

3. The year is 2010. If you had the power to decide how our health care system utilizes health educators, what duties might you assign to them in the clinical setting? How might your choices influence the goal of eliminating health disparities in the United States within the next ten years?

4. Assume that it is at least the year 2030 and after many years as a practicing health educator you are retiring. At your retirement banquet, you have been asked to spend five minutes summarizing the accomplishments of your profession. What will you say?

5. What are some ways that the health education/health promotion community can make prevention more palatable to the public? How might you implement your choices?

ACTIVITIES

1. Make a list of five of your strongest attributes. Make a second list of five tasks you most like to do. Using these lists and what you know about health education, write a paragraph description of the "perfect" health education job for you.

2. Construct and administer a short survey to the health education faculty at your institution on what they see as major influences on the future practice of health education. Compile your results and share them with the class.

3. Interview two graduates from the health education program in which you are studying who are now practicing in the field of health education. Make certain they are in different settings—for instance, one in a school, one in community/public health. Try to ascertain their feelings about their jobs and the influences they see impacting the way they practice, both now and in the future.

4. Assume the year is 2010. You are responsible for writing a job description that will be used to advertise for a new community/public health educator position. Write out the description, making sure to include the qualifications and duties the applicant will have to possess.

WEBLINKS

1. **http://www.healthypeople.gov/data**

   Healthy People 2010 Data Section

   This site includes a listing of the indicators and a short explanation about the indicators, a link to data used to update progress toward meeting the 467 objectives, and links to other data sources that measure health indicators of the population.

2. **http://www.healthypeople.gov/Publications/HealthyCommunities2001/default.htm**

   This link is for an online guide for building community coalitions, creating a vision, measuring results, and creating partnerships dedicated to improving the health of a community. The MAP-IT paradigm is featured. It includes "Strategies for Success" to help in starting community activities.

3. **http://www.kaiseredu.org**

   Kaiser Family Foundation

   The link to the Kaiser Family Foundation Web site highlighting health policy issues enables access to background information on several current policy topics, and includes modules covering specific policy issues.

4. **http://www.hsc.usf.edu/CFH/cnheo/21st_century.htm**

   Coalition of National Health Education Organizations

   This is a link to the reports on health education in the twenty-first century. Reports from both the 2001 and 2002 meetings are included in a PDF format. The Coalition exists to mobilize the resources of the health education profession in order to expand and improve health education, regardless of the setting.

5. **http://www.nap.edu/catalog/10759.html**

   National Academies Press

   This Web site contains a link to the workshop entitled "Who Will Keep the Nation Healthy? A Summary." The entire document is available free in PDF. The document includes the results of deliberations and recommendations from members of the Committee on Educating Public Health Professionals for the twenty-first century that was convened by the Institute of Medicine for the purpose of exploring this vital topic.

CASE STUDY

One day while leaving the health education office on your campus, you notice an announcement posted on the message board that the health education program in which you are enrolled is seeking national accreditation. The announcement includes information from the department chair on the reasons for accreditation along with a request for student assistance in working with faculty to prepare the necessary self-study documentation prior to the visit from an outside review team. Because you are entering the second semester of your junior year, you decide that a great way to learn more about the health education program and the field of health education in general would be to volunteer to serve in this capacity.

You notify the department chair of your willingness to help, and she appoints you to one of the program study committees, specifically the committee dealing with how Web-based teaching is used in delivering the health education curriculum. You are excited about that committee because you have some opinions on the value of Web-based courses. Although you have never enrolled in a Web-based course yourself, you know people who have, and they seem to have mixed feelings about the courses they have taken. The ambivalence of your classmates has led you to believe that Web-based courses are not as rigorous as courses offered by more traditional methods.

At the first meeting of the study committee, the committee chair outlines tasks that will need to be accomplished and suggests a timeline for completion. One of the major tasks is to determine if the Web-based courses offered by the department are meeting the goals for which they are designed. How might that task be accomplished? What questions would you need to ask to obtain that information? What methods would you use to collect the necessary data? How might the findings be used by health education programs in planning for the future?

REFERENCES

Acock, A. C., & Demo, D. H. (1994). *Family diversity and well-being.* Thousand Oaks, CA: Sage.

Allensworth, D. D., & Kolbe, L. J. (1987). The comprehensive school health program: Exploring an expanded concept. *Journal of School Health, 57*(10), 409–412.

Butler, J. T. (1997). *Principles of health education and health promotion* (2nd ed.). Englewood, CO: Morton.

Cheal, D. (1991). *The family and the state of theory.* Toronto: University of Toronto Press.

Clark, N. M. (1994). Health educators and the future: Lead, follow, or get out of the way. *Journal of Health Education, 25*(3), 136–141.

Clark, N. M., & McLeroy, K. R. (1995). Creating capacity through health education: What we know and what we don't. *Health Education Quarterly, 22*(3), 273–289.

Davies, J., Smith, G., & Gustafson, D. (2001). Public health informatics transforms the notifiable condition system. *Northwest Public Health, Spring/Summer,* 14–17.

English, G. M., & Videto, D. M. (1997). The future of health education: The knowledge to practice paradox. *Journal of Health Education, 28*(1), 4–8.r

Epperly, T. (2004). Personal communication, Family Practice Residency program of Idaho, Boise.

Fullerton, H. N., & Toossi, M. (2001). Labor force projections to 2010: Steady growth and changing composition. *Monthly Labor Review, 124*(11), 21–38.

Gheisar, B., & Clark, C. J. (2000). New immigrant and refugee communities mean new challenges for public health. *Washington Public Health, Fall,* University of Washington, 2.

Glasgow, R. E., McCaul, K. D., & Fisher, K. J. (1993). Participation in worksite health promotion: A critique of the literature and recommendations for future practice. *Health Education Quarterly, 20*(3), 391–408.

Gold, R. (1997, November). Address at the American Public Health Association Convention, Indianapolis, IN.

Goodman, R. M. (2000). On contemplation at 50: SOPHE Presidential Address. *Health Education and Behavior, 27*(4), 423–429.

Green, L. W., & Kreuter, M. W. (1991). *Health promotion planning: an educational and environmental approach* (2nd ed.). Mountain View: Mayfield.

Hale, C. (2000). Demographic trends influencing public health practice. *Washington Public Health, Fall,* University of Washington, 1–3.

Idaho Blue Shield Human Resources Department. (2004, March). Personal conversation.

Kids Count Data Book. (2003). New York: Annie E. Casey Foundation.

Kolbe, L. J., et al. (1995). The School Health Policies and Programs Study (SHPPS): Context, methods, general findings, and future efforts. *Journal of School Health, 65*(8), 339–343.

Lorig, K. R., Manzonson, D. P., & Holman, H. R. (1993). Evidence suggesting that health education for self-management in patients with chronic arthritis has sustained benefits while reducing health care costs. *Arthritis and Rheumatism, 36*(4), 439–446.

McDermott, R. J. (2000). Health education research: Evolution or revolution (or maybe both)? *Journal of Health Education, 31*(5), 264–271.

McGinnis, J. M., & DeGraw, C. (1991). Healthy Schools 2000: Creating partnerships for the decade. *Journal of School Health, 61*(7), 292–296.

McGinnis, J. M., & Foege, W. H. (1993). Actual causes of death in the United States. *Journal of the American Medical Association, 270*(18), 2207–2212.

McKenzie, J. F. (2004). Professional preparation: Is a generic health educator really possible? *American Journal of Health Education, 35*(1), 46–48.

McKenzie, J. F., Kotecki, J. E., & Pinger, R. R. (2002). *An introduction to community health.* (4th ed.). Boston: Jones and Bartlett.

Mokdad, A. H., Marks, J. S., Stroup, D. F., & Gerberding, J. L. (2004). Actual causes of death in the United States, 2000. *Journal of the American Medical Association, 291*(10), 1238–1245.

Motawani, J., Hodge, J., & Crampton, S. (1995). Managing diversity in the health care industry: A conceptual model and an empirical investigation. *Health Care Supervisor, 13*(3), 16–23.

Mullen, P. D., et al. (1995). Settings as an important dimension in health education/ promotion policy, programs, and research. *Health Education Quarterly, 22*(3), 329–345.

National Commission for Health Education Credentialing (2004). CHES Requirements. Available at: http://www.nchec.org/

O'Rourke, T. (1989). Reflections on directions in health education: Implications for policy and practice. *Health Education, 20*(6), 4–14.

Rankin, S. H., & Stallings, K. D. (1996). *Patient education issues, principles, and practices.* New York: Lippincott.

Redman, B. K. (1993). *The process of patient education.* St. Louis: Mosby.

Schuster, C. (1995). Have we forgotten the older adults? An argument in support of more health promotion programs for and research directed toward people 65 years and older. *Journal of Health Education, 26*(6), 338–344.

Seffrin, J. R. (1994). America's interest in comprehensive school health education. *Journal of School Health, 64*(10), 397–399.

Seffrin, J. R. (1997, March). *AAHE scholar's address.* St. Louis: American Alliance for Health, Physical Education, Recreation, and Dance Convention.

Simons-Morton, B. G., Greene, W. H., & Gottlieb, N. H. (1995). *Introduction to health education and health promotion* (2nd ed.). Prospect Heights, IL: Waveland Press.

Stacy, J. (1991). *Brave new families.* New York: Basic Books.

U.S. Bureau of the Census. (2002). *Population briefs.* Available at: http://www.census.gov/population/www/cen2000/briefs.html

U.S. Bureau of the Census. (2004). *P25-1130 Population projections of the United States by age, sex, race, and Hispanic origin.* Available at: http://www.census.gov/prod/1/ pop/p25-1130/

U.S. Department of Health and Human Services (USDHHS). (1993). *1992 national survey of worksite health promotion activities summary report.* Washington, DC: Public Health Services.

Warner, K. E. (1996, April). All that is gold does not glitter: The economics of health education and health promotion. Washington, D.C.: National Conference on Health Promotion and Health Education.

Development of a Unified Code of Ethics for the Health Education Profession*

The earliest code of ethics for health educators appears to be the 1976 SOPHE Code of Ethics, developed to guide professional behaviors toward the highest standards of practice for the profession. Following member input, Ethics Committee Chair Elizabeth Bernheimer and Paul Mico refined the Code in 1978. Between 1980 and 1983 renewed attention to the code of ethics resulted in a revision that was to be reviewed by SOPHE Chapters and, if accepted, then submitted to other health education professional associations to serve as a guide for the profession (Bloom, 1999). The 1983 SOPHE Code of Ethics was a combination of standards and principles but no specific rules of conduct at that time (Taub et al., 1987).

Following the earlier recommendation of SOPHE President, Lawrence Green, that SOPHE, AAHE, and the Public Health Education section of APHA consider appointing joint committees, a SOPHE–AAHE Joint Committee was appointed by then AAHE president Peter Cortese and then SOPHE president Ruth Richards in 1984. This committee was charged with developing a profession-wide code of ethics (Bloom, 1999). Between August 1984 and November 1985 the Committee, chaired by Alyson Taub, carried out its charge to (1) identify and use all existing health education ethics statements, (2) determine the appropriate relationship between the code of ethics and the Role Delineation guidelines, including recommendations for enforcement, and (3) to prepare an ethics document for approval as a profession-wide code of ethics. The Joint Committee found that the only health education organization to work on ethics, other than SOPHE, was the American College Health Association, which included a section on ethics in their *Recommended Standards and Practices for a College Health Education Program*. The committee concluded that it was premature to describe how the Code might relate to the Role Delineation guidelines and further recommended that individual responsibility for adhering to the Code of Ethics be the method of enforcement. Finally, the Joint Committee recommended that in the absence of resources to retain expert consultation in development of ethical codes of conduct, the 1983 SOPHE Code of Ethics be adopted profession-wide and serve as a basis for the next step involving development of rules of conduct (Taub et al., 1987). While SOPHE accepted the Joint Committee's recommendation, there was no similar action by AAHE (Bloom, 1999). The AAHE Board chose not to accept the suggestion of adopting the SOPHE Code on behalf

*This introduction was prepared through the joint efforts of Ellen Capwell (SOPHE), Becky Smith (AAHE), Janet Shirreffs (AAHE), and Larry K. Olsen (ASHA). Prepared 11/14/99.

of the profession because they realized that the membership of AAHE needed to be more completely involved in discussing and formulating a Code of Ethics before the AAHE Board could adequately represent the interests and needs of AAHE members in collaborative work on ethics with other professional societies.

In September of 1991 an ad hoc AAHE Ethics Committee, chaired by Janet Shirreffs, was charged by President Thomas O'Rourke to develop a code of ethics that represented the professional needs of the variety of health education professionals in the membership of AAHE. They were to review the literature, including other professional codes of ethics, and conduct in-depth surveys of AAHE members. For the next two years, the AAHE Ethics Committee executed its charge through a variety of venues, including correspondence, surveys, face-to-face meetings, presentations and discussion sessions at the national conventions of AAHE, ASHA, and APHA, and through conducting focus group sessions at strategic locations around the country. Based upon the work of this committee, an AAHE Code of Ethics was adopted by the AAHE Board of Directors in April 1993 (AAHE, 1994). Subsequently, both AAHE and SOPHE continued to focus on ethical issues. SOPHE has promoted programming in ethics through its annual and midyear meetings. In December 1992 a summary of the 1983 SOPHE Code of Ethics was prepared by Sarah Olson and distributed as a promotional piece. The SOPHE Board of Trustees supported the summary Code of Ethics in 1994. Since 1993 AAHE has had a standing committee on ethics that recently proposed convention programming and publications in the area of ethics. Recognizing the need to work with other organizations toward a profession-wide Code of Ethics, the SOPHE Board requested that the Coalition of National Health Education Organizations (CNHEO) propose a strategy for accomplishing this goal. In July 1994 the Board adopted a motion that SOPHE support a profession-wide Code of Ethics based on ethical principles and that AAHE should be contacted for support in the effort (Bloom, 1999).

In 1995, the National Commission for Health Education Credentialing, Inc. (NCHEC) and CNHEO co-sponsored a conference, The Health Education Profession in the Twenty-First Century: Setting the Stage (Brown et al., 1996). During that conference, it was recommended that efforts be expanded to develop a profession-wide Code of Ethics.

Shortly thereafter, delegates to the Coalition of National Health Education Organizations pledged to work toward development of a profession-wide Code of Ethics using the existing SOPHE and AAHE Codes as a starting point (Bloom, 1999). A National Ethics Task Force was subsequently developed, with representatives from the various organizations represented on the coalition. It was decided that the coalition delegates would not be the Task Force. As a result, the various member organizations of the coalition were asked to recommend individuals for inclusion on this important Task Force.

During the November 1996 APHA meeting, Larry Olsen, who was the coordinator of the Coalition of National Health Education Organizations and delegate to the coalition from ASHA, William Livingood (SOPHE), and Beverly Mahoney (AAHE) led a session on ethics sponsored by the CNHEO. At that meeting, the basic conceptual plan that had been developed by the coalition's Ethics Task Force was presented. Those attending the session were asked to provide input, both for the process and the content of the "new" Code of Ethics. Those in attendance were strong in their support for the importance of having a Code of Ethics for the profession that would provide an ethical framework for health educators, regardless of the setting in which health education was practiced.

The Ethics Task Force of the Coalition reviewed the two existing codes (SOPHE and AAHE) along with the supporting documents for both, and decided that they would enlist the support of a consultant to assist in the unification process. Claire Stiles of Eckerd College was subsequently retained to offer comments about the proposals of the Task Force, as well as the various drafts that would be developed.

A presentation on behalf of the Ethics Task Force was made in November 1997 at the national APHA meeting in Indianapolis, and the first draft of the "Unified Code of Ethics" was presented. Attendees were asked to comment about the draft document and were asked to take copies of the draft document to distribute among their constituencies. Comments from professionals in the field were returned to and considered by the Task Force.

A second (revised) draft of the Unified Code was presented during the March 1998 AAHE meeting in Reno. Comments received from the APHA Indianapolis meeting and field distribution had been incorporated into the document. In addition, the AAHE Ethics Committee had the opportunity to comment about the "new" document. During the presentation in Reno, participants were put into small groups to discuss and comment on each of the articles included in the draft document. These comments were subsequently incorporated into the document and the stage was set for a series of meetings designed to elicit commentary from professionals in the field, as well as those who attended the meetings of national professional health education organizations.

Following yet another revision of the emerging code, presentations on behalf of the Task Force were made in San Antonio in May 1998 at the joint SOPHE/ASTDHPPHE meeting; in San Diego in June 1998 at the national meeting of ACHA; and in Colorado Springs in October 1998 at the national meeting of ASHA. Throughout this process, comments and suggestions about the code were received and examined by the Task Force. Throughout this process of revision and refinement, care was taken to retain the context and concepts present in the "parent" SOPHE and AAHE documents.

The "first final draft" of the Unified Code of Ethics was presented in Washington, DC, at the November 1998 meeting of the APHA. The coalition also met in conjunction with APHA and it was decided that the final draft of the Unified Code would be prepared for presentation to the field in 1999.

In April 1999 the Unified Code of Ethics was presented in Boston at the national AAHE meeting. During that meeting the coalition also met and it was decided that all delegates to the coalition, as well as the Ethics Task Force members, would examine closely the work that had been done and offer comments and suggestions. It was further decided that coalition delegates would be sent a copy of the entire document (both the long and short forms), so that the documents could be discussed during the coalition's May 1999 conference call. During that conference call, the delegates voted to present the Code of Ethics to their respective organizations, for ratification during the remainder of 1999.

On November 8, 1999, the coalition delegates met in Chicago in conjunction with the American Public Health Association's annual meeting. At that meeting, the Code of Ethics was a topic of discussion. Letters had been received from all the delegate organizations indicating that they had approved the document. It was moved and seconded that the Code of Ethics be approved and distributed to the profession. There being no further comments by the CNHEO delegates, the Code of Ethics was approved, unanimously, as a Code of Ethics for the profession of Health Education.

The Code of Ethics that has evolved from this long and arduous process is not seen as a completed project. Rather, it is envisioned as a living document that will continue to evolve as the practice of Health Education changes to meet the challenges of the new millennium.

References

Association for the Advancement of Health Education (1994). Code of ethics for health educators. *Journal of Health Education, 25*(4), 197–200.

Bloom, F. K. (1999). The Society for Public Health Education: Its development and contributions: 1976–1996. Unpublished doctoral dissertation, Columbia University.

l., Cissell, W., DuShaw, M., Good-McDermott, R., Middleton, K., , & Welsh, V. (1996). The health profession in the twenty-first cenng the stage. *Journal of Health Education, 27*(6), 357–364.

Taub, A., Kreuter, M., Parcel, G., & Vitello, E. (1987). Report from the AAHE/SOPHE Joint Committee on Ethics. *Health Education Quarterly, 14*(1), 79–90.

Members of the Ethics Task Force

Mal Goldsmith (ASHA)
Alyson Taub (SHES Section, APHA)
June Gorski (SOPHE)
Ken McLeroy (PHEHP Section, APHA)
Larry K. Olsen (ASHA), Committee Chair
Wanda Jubb (SSDHPER)

Code of Ethics for the Health Education Profession

*Long Version**

Preamble

The health education profession is dedicated to excellence in the practice of promoting individual, family, organizational, and community health. Guided by common ideals, health educators are responsible for upholding the integrity and ethics of the profession as they face the daily challenges of making decisions. By acknowledging the value of diversity in society and embracing a cross-cultural approach, health educators support the worth, dignity, potential, and uniqueness of all people.

The Code of Ethics provides a framework of shared values within which health education is practiced. The Code of Ethics is grounded in fundamental ethical principles that underlie all health care services: respect for autonomy, promotion of social justice, active promotion of good, and avoidance of harm. The responsibility of each health educator is to aspire to the highest possible standards of conduct and to encourage the ethical behavior of all those with whom they work.

Regardless of job title, professional affiliation, work setting, or population served, health educators abide by these guidelines when making professional decisions.

Article I: Responsibility to the Public

A health educator's ultimate responsibility is to educate people for the purpose of promoting, maintaining, and improving individual, family, and community health. When a conflict of issues arises among individuals, groups, organizations, agencies, or institutions, health educators must consider all issues and give priority to those that promote wellness and quality of living through principles of self-determination and freedom of choice for the individual.

Section 1 Health educators support the right of individuals to make informed decisions regarding health, as long as such decisions pose no threat to the health of others.

Section 2 Health educators encourage actions and social policies that support and facilitate the best balance of benefits over harm for all affected parties.

Section 3 Health educators accurately communicate the potential benefits and consequences of the services and programs with which they are associated.

Section 4 Health educators accept the responsibility to act on issues that can adversely affect the health of individuals, families, and communities.

Section 5 Health educators are truthful about their qualifications and the limitations of their expertise and provide services consistent with their competencies.

*Used with the permission of the Coalition of National Health Education Organizations.

Section 6   Health educators protect the privacy and dignity of individuals.

Section 7   Health educators actively involve individuals, groups, and communities in the entire educational process so that all aspects of the process are clearly understood by those who may be affected.

Section 8   Health educators respect and acknowledge the rights of others to hold diverse values, attitudes, and opinions.

Section 9   Health educators provide services equitably to all people.

Article II: Responsibility to the Profession

Health educators are responsible for their professional behavior, for the reputation of their profession, and for promoting ethical conduct among their colleagues.

Section 1   Health educators maintain, improve, and expand their professional competence through continued study and education; membership, participation, and leadership in professional organizations; and involvement in issues related to the health of the public.

Section 2   Health educators model and encourage nondiscriminatory standards of behavior in their interactions with others.

Section 3   Health educators encourage and accept responsible critical discourse to protect and enhance the profession.

Section 4   Health educators contribute to the development of the profession by sharing the processes and outcomes of their work.

Section 5   Health educators are aware of possible professional conflicts of interest, exercise integrity in conflict situations, and do not manipulate or violate the rights of others.

Section 6   Health educators give appropriate recognition to others for their professional contributions and achievements.

Article III: Responsibility to Employers

Health educators recognize the boundaries of their professional competence and are accountable for their professional activities and actions.

Section 1   Health educators accurately represent their qualifications and the qualifications of others whom they recommend.

Section 2   Health educators use appropriate standards, theories, and guidelines as criteria when carrying out their professional responsibilities.

Section 3   Health educators accurately represent potential service and program outcomes to employers.

Section 4   Health educators anticipate and disclose competing commitments, conflicts of interest, and endorsement of products.

Section 5   Health educators openly communicate to employers expectations of job-related assignments that conflict with their professional ethics.

Section 6   Health educators maintain competence in their areas of professional practice.

Article IV: Responsibility in the Delivery of Health Education

Health educators promote integrity in the delivery of health education. They respect the rights, dignity, confidentiality, and worth of all people by adapting strategies and methods to meet the needs of diverse populations and communities.

Section 1   Health educators are sensitive to social and cultural diversity and are in accord with the law when planning and implementing programs.

Section 2   Health educators are informed of the latest advances in theory, research, and practice, and use strategies and methods that are grounded in and contribute to development of professional standards, theories, guidelines, statistics, and experience.

Section 3   Health educators are committed to rigorous evaluation of both program effectiveness and the methods used to achieve results.

Section 4   Health educators empower individuals to adopt healthy lifestyles through informed choice rather than by coercion or intimidation.

Section 5   Health educators communicate the potential outcomes of proposed services, strategies, and pending decisions to all individuals who will be affected.

Article V: Responsibility in Research and Evaluation

Health educators contribute to the health of the population and to the profession through research and evaluation activities. When planning and conducting research or evaluation, health educators do so in accordance with federal and state laws and regulations, organizational and institutional policies, and professional standards.

Section 1   Health educators support principles and practices of research and evaluation that do no harm to individuals, groups, society, or the environment.

Section 2   Health educators ensure that participation in research is voluntary and is based upon the informed consent of the participants.

Section 3   Health educators respect the privacy, rights, and dignity of research participants, and honor commitments made to those participants.

Section 4   Health educators treat all information obtained from participants as confidential unless otherwise required by law.

Section 5   Health educators take credit, including authorship, only for work they have actually performed and give credit to the contributions of others.

Section 6   Health educators who serve as research or evaluation consultants discuss their results only with those to whom they are pro-

viding service, unless maintaining such confidentiality would jeopardize the health or safety of others.

Section 7   Health educators report the results of their research and evaluation objectively, accurately, and in a timely fashion.

Article VI: Responsibility in Professional Preparation

Those involved in the preparation and training of health educators have an obligation to accord learners the same respect and treatment given other groups by providing quality education that benefits the profession and the public.

Section 1   Health educators select students for professional preparation programs based upon equal opportunity for all, and the individual's academic performance, abilities, and potential contribution to the profession and the public's health.

Section 2   Health educators strive to make the educational environment and culture conducive to the health of all involved, and free from sexual harassment and all forms of discrimination.

Section 3   Health educators involved in professional preparation and professional development engage in careful preparation; present material that is accurate, up-to-date, and timely; provide reasonable and timely feedback; state clear and reasonable expectations; and conduct fair assessments and evaluations of learners.

Section 4   Health educators provide objective and accurate counseling to learners about career opportunities, development, and advancement, and assist learners to secure professional employment.

Section 5   Health educators provide adequate supervision and meaningful opportunities for the professional development of learners.

Code of Ethics for the Health Education Profession

Short Version*

Preamble

The health education profession is dedicated to excellence in the practice of promoting individual, family, organizational, and community health. The Code of Ethics provides a framework of shared values within which health education is practiced. The responsibility of each health educator is to aspire to the highest possible standards of conduct and to encourage the ethical behavior of all those with whom they work.

Article I: Responsibility to the Public

A health educator's ultimate responsibility is to educate people for the purpose of promoting, maintaining, and improving individual, family, and community health. When a conflict of issues arises among individuals, groups, organizations, agencies, or institutions, health educators must consider all issues and give priority to those that promote wellness and quality of living through principles of self-determination and freedom of choice for the individual.

Article II: Responsibility to the Profession

Health educators are responsible for their professional behavior, for the reputation of their profession, and for promoting ethical conduct among their colleagues.

Article III: Responsibility to Employers

Health educators recognize the boundaries of their professional competence and are accountable for their professional activities and actions.

Article IV: Responsibility in the Delivery of Health Education

Health educators promote integrity in the delivery of health education. They respect the rights, dignity, confidentiality, and worth of all people by adapting strategies and methods to meet the needs of diverse populations and communities.

Article V: Responsibility in Research and Evaluation

Health educators contribute to the health of the population and to the profession through research and evaluation activities. When planning and conducting research or evaluation, health educators do so in accordance with federal and state laws and regulations, organizational and institutional policies, and professional standards.

Article VI: Responsibility in Professional Preparation

Those involved in the preparation and training of health educators have an obligation to accord learners the same respect and treatment given other groups by providing quality education that benefits the profession and the public.

*Used with the permission of the Coalition of National Health Education Organizations.

Responsibilities and Competencies for Entry-Level Health Educators

Responsibility I—Assessing Individual and Community Needs for Health Education

Competency A

Obtain health-related data about social and cultural environments, growth and development factors, needs, and interests.

Sub-Competencies

1. Select valid sources of information about health needs and interests.
2. Utilize computerized sources of health-related information.
3. Employ or develop appropriate data-gathering instruments.
4. Apply survey techniques to acquire health data.

Competency B

Distinguish between behaviors that foster, and those that hinder, well-being.

Sub-Competencies

1. Investigate physical, social, emotional, and intellectual factors influencing health behaviors.
2. Identify behaviors that tend to promote or compromise health.
3. Recognize the role of learning and affective experience in shaping patterns of health behavior.

Competency C

Infer needs for health education on the basis of obtained data.

Sub-Competencies

1. Analyze needs assessment data.
2. Determine priority areas of need for health education.

Responsibility II—Planning Effective Health Education Programs

Competency A

Recruit community organizations, resource people, and potential participants for support and assistance in program planning.

Sub-Competencies

1. Communicate need for the program to those who will be involved.
2. Obtain commitments from personnel and decision makers who will be involved in the program.
3. Seek ideas and opinions of those who will affect, or be affected by, the program.
4. Incorporate feasible ideas and recommendations into the planning process.

Source: From *A Competency-Based Framework for Professional Development of Certified Health Education Specialists,* NCHEC, New York, 1996.

Competency B

Develop a logical scope and sequence plan for a health education program.

Sub-Competencies

1. Determine the range of health information requisite to a given program of instruction.
2. Organize the subject areas comprising the scope of a program in logical sequence.

Competency C

Formulate appropriate and measurable program objectives.

Sub-Competencies

1. Infer educational objectives facilitative of achievement of specified competencies.
2. Develop a framework of broadly stated, operational objectives relevant to a proposed health education program.

Competency D

Design educational programs consistent with specified program objectives.

Sub-Competencies

1. Match proposed learning activities with those implicit in the stated objectives.
2. Formulate a wide variety of alternative educational methods.
3. Select strategies best suited to implementation of educational objectives in a given setting.
4. Plan a sequence of learning opportunities building upon, and reinforcing mastery of, preceding objectives.

Responsibility III— Implementing Health Education Programs

Competency A

Exhibit competence in carrying out planned educational programs.

Sub-Competencies

1. Employ a wide range of educational methods and techniques.
2. Apply individual or group process methods as appropriate to given learning situations.
3. Utilize instructional equipment and other instructional media effectively.
4. Select methods that best facilitate practice of program objectives.

Competency B

Infer enabling objectives as needed to implement instructional programs in specified settings.

Sub-Competencies

1. Pretest learners to ascertain present abilities and knowledge relative to proposed program objectives.
2. Develop subordinate measurable objectives as needed for instruction.

Competency C

Select methods and media best suited to implement program plans for specific learners.

Sub-Competencies

1. Analyze learner characteristics, legal aspects, feasibility, and other considerations influencing choices among methods.
2. Evaluate the efficacy of alternative methods and techniques capable of facilitating program objectives.
3. Determine the availability of information, personnel, time, and equipment needed to implement the program for a given audience.

Competency D

Monitor educational programs, adjusting objectives and activities as necessary.

Sub-Competencies

1. Compare actual program activities with the stated objectives.
2. Assess the relevance of existing program objectives to current needs.
3. Revise program activities and objectives as necessitated by changes in learner needs.
4. Appraise applicability of resources and materials relative to given educational objectives.

Responsibility IV—Evaluating Effectiveness of Health Education Programs

Competency A

Develop plans to assess achievement of program objectives.

Sub-Competencies
1. Determine standards of performance to be applied as criteria of effectiveness.
2. Establish a realistic scope of evaluation efforts.
3. Develop an inventory of existing valid and reliable tests and survey instruments.
4. Select appropriate methods for evaluating program effectiveness.

Competency B

Carry out evaluation plans.

Sub-Competencies
1. Facilitate administration of the tests and activities specified in the plan.
2. Utilize data-collecting methods appropriate to the objectives.
3. Analyze resulting evaluation data.

Competency C

Interpret results of program evaluation.

Sub-Competencies
1. Apply criteria of effectiveness to obtained results of a program.
2. Translate evaluation results into terms easily understood by others.
3. Report effectiveness of educational programs in achieving proposed objectives.

Competency D

Infer implications from findings for future program planning.

Sub-Competencies
1. Explore possible explanations for important evaluation findings.
2. Recommend strategies for implementing results of evaluation.

Responsibility V—Coordinating Provision of Health Education Services

Competency A

Develop a plan for coordinating health education services.

Sub-Competencies
1. Determine the extent of available health education services.
2. Match health education services to proposed program activities.
3. Identify gaps and overlaps in the provision of collaborative health services.

Competency B

Facilitate cooperation between and among levels of program personnel.

Sub-Competencies
1. Promote cooperation and feedback among personnel related to the program.
2. Apply various methods of conflict reduction as needed.
3. Analyze the role of health educator as liaison between program staff and outside groups and organizations.

Competency C

Formulate practical modes of collaboration among health agencies and organizations.

Sub-Competencies
1. Stimulate development of cooperation among personnel responsible for community health education program.
2. Suggest approaches for integrating health education within existing health programs.
3. Develop plans for promoting collaborative efforts among health agencies and organizations with mutual interests.

Competency D

Organize in-service training programs for teachers, volunteers, and other interested personnel.

Sub-Competencies

1. Plan an operational, competency-oriented training program.
2. Utilize instructional resources that meet a variety of in-service training needs.
3. Demonstrate a wide range of strategies for conducting in-service training programs.

Responsibility VI—Acting as a Resource Person in Health Education

Competency A

Utilize computerized health information retrieval systems effectively.

Sub-Competencies

1. Match an information need with the appropriate retrieval system.
2. Access principal on-line and other database health information resources.

Competency B

Establish effective consultative relationships with those requesting assistance in solving health-related problems.

Sub-Competencies

1. Analyze parameters of effective consultative relationships.
2. Describe special skills and abilities needed by health educators for consultation activities.
3. Formulate a plan for providing consultation to other health professionals.
4. Explain the process of marketing health education consultative services.

Competency C

Interpret and respond to requests for health information.

Sub-Competencies

1. Analyze general processes for identifying the information needed to satisfy a request.

2. Employ a wide range of approaches in referring requesters to valid sources of health information.

Competency D

Select effective educational resource materials for dissemination.

Sub-Competencies

1. Assemble educational material of value to the health of individuals and community groups.
2. Evaluate the worth and applicability of resource materials for given audiences.
3. Apply various processes in the acquisition of resource materials.
4. Compare different methods for distributing educational materials.

Responsibility VII—Communicating Health and Health Education Needs, Concerns, and Resources

Competency A

Interpret concepts, purposes, and theories of health education.

Sub-Competencies

1. Evaluate the state of the art of health education.
2. Analyze the foundations of the discipline of health education.
3. Describe major responsibilities of the health educator in the practice of health education.

Competency B

Predict the impact of societal value systems on health education programs.

Sub-Competencies

1. Investigate social forces causing opposing viewpoints regarding health education needs and concerns.
2. Employ a wide range of strategies for dealing with controversial health issues.

Competency C

Select a variety of communication methods and techniques in providing health information.

Sub-Competencies

1. Utilize a wide range of techniques for communicating health and health education information.
2. Demonstrate proficiency in communicating health information and health education needs.

Competency D

Foster communication between health care providers and consumers.

Sub-Competencies

1. Interpret the significance and implications of health care providers' messages to consumers.
2. Act as liaison between consumer groups and individuals and health care provider organizations.

Eta Sigma Gamma Chapters:
Locations and Dates of Installation

Chapter	Location	Date of Installation
Alpha	Ball State University, Muncie, IN	1968
Beta	Eastern Kentucky University, Richmond, KY	1969
Gamma	California State University, Long Beach, CA	1970
Delta	California State University, San Diego, CA	1970
Epsilon	University of Maryland, College Park, MD	1970
Zeta*	Trenton State College, Trenton, NJ	1970
Eta	Central Michigan University, Mt. Pleasant, MI	1970
Theta	University of Nebraska, Lincoln, NE	1972
Iota	University of Toledo, Toledo, OH	1973
Kappa	SUNY College of Cortland, Cortland, NY	1973
Lambda	Indiana State University, Terre Haute, IN	1974
Mu	Western Kentucky University, Bowling Green, KY	1974
Nu	Indiana University, Bloomington, IN	1974
Xi	Purdue University, West Lafayette, IN	1974
Omicron*	Slippery Rock University, Slippery Rock, PA	1974
Pi	Western Illinois University, Macomb, IL	1974
Rho	Kent State University, Kent, OH	1974
Sigma	James Madison University, Harrisonburg, VA	1974
Tau	University of Illinois, Champaign-Urbana, IL	1975
Upsilon*	Russell Sage College, Albany, NY	1975
Phi	University of Northern Colorado, Greeley, CO	1976
Chi	University of Utah, Salt Lake City, UT	1976
Psi	Brigham Young University, Provo, UT	1976
Omega	Illinois State University, Normal, IL	1976
Alpha Alpha	Southern Illinois University, Carbondale, IL	1976
Alpha Beta*	Kansas State University, Manhattan, KS	1976
Alpha Gamma	University of North Florida, Jacksonville, FL	1976
Alpha Delta*	Florida State University, Tallahassee, FL	1976
Alpha Epsilon*	University of New Mexico, Albuquerque, NM	1977
Alpha Zeta*	California State University, Northridge, CA	1977
Alpha Eta*	Texas Tech University, Lubbock, TX	1977
Alpha Theta	Adelphi University, Garden City, NY	1977
Alpha Iota	University of Southern Mississippi, Hattiesburg, MS	1977
Alpha Kappa	University of Central Arkansas, Conway, AK	1977
Alpha Lambda	University of Florida, Gainesville, FL	1977
Alpha Mu	University of Tennessee, Knoxville, TN	1978
Alpha Nu	University of North Carolina, Greensboro, NC	1978
Alpha Xi*	Penn State University, University Park, PA	1978

Chapter	Location	Date of Installation
Alpha Omicron	Temple University, Philadelphia, PA	1978
Alpha Pi	Texas A & M University, College Station, TX	1978
Alpha Rho*	Montclair State University, Montclair, NJ	1978
Alpha Sigma*	Arizona State University, Tempe, AZ	1978
Alpha Tau	Oregon State University, Corvallis, OR	1979
Alpha Upsilon	Central Washington University, Ellensburg, WA	1979
Alpha Phi	Texas Women's University, Denton, TX	1979
Alpha Chi*	St. Francis College, Brooklyn, NY	1979
Alpha Psi*	The Ohio State University, Columbus, OH	1980
Alpha Omega	University of Nebraska, Omaha, NE	1980
Beta Alpha	University of Minnesota, Duluth, MN	1980
Beta Beta*	University of South Carolina, Columbia, SC	1980
Beta Gamma*	Bowling Green State University, Bowling Green, OH	1980
Beta Delta	Eastern Michigan University, Ypsilanti, MI	1980
Beta Epsilon	University of Maine, Farmington, ME	1980
Beta Zeta	Towson State University, Towson, MD	1980
Beta Eta	Sam Houston State University, Huntsville, TX	1980
Beta Theta	Eastern Carolina University, Greenville, NC	1980
Beta Iota*	Eastern Tennessee State University, Johnson City, TN	1980
Beta Kappa	Mankato State University, Mankato, MN	1981
Beta Lambda*	University of Oregon, Eugene, OR	1981
Beta Mu*	Northeastern University, Boston, MA	1981
Beta Nu	Eastern Illinois University, Charleston, IL	1982
Beta Xi*	West Chester University, West Chester, PA	1982
Beta Omicron	Worcester State College, Worcester, MA	1982
Beta Pi*	University of Georgia, Athens, GA	1983
Beta Rho*	Louisiana State University, Baton Rouge, LA	1983
Beta Sigma*	Wayne State University, Detroit, MI	1983
Beta Tau*	University of Arkansas, Fayetteville, AK	1983
Beta Upsilon*	Texas A & I University, Kingsville, TX	1983
Beta Phi	University of Wisconsin, La Crosse, WI	1983
Beta Chi*	University of Alabama–Birmingham, Birmingham, AL	1984
Beta Psi	State University of New York, Brockport, NY	1984
Beta Omega	New Mexico State University, Las Cruces, NM	1984
Gamma Alpha	Western Washington University, Bellingham, WA	1984
Gamma Beta*	University of Richmond, Richmond, VA	1984
Gamma Gamma*	Virginia Tech, Blacksburg, VA	1986
Gamma Delta	Southern Illinois University, Edwardsville, IL	1987
Gamma Epsilon*	Utah State University, Logan, UT	1987
Gamma Zeta	Plymouth State University, Plymouth, NH	1988
Gamma Eta	University of Cincinnati, Cincinnati, OH	1988
Gamma Theta*	Youngstown State University, Youngstown, OH	1991
Gamma Iota	Georgia College, Milledgeville, GA	1991
Gamma Kappa	Liberty University, Lynchberg, VA	1992
Gamma Lambda	University of Texas–El Paso, El Paso, TX	1993
Gamma Mu	Western Michigan University, Kalamazoo, MI	1993
Gamma Nu*	University of Nevada–Reno, Reno, NV	1993
Gamma Xi*	East Stroudsburg University, East Stroudsburg, PA	1995
Gamma Omicron	Springfield College, Springfield, MA	1995
Gamma Pi	Hofstra University, Hempstead, NY	1995
Gamma Rho	Truman State University, Kirksville, MO	1996
Gamma Sigma	Appalachian State University, Boone, NC	1996
Gamma Tau	University of North Texas, Denton, TX	1996

Chapter	Location	Date of Installation
Gamma Upsilon	Georgia Southern University, Statesboro, GA	1996
Gamma Phi*	North Carolina Central University, Durham, NC	1998
Gamma Chi	Clemson University, Clemson, SC	1997
Gamma Psi*	Western Oregon State University, Monmouth, OR	1997
Gamma Omega	William Paterson College, Wayne, NJ	1997
Delta Alpha	Iowa State University, Ames, IA	1997
Delta Beta	University of Montana, Missoula, MT	1998
Delta Gamma*	Cleveland State University, Cleveland, OH	1998
Delta Delta	California State University, San Bernardino, CA	1998
Delta Epsilon	Morgan State University, Baltimore, MD	1999
Delta Zeta	Coastal Carolina University, Conway, SC	1999
Delta Eta	Ohio University, Athens, OH	2000
Delta Theta	SUNY College at Potsdam, Potsdam, NY	2000
Delta Iota	Southern Connecticut State University, New Haven, CT	2001
Delta Kappa	University of South Florida, Tampa, FL	2002
Delta Lambda	Malone College, Canton, OH	2002
Delta Mu	Morehead State University, Morehead, KY	2002
Delta Nu	Idaho State University, Pocatello, ID	2002
Delta Xi	University of Alabama, Tuscaloosa, AL	2003
Delta Omicron	Lamar University, Beaumont, TX	2003
Delta Pi	Bridgewater State College, Bridgewater, MA	2004
Delta Rho	California State University, Fullerton, CA	2004

Source: Reprinted by permission of the National Office of Eta Sigma Gamma.
*These chapters were inactive at the time of this writing.

Glossary

A New Perspective on the Health of Canadians the Canadian publication that presented the epidemiological evidence supporting the importance of lifestyle and environmental factors on health and sickness and called for numerous national health promotion strategies to encourage Canadians to become more responsible for their own health.

abstracts short summaries of research studies that have appeared in selected journals.

accreditation "the process by which a recognized professional body evaluates an entire college or university professional preparation program" (Cleary, 1995, p. 39) (Chapter 6).

action stage a stage of the transtheoretical model in which a person is overtly making changes.

adjusted rate a rate that is statistically adjusted for a certain characteristic such as age, expressed for a total population.

administrative assessment "an analysis of the policies, resources, and circumstances prevailing in an organization to facilitate or hinder the development of the health promotion program" (Green & Kreuter, 1999, p. 503) (Chapter 4).

advocacy "the actions or endeavors individuals or groups engage in in order to alter public opinion in favor or in opposition to a certain policy" (Pinzon-Perez & Perez, 1999, p. 29) (Chapter 1).

American Academy of Health Behavior (AAHB) society of researchers and scholars in the areas of human behavior, health education, and health promotion.

American Alliance for Health, Physical Education, Recreation and Dance (AAHPERD) a professional alliance of six national associations (American Association for Active Lifestyles and Fitness, American

Association for Health Education, American Association for Leisure and Recreation, National Association for Girls' and Women's Sports, National Association for Sport and Physical Education, National Dance Association) and six district associations (Central, Eastern, Midwest, Northwest, Southern, and Southwest).

American Association for Health Education (AAHE) a professional association within AAHPERD.

American College Health Association (ACHA) a professional association comprised mostly of individuals who work in colleges and universities.

American Public Health Association (APHA) a professional association for those individuals working in the fields of public health.

American Red Cross (ARC) a quasi-governmental organization.

American School Health Association (ASHA) a professional association comprised of individuals interested in coordinated school health programs.

anonymity exists when no one, including those conducting the program, can relate a participant's identity to any information pertaining to the program.

Asclepiads a brotherhood of men associated with the Asclepian temples who first began the practice of medicine based on a more rational basis.

Asclepios the Greek god of medicine, for whom many temples were built.

assessment the estimation of the relative magnitude, importance, or value of objects observed.

atomic theory Hippocrates' theory of disease causation.

attitude toward the behavior an attitude about a certain behavior; a construct of the theory of planned behavior.

bacteriological period of public health the period of 1875 to 1900, during which great advancements in the study of bacteria occurred.

behavioral assessment "delineation of the specific health-related actions that will most likely cause a health outcome" (Green & Kreuter, p. 503) (Chapter 4).

behavioral capability the knowledge and skills necessary to perform a behavior.

behavior change philosophy involves a health educator using behavioral contracts, goal setting, and self-monitoring to help foster and motivate the modification of an unhealthy habit in an individual with whom the health educator is working.

beneficence "simply doing good" (Balog et al., 1985, p. 91) (Chapter 4).

benevolence see beneficence.

browser a software package used for exploring the World Wide Web—Netscape®, for example.

caduceus the serpent and staff symbol of medicine, which was the symbol of the Asclepian Temples.

certification "a process by which a professional organization grants recognition to an individual who, upon completion of a competency-based curriculum, can demonstrate a predetermined standard of performance" (Cleary, 1995, p. 39) (Chapter 6).

Certified Health Education Specialist (CHES) a health educator who has met all necessary requirements and has been certified by the National Commission for Health Education Credentialing, Inc.

chain of infection a model used to help explain the spread of a communicable disease from one host to another.

change process theories theories that focus on behavior change.

Coalition of National Health Education Organizations, USA (CNHEO) a coalition made up of representatives from eight professional associations, of which health educators are members.

code of ethics "document that maps the dimensions of the profession's collective social responsibility and acknowledges the obligations individual practitioners share in meeting the profession's responsibilities" (Feeney & Freeman, 1999, p. 6) (Chapter 5)

Code of Hammurabi the earliest written record concerning public health.

cognitive-based philosophy a philosophy that focuses on the acquisition of content and factual information to increase knowledge so a person is better equipped to make health-related decisions.

communicable disease model a model used to help explain the spread of a communicable disease from one host to another via the elements of agent, host, and environment.

communicable diseases "those diseases for which biological agents or their products are the cause and that are transmissible from one individual to another" (McKenzie et al., 2005, pp. 92–93) (Chapter 1)

community health "the health status of a defined group of people and the actions and conditions to protect and improve the health of the community" (Green & McKenzie, 2002, p. 247) (Chapter 1).

community health education health education programs conducted in departments of health, voluntary agencies, hospitals, religious organizations, and so on.

competencies "reflects the ability of the student to understand, know, etc." (National Commission for Health Education Credentialing, Inc., 1996b, p. 12) (Chapter 6).

Competencies Update Project (CUP) a project to review and update both entry-level and advanced-level health education competencies.

comprehensive school health instruction the development, delivery, and evaluation of a planned curriculum, preschool through grade 12, with goals, objectives, content sequence, and specific classroom lessons that include, but are not limited to, the following major content areas: community health, consumer health, environmental health, family life, mental and emotional health, injury prevention and safety, nutrition, personal health, prevention and control of disease, and substance use and abuse (Joint Committee on Health Education Terminology, 1991a, p. 102).

computerized databases computerized storage disks containing a large compilation of references; each database is specific to a general subject area (e.g., education, medicine) and provides access to the cumulative information found in several index or abstract sources on that subject area.

concepts the primary elements, building blocks, or major components of theories.

confidentiality exists when only those responsible for conducting a program can link information about a participant with that person and have promised not to reveal such to others.

consequentialism theories that evaluate the moral status of an act by looking at its consequences (White, 1988) (Chapter 5).

conservative a person who generally distrusts governmental regulations and tax-supported programs for addressing social or economic problems.

construct a concept that has been developed, created, or adopted for use with a specific theory.

contemplation stage a stage of the transtheoretical model in which a person is seriously thinking about change in the next six months.

continuum theories "those behavior change theories that identify variables that influence action and combine them to predict the likelihood of action" (Weinstein, Rothman, & Sutton, 1998) (Chapter 4).

coordinated school health program "an organized set of policies, procedures, and activities designed to protect, promote, and improve the health and well-being of students and staff, thus improving a student's ability to learn. It includes, but is not limited to, comprehensive school health education; school health services; a healthy school environment; school counseling; psychological and social services; physical education; school nutrition services; family and community involvement in school health; and school-site health promotion for staff" (Joint Terminology Committee, 2001, p. 99).

credentialing a process whereby an individual or a professional preparation program meets the specified standards established by the credentialing body and is thus recognized for having done so.

crude rate the rate expressed for a total population.

cue to action a construct of the health belief model that motivates a person to act.

cultural sensitivity having and showing respect for cultures other than one's own.

culturally competent having the knowledge and interpersonal skills to understand, appreciate, and work with individuals from cultures other than one's own; it involves an awareness and acceptance of cultural differences, self-awareness, knowledge of the culture of those in the priority population, and the adaptation of professional skills to respond to the priority population's cultural differences (McManus, 1988) (Chapter 1).

death rates the number of deaths per 100,000 resident population, sometimes referred to as mortality or fatality rates.

decision-making philosophy the belief that the use of scenarios, case studies, and simulated problems is the best method to motivate persons to adopt positive health behaviors.

demographic profile a statistical breakdown of the population of a country, region, state, or city by age group, sex, race, and ethnicity.

diffusion theory a theory that provides an explanation for the movement of an innovation through a population.

Directors of Health Promotion and Public Health Education (DHPE) a professional association comprised of individuals who, by position, head their state or territory public health education efforts.

disability-adjusted life expectancy (DALE) synonym for health-adjusted life expectancy (HALE) (see HALE).

disability-adjusted life years (DALYs) a measure of health that takes into effect the severity of the health condition, age, and impact on the future.

discipline "a branch of knowledge or learning" (Agnes, 2001, p. 410) (Chapter 1).

disease prevention "the process of reducing risks and alleviating disease to promote, preserve, and restore health and minimize suffering and distress" (Joint Terminology Committee, 2001, p. 99).

early adopters a group of people who are very interested in innovation, but who do not want to be the first involved.

early majority a group of people who may be interested in an innovation but will need some external motivation to get involved.

eclectic health education philosophy a philosophical approach held by health educators that no one philosophy is "right" for all times and circumstances and that the best philosophy involves blending the various philosophical approaches or using different approaches depending on the setting (school, community, worksite).

ecological "refers to the social, political, economic, organizational, policy, regulatory, and other environmental circumstances interacting with behavior in affecting health" (Green & Kreuter, 1999, p. 27) (Chapter 1).

ecological perspective a means of examining the influences on health-related behaviors and conditions via five levels: intrapersonal (individual) factors, interpersonal factors, institutional (organizational) factors, community factors, and public policy factors.

educational assessment "the delineation of factors that predispose, enable, and reinforce a specific behavior or that through behavior affect environmental changes" (Green & Kreuter, 1999, p. 505) (Chapter 4).

emerging profession an occupation that does not rank so clearly high or so clearly low on the attributes that distinguish an occupation from a profession (Barber, 1988) (Chapter 1).

emotional-coping response to learn, a person must be able to deal with the sources of anxiety that surround a behavior.

EMPOWER an acronym for a computer program that stands for Expert Methods for Planning and Organization Within Everyone's Reach.

empowerment "a social action process that promotes participation of people, organizations and communities in gaining control over their lives in their community and larger society. With this perspective, empowerment is not characterized as achieving power to dominate others, but rather power to act with others to effect change" (Wallerstein & Bernstein, 1988, p. 380) (Chapter 1).

enabling factor "any characteristic of the environment that facilitates action and any skill or resource required to attain a specific behavior" (Green & Kreuter, 1999, p. 505) (Chapter 4).

endemic occurs regularly in a population as a matter of course.

environment "all those matters related to health which are external to the human body and over which the individual has little or no control" (Lalonde, 1974, p. 32) (Chapter 1).

environmental assessment "a systematic assessment of factors in the social and physical environment that interact with behavior to produce health effects or quality-of-life outcomes. Also referred to as **ecological assessment**" (Green & Kreuter, 1999, p. 505) (Chapter 4).

epidemic an unexpectedly large number of cases of disease in a population.

epidemiological assessment "the delineation of the extent, distribution, and causes of a health problem in a defined population" (Green & Kreuter, 1999, p. 505) (Chapter 4).

epidemiological data information gathered when measuring health and ill health.

epidemiology "the study of the distribution and determinants of diseases and injuries in human populations" (Mausner & Kramer, 1985, p. 1) (Chapter 1).

epistemology the study of knowledge (Thiroux, 1995) (Chapter 1).

Eta Sigma Gamma (ESG) the national health education honorary society.

ethical good/bad, and right/wrong.

ethics "the study of morality, one of the three major areas of philosophy, also referred to as moral philosophy" (Thiroux, 1995) (Chapter 5).

expectancies values people place on expected outcomes.

expectations beliefs about the likely outcomes of certain behaviors.

formalism (deontological or nonconsequentialism) "theories which look at the nature of the individual act and determine morality from whether that act is right or wrong in itself" (Mellert, 1995, p. 130) (Chapter 5).

freeing/functioning philosophy proponents of this philosophy help the person make the best health choices possible for that person, based on the individual's needs and interests, not on societal expectations.

goodness (rightness) a state or quality of being good; one of the five principles of common moral ground.

government documents unclassified publications authored and disseminated by federal, state, or local agencies intended for public use.

graduate research assistantship an award given a graduate student who works closely with one or more faculty members on a research project; the student is usually granted tuition assistance and a stipend in return for the work.

graduate teaching assistantship an award given a graduate student who teaches for the program and in return is usually granted tuition assistance and a stipend.

governmental health agencies agencies designated as having authority for certain specific duties or tasks outlined by the governmental bodies that oversee them.

hard money funds used to support health education positions and programs that are part of the regular budget of an employer.

health "the state of complete mental, physical, and social well-being, not merely the absence of disease or infirmity" (WHO, 1947) (Chapter 1).

health-adjusted life expectancy (HALE) "any of a number of summary measures which use explicit weights to combine health expectancies for a set of discrete health states into a single indicator estimating the expectation of equivalent years of good health" (Murray, Salomon, Mathers, & Lopez, 2002, p. 759) (Chapter 1).

health behavior see lifestyle.

health belief model an intrapersonal theory that "addresses a person's perceptions of the threat of a health problem and the accompanying appraisal of a recommended behavior for preventing or managing the problem" (Glanz & Rimer, 1995, p. 17).

health care organization "consists of the quantity, quality, arrangement, nature and relationships of people and resources in the provision of health care" (Lalonde, 1974, p. 32), also referred to as the health care system.

health care settings locations for health education programs, including public and for-profit hospitals, free-standing medical care clinics, home health agencies, and physician organizations such as health maintenance organizations (HMOs) and preferred provider organizations (PPOs).

health education "any combination of planned learning experiences based on sound theories that provide individuals, groups, and communities the opportunity to acquire information and the skills needed to make quality health decisions" (Joint Committee, 2001, p. 99) (Chapter 1).

health field a term that includes all matters that affect health; far more encompassing than the health care system.

Health Field Concept a framework that was developed in Canada to study health; it has four elements: human biology, environment, lifestyle, and health care organization.

health literacy the capacity of individuals to access, interpret, and understand basic health information and services and the skills to use the information and services to promote health.

health promotion "any planned combination of educational, political, environmental, regulatory, or organizational mechanisms that support actions and conditions of living conducive to the health of individuals, groups, and communities" (Joint Committee, 2001, p. 101) (Chapter 1).

Healthy People the first major U.S. government document recognizing the importance of lifestyle in promoting health and well-being.

Healthy People 2000 a document that contains the health objectives for the United States during the 1990s.

Healthy People 2010 the latest listing of National Health Objectives for the United States through the year 2010.

health-related quality of life (HRQOL) those aspects of people's quality of life that can be clearly shown to affect their health, either physically or mentally (McHorney, 1999) (Chapter 1).

Hippocrates a Greek physician from the Asclepian tradition who eventually became known as the father of medicine.

holistic philosophy the philosophy that the mind and body blend into a single unit; the person is a unified being.

home page analogous to a combination of a cover and table of contents in a book, a home page names a specific Web site and directs the user to options within that site.

human biology "all those aspects of health, both physical and mental, which are developed within the human body as a consequence of the basic biology of man [sic] and the organic make-up of an individual" (Lalonde, 1974, p. 31) (Chapter 1).

humanism a philosophy characterized by having a concern for humanity; it also promotes the basic premise of the worth of human life and that individuals can achieve self-fulfillment.

Hygeia the daughter of Asclepios granted the power to prevent disease.

hypertext a type of document that allows convenient links to other documents found on the World Wide Web; it is a simple way of cross-referencing words or phrases with additional information; words or symbols that appear in color are hypertext words, and clicking on them provides links to related documents in the field (Rivard & Olpin, 1998).

hypertext markup language the programming language used on the Internet.

hypertext transfer protocol the protocol for exchanging hypertext documents between sites on the Web.

impact evaluation "the assessment of program effects on intermediate objectives including changes in predisposing, enabling, and reinforcing factors, as well as behavioral and environmental changes" (Green & Kreuter, 1999, p. 507) (Chapter 4).

implementation "the act of converting program objectives into actions through policy changes, regulation and organization" (Green & Kreuter, 1999, p. 507) (Chapter 4).

indexes reference books that provide links to articles from many refereed journals, books, and selected reports; each index is written to target specific subject headings, so one index is not all-encompassing for all subjects.

individual freedom (equality principle, or principle of autonomy) people, being individuals with individual differences, must have the freedom to choose their own ways and means of being moral within the framework of value of life, goodness, justice, and truth-telling (Thiroux, 1995) (Chapter 5).

informed consent requires: a) disclosure of relevant information to prospective participants about the program; b) their comprehension of the information; and c) their voluntary agreement, free from coercion and undue influence, to participate (OHSR, n. d.) (Chapter 5).

innovators the first people to adopt an innovation.

International Union for Health Promotion and Education (IUHPE) a professional association open to individuals who are interested in health education worldwide.

Internet an integrated network of computers that spans the entire world; the computers can transfer data to one another via phone lines, microwaves, fiber optics, and satellites (Kittleson, 1997) (Chapter 9).

justice (fairness) "human beings should treat other human beings fairly and justly in distributing goodness and badness among them" (Thiroux, 1995, p. 184) (Chapter 5); a basic principle of ethics.

laggards the last group of people to get involved in an innovation, if they get involved at all.

late majority a group of people who are skeptical and will not adopt an innovation until most people in the social system have done so.

liberal generally, a person who favors governmental programs to address perceived social and economic inequities between segments of society.

licensure "a process by which an agency or government (usually a state) grants permission to individuals to practice a given profession by certifying that those licensed have attained specific standards of competence" (Cleary, 1995, p. 39) (Chapter 6).

life expectancy "the average number of years of life remaining to a person at a particular age and based on a given set of age-specific death rates, generally the mortality conditions existing in the period mentioned. Life expectancy may be determined by race, sex, or other characteristics using age-specific death rates for the population with that characteristic" (Freid et al., 2003, p. 434) (Chapter 1).

lifestyle "an aggregation of decisions by individuals which affect their health and over which they more or less have control" (Lalonde, 1974, p. 32) (Chapter 1).

likelihood of taking action chances that a person will behave in a particular way; a construct of the health belief model.

local public health agency (LPHA) a governmental organization that is located in a city or county.

locus of control one's perception of the center of control over reinforcement.

macrolevel having health education interventions targeted to the community as a whole, instead of to individuals.

maintenance the stage of the transtheoretical model in which a person is taking steps to sustain change and resist temptation to relapse.

MATCH an acronym for Multilevel Approach To Community Health.

M.Ed., M.P.H., M.S. degree designations available to master's-level health education students, depending on the institution they attend and their area of emphasis.

Medicaid government health insurance for the poor.

Medicare government health insurance for the elderly and disabled.

mental health (termed *psychological health* by Goodstadt, Simpson, & Loranger, 1987) may include emotional health; may make explicit reference to intellectual capabilities; the sub-jective sense of well-being (Goodstadt, Simpson, & Loranger, 1987, p. 59) (Chapter 1).

metaphysics the study of the nature of reality (Thiroux, 1995) (Chapter 5).

miasmas theory a belief that vapors, or miasmas, rising from rotting refuse could travel through the air for great distances and result in disease when inhaled.

microlevel targeting health education interventions to individuals.

model a subclass of a theory.

moderate a person who acts in a more situationally specific manner in regard to using tax-supported programs to solve social problems.

modifiable risk factors changeable or controllable risk factors.

moral good/bad, and right/wrong.

moral philosophy see ethics.

multicausation disease model a model that explains the onset of disease caused by more than one factor.

multitasking the skill of coordinating and completing multiple health education projects at the same time.

National Commission for Health Education Credentialing, Inc. the organization that oversees the health education certification process.

National School Health Education Coalition (NaSHEC) a coalition of more than ninety associations and organizations that supports coordinated school health programs.

National Task Force on the Preparation and Practice of Health Educators the group that oversaw development of the roles and responsibilities of health educators and ultimately the CHES credentialing system.

National Wellness Institute, Inc. a professional association for those interested in wellness programs.

networking establishing and maintaining a wide range of contacts in the field that may be of help when looking for a job and in carrying out one's job responsibilities once hired.

noncommunicable diseases "those that cannot be transmitted from an infected person to a susceptible, healthy one" (McKenzie et al., 2005, p. 93) (Chapter 1).

nongovernmental agency those that operate, for the most part, free from governmental interference as long as they comply with the Internal Revenue Service's guidelines for their tax status (McKenzie et al., 2005) (Chapter 8).

nonmaleficence "the non-infliction of harm to others" (Balog et al., 1985, p. 91) (Chapter 5).

nonmodifiable risk factors nonchangeable or noncontrollable risk factors.

objective statement describing specific, measurable cognitive or affective changes in the learner. An objective establishes a performance standard for the learner.

outcome evaluation "assessment of the effects of a program on its ultimate objectives, including changes in health and social benefits or quality of life" (Green & Kreuter, 1999, p. 508) (Chapter 4).

ownership a feeling of responsibility for program outcomes.

Panacea the daughter of Asclepios granted the power to treat disease.

pandemic an outbreak of a disease over a wide geographical area, such as a continent.

participation the active involvement of those in the priority population in helping identify, plan, and implement programs to address the health problems they face.

perceived barriers the cost of engaging in a health behavior; a construct of the health belief model.

perceived behavioral control a belief held by people that they have control over a behavior; a construct of the theory of planned behavior.

perceived benefits a belief that a particular health recommendation would be beneficial in reducing a perceived threat; a construct of the health belief model.

perceived seriousness/severity a belief that a health problem is serious; a construct of the health belief model.

perceived susceptibility a belief that one is vulnerable to a health problem; a construct of the health belief model.

perceived threat a belief that one is vulnerable to a serious health problem or to the sequelae of that illness or condition; a construct of the health belief model.

philanthropic foundations "endowed institutions that donate money for the good of humankind" (McKenzie et al., 2005, p. 54) (Chapter 8).

philosophy a statement summarizing the attitudes, principles, beliefs, values, and concepts held by an individual or a group.

philosophy of symmetry a philosophy of health with physical, emotional, spiritual, and social components of health.

physical health the absence of disease and disability; functioning adequately from the perspective of physical and physiological abilities; the biological integrity of the individual (Goodstadt, Simpson, & Loranger, 1987, p. 59) (Chapter 1).

popular press publications publications ranging from weekly summary magazines (e.g., *Newsweek*) to monthly magazines (e.g., *Better Homes and Gardens*); often, articles include editorials; information from these sources should be heavily scrutinized before using.

population-based approaches community health methods that are used to help change behavior in groups of people. Examples include policy development, policy advocacy, organizational change, community development, empowerment of individuals, and economic supports.

portfolio a collection of evidence that enables students to demonstrate mastery of desired course or program outcomes.

postmodern family any family structure that differs from a family composed of two parents and their children.

postsecondary institution in the United States, an institution that provides further education after high school.

PRECEDE-PROCEED an acronym for a theory of implementation that stands for Predisposing, Reinforcing, and Enabling Constructs in Educational/Environmental Diagnosis and Evaluation and Policy, Regulatory, and Organizational Constructs in Educational and Environmental Development.

precontemplation stage the stage of the transtheoretical model in which a person is not thinking about change in the next six months.

predisposing factor "any characteristic of a person or population that motivates behavior prior to the occurrence of the behavior" (Green & Kreuter, 1999, p. 508) (Chapter 4).

preparation stage the stage of the transtheoretical model in which a person is actively planning change.

prevention the planning for and measures taken to forestall the onset of, limit the spread of, and rehabilitate after pathogenesis or other health problems.

primary data original data gathered by the health educator as part of a needs assessment; this includes data gathered from telephone surveys, focus groups, and interviews.

primary prevention preventive measures that forestall the onset of illness or injury during the prepathogenesis period.

primary sources published studies or eyewitness accounts written by the person(s) who actually conducted the study or observed the event.

privacy "the claim of individuals, groups, or institutions to determine for themselves when, how, and to what extent information about them is communicated to others" (Westin, 1968, p. 7) (Chapter 5).

process evaluation "the assessment of policies, materials, personnel, performance, quality of practice or services, and other inputs and implementation experiences" (Green & Kreuter, 1999, p. 508) (Chapter 4).

profession "the sociological construct for an occupation that has special status" (Livingood, 1996, p. 421) (Chapter 1).

professional ethics "actions that are right and wrong in the workplace and are of public matter. Professional moral principles are not statements of taste or preference; they tell practitioners what they ought to do and what they ought not to do" (Feeney & Freeman, 1999, p. 6) (Chapter 5).

professional health associations/organizations "organizations that promote the high standards of professional practice for their respective professions, thereby improving the health of society by improving the people in the professions" (McKenzie, et al., 2005) (Chapter 8).

Promoting Health/Preventing Disease: Objectives for the Nation a document containing 226 health objectives for the United States to be accomplished during the 1980s.

public health "the health status of a defined group of people and the governmental actions and conditions to promote, protect, and preserve their health" (McKenzie et al., 2005, p. 6) (Chapter 1).

public health agencies also called "official governmental health agencies"; agencies usually financed through public tax monies and typically offering health promotion and education programs.

quasi-governmental health agencies agencies that possess some of the characteristics of a governmental health agency but also possess some of the characteristics of nongovernmental agencies.

rate "a measure of some event, disease, or condition in relation to a unit of population, along with some specification of time" (Freid, Prager, MacKay, & Xia, 2003, p. 449) (Chapter 1).

reciprocal determinism "behavior changes result from an interaction between the person and the environment; change is bidirectional" (Glanz & Rimer, 1995) (Chapter 4).

reduction of threat a belief that a particular health recommendation would be beneficial in reducing a threat at a subjectively acceptable cost; a construct of the health belief model.

refereed journal a journal that publishes original manuscripts only after they have been read and critiqued by a panel of experts in the field.

reinforcement a response to behavior that increases the chance of recurrence.

reinforcing factor "any reward or punishment following or anticipated as a consequence of a behavior, serving to strengthen the motivation for or against the behavior" (Green & Kreuter, 1999, p. 508) (Chapter 4).

responsibilities the seven major responsibilities of all entry-level health educators.

risk factors inherited, environmental, and behavioral influences "capable of provoking ill health with or without previous disposition" (USDHEW, 1979, p. 13) (Chapter 1).

role delineation the process of identifying the specific responsibilities, competencies, and sub-competencies associated with the practice of health education.

School Health Advisory Council (SHAC) community members such as parents; medical, health, and safety professionals; and political, religious, and corporate or business leaders who assist with the planning and promotion of school health initiatives.

school health education health education programs that instruct school-age children about health and health-related behaviors.

School Health Education Evaluation Study a landmark study that examined the entire health program of selected schools in the Los Angeles area.

School Health Education Study a nationwide study that examined the status of health education and resulted in the development of an important curriculum.

search engine site on the World Wide Web specifically designed to search for all links associated with a word or phrase that the user wants information on; the search engines greatly decrease the time it takes to search for information on the Web; examples are Yahoo®, AltaVista®, and Hotbot®.

secondary data preexisting data used by a health educator in a needs assessment.

secondary prevention preventive measures that lead to early diagnosis and prompt treatment of a disease or an injury to limit disability, impairment, or dependency and to prevent more severe pathogenesis.

secondary sources articles that often provide an overview or a summary of several related studies or that chronicle the history of several related events, written by someone who did not conduct the study or observe firsthand the event that is written about.

self-control (self-regulation) gaining control over one's own behavior by monitoring and adjusting it.

self-efficacy people's confidence in their ability to perform a certain desired task or function.

septicemia "the presence of bacteria in the blood (bacteremia), often associated with severe disease" (NLM & NIH, 2003, p.1).

service learning course credit for students to work with a community agency to meet an identified community need.

social assessment "the assessment in both objective and subjective terms of high-priority problems or aspirations for the common good, defined for a population by economic and social indicators and by individuals in terms of their quality of life" (Green & Kreuter, 1999, p. 509) (Chapter 4).

social change philosophy a philosophy emphasizing the role of health education in creating social, economic, and political change that benefits the health of individuals and groups.

social ecology an approach to health education that goes beyond individual behavior change to examine and modify the social, political, and economic factors impacting health behavior decisions.

social health the ability to interact effectively with other people and the social environment; satisfying interpersonal relationships; role fulfillment.

Society for Public Health Education, Inc. (SOPHE) a professional association for health educators.

Society of State Directors of Health, Physical Education, and Recreation (SSDHPER) a professional association comprised of individuals who, by position in a state/territorial department of education, represent their state/territory.

soft money funds to support health education positions and programs secured through grants or contracts, which may be discontinued at the end of a designated period.

Smith Papyri the oldest written document related to health, which describes various surgical techniques and dates back to 1600 B.C.

specific rate a rate for a particular population subgroup, such as for a particular disease (i.e., disease-specific) or for a particular age of people (i.e., age-specific) (Mausner & Kramer, 1985) (Chapter 1).

spiritual health a form of health associated with the concept of self-actualization; it sometimes reflects a concern for issues related to one's value system; alternatively, it may be concerned with a belief in a transcending unifying force (whether its basis is in nature, scientific law, or a godlike source) (Goodstadt, Simpson, & Loranger, 1987, p. 59) (Chapter 1).

stage theories those behavior change theories that are comprised of an ordered set of categories into which people can be classified, and for which factors could be identified that could induce movement from one category to the next (Weinstein & Sandman, 2002b) (Chapter 4).

sub-competencies "reflects the ability of the student to list, describe, etc." (National Commission for Health Education Credentialing, Inc. 1996b, p. 12) (Chapter 6).

subjective norm a belief held by people that others (individuals or groups) think they should do something and that they care about what others think; a construct of the theory of planned behavior.

technology any device used by society to increase access to or opportunity for people to be exposed to that device—for example, computers and television have increased educational access and opportunities for many people; thus, they are examples of technology.

termination zero chance of relapse

tertiary prevention preventive measures aimed at rehabilitation following significant pathogenesis.

theories/models of implementation theories and models used in planning, implementing, and evaluating health education/promotion programs.

theory "a set of interrelated concepts, definitions, and propositions that presents a systematic view of events or situations by specifying relations among variables in order to explain and predict the events of the situations" (Glanz et al., 2002b, p. 25) (Chapter 4).

theory of planned behavior an intrapersonal theory that addresses individuals' intentions to perform a given behavior as a function of their attitude toward performing the behavior, their beliefs about what is relevant, what others think they should do, and their perception of the ease or difficulty in performing the behavior.

traditional family a family having two parents and their children.

transtheoretical model also known as the stages of change model, it is an intrapersonal theory that addresses an "individual's readiness to change or attempt to change toward healthy behaviors" (Glanz & Rimer, 1995, p. 17) (Chapter 4).

truth telling (honesty) to tell the truth; one of the five principles of common moral ground.

Uniform Resource Locator (URL) identifier for a site on the World Wide Web; specifies locations, or addresses.

value of life a basic principle of ethics: no life should be ended without very strong justification.

variable the operational (practical use) form of a construct.

voluntary health agencies "organizations that are created by concerned citizens to deal with health needs not met by governmental agencies" (McKenzie et al., 2005, p. 51) (Chapters 7 and 8); these organizations rely heavily on volunteer help and donations to function.

wellness "an approach to health that focuses on balancing the many aspects, or dimensions, of a person's life through increasing the adoption of health enhancing conditions and behaviors rather than attempting to minimize conditions of illness" (Joint Terminology Committee, 2001, p. 103).

worksite health promotion health promotion and education programs offered by business and industry entities for their employees.

World Wide Web an interactive information delivery service that includes a repository of resources about most subjects; documents are related by subject area and linked together, thus creating a "web" (Larsson, 1996) (Chapter 9).

years of potential life lost (YPLL) a measure of premature mortality calculated by subtracting a person's age at death from seventy-five years (Freid et al., 2003, p. 454).

Credits

Figure 1.5 J. F. McKenzie, R. R. Pinger, and J. E. Kotecki. *An Introduction to Community Health.* 5th ed. Copyright © 2005, Jones and Bartlett Publishers, Sudbury, MA. Reprinted wth permission. **Box 1.1** Reprinted by permission of Jean Woodward, Health Education Specialist, Idaho Department of Health and Welfare. **Table 1.7** Reprinted from *Research in Personnel and Human Resource Management, Volume 4*, J. R. Terborg, Health promotion at the worksite, copyright © 1986 JAI Press, with permission from Elsevier.

Figure 4.9 From The precaution adoption process model (PAPM) by Weinstein and Sandman in K. Glanz, B. K. Rimer and F. M. Lewis (eds.), *Health Behavior and Health Education: Theory, Research, and Practice*, 3e. Copyright © 2002 Jossey Bass. This material is used by permisison of John Wiley & Sons, Inc. **Box 4.2** Reprinted by permission of Maggie Mann, Health Promotion Director, Southeastern District Health Department, Idaho.

Box 5.1 From R. B. Mellert, *Seven Ethical Principles.* Copyright © 1995 by Kendall Hunt Publishing Company. Reprinted by permission of R. B. Mellert. **Box 5.4** Reprinted by permission of Brittany Mathers, Hepatitis C Surveillance Employee, Indiana State Department of Health, Ball State University.

Box 6.1 Reprinted by permission of Julia A. Eminger, Regional Program Director, Indiana Tobacco Prevention and Cessation Agency. **Box 6.2** A Cooperative Project of the American Association for Health Education, American Public Health Association (Public Health Education & Health Promotion Section and School Health Education & Services Section), American School Health Association, Association of Schools of Public Health, Association of State & Territorial Directors of Health Promotion & Public Health Education, Coalition of National Health Education Organizations, Council on Education for Public Health, Eta Sigma Gama, National Commission for Health Education Credentialing, Society for Public Health Education, Society of State Directors of Health, Physical Education, & Recreation. Reprinted by permission.

Box 6.3 From the final report of the national task force on accreditation in health education by the Society for Public Health Education (SOPHE) and the American Association for Health Education (AAHE), in *Health Education and Behavior* October/November 2004 Quarterly Journal. Copyright © 2004 Sage Publications, Inc. **Box 6.5** Reprinted by permission of Jaime Holbrook, Health Educator, Hamilton County General Health District, Ohio.

Box 7.1 Reprinted by permission of Kate Mathay, Health Teacher, Centerville City Schools, Ohio. **Box 7.2** Reprinted by permission of Sarah Kirsch, Health Promotions Director, American Cancer Society. **Box 7.3** Reprinted by permission of Melissa Schulte, Health Education Specialist, County of Fresno, Department of Community Health. **Box 7.4** Reprinted by permission of Tajuan Stoker, Health and Fitness Coordinator, TriHealth Corporation, Luxottica Retail. **Box 7.5** Jennifer R. Flanagan, Health Educator, Ball Memorial Hospital Family Medicine Residency Center **Box 7.6** Reprinted by permission of Christina Berg, Director of Wellness Services, Boise State University. **Box 7.7** Reprinted by permission of Mary Singler, Health Promotion Manager, Northern Kentucky Health Department.

American Heart Association logo, American Heart Association. **Box 8.2** Reprinted by permission of Cheryl Castillejos, Assistant Wellness Director, Health Solutions, Inc. **Box 8.3** Reprinted by permission of Suzanne Batdorff, Health Educator, Delaware County Health Department, Indiana.

Chapter 9 Screen capture of Cinahl homepage ©2005 Cinahl Information Systems. Reprinted by permission. **Figure 9.2** and **Figure 9.3** Reprinted with permission. Google Brand Features are trademarks or distinctive brand features of Google Technology, Inc.

Appendix A Reprinted with permission from the Society for Public Health Education, Washington, DC.

Index

Note: A page number followed by *f* indicates a figure or photograph, by *t* indicates a table, and by *b* indicates boxed material. Page numbers for Key Terms are in boldface.